The Case against
Assisted Suicide

The Case against Assisted Suicide

For the Right to End-of-Life Care

Edited by

Kathleen Foley, M.D.

Professor, Department of Neurology, Weill Medical College of Cornell
University
Attending Neurologist, Pain and Palliative Care Service, Memorial
Sloan-Kettering Cancer Center
Director, Project on Death in America, Open Society Institute, Soros
Foundation
New York, New York

and

Herbert Hendin, M.D.

Professor, Department of Psychiatry and Behavioral Sciences,
New York Medical College
Medical Director, American Foundation for Suicide Prevention
New York, New York

The Johns Hopkins University Press

Baltimore and London

© 2002 The Johns Hopkins University Press
All rights reserved. Published 2002
Printed in the United States of America on acid-free paper
9 8 7 6 5 4 3 2 1

The Johns Hopkins University Press
2715 North Charles Street
Baltimore, Maryland 21218-4363
www.press.jhu.edu

Library of Congress Cataloging-in-Publication Data

The case against assisted suicide : for the right to end-of-life care /
    edited by Kathleen Foley and Herbert Hendin
        p. ; cm.
Includes bibliographical references and index.
ISBN 0-8018-6792-4 (hardcover : alk. paper)
1. Assisted suicide.
    [DNLM: 1. Suicide, Assisted—legislation & jurisprudence—
United States. 2. Terminal Care—United States. W32.5 AA1 C337
2002] I. Foley, Kathleen M., 1944– II. Hendin, Herbert.
    R726.C355 2002
    174'.24—dc21
    2001000823

A catalog record for this book is available from the British Library.

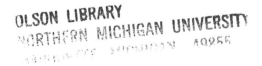

Contents

Reason to Be Concerned

A Better Way

Preface

The debate over physician-assisted suicide has drawn attention to the complex issues of end-of-life care. This edited text brings together a group of authors—ethicists, lawyers, clinicians, health care policy experts—who have argued thoughtfully and cogently against physician-assisted suicide as a social policy. We hope that this book serves as a resource for facts, opinions, and general discourse while offering a comprehensive perspective on the case against physician-assisted suicide and for palliative care. To date there is no such book.

One of our major goals is to draw attention to the vulnerability of the dying population and the evidence that legalizing assisted suicide increases that vulnerability. That evidence is drawn largely from the Dutch and Oregon experiences with physician-assisted suicide.

A driving force in this publication is our own clinical experience in caring for patients with serious life-threatening illnesses such as cancer and suicidal depression. Such patients, who are often elderly, are profoundly vulnerable in our current social and health care system, which devalues their quality of life and inadequately assesses and treats their pain, their psychological symptoms, their emotional distress, and the associated burden to their caregivers. We join with each of the authors in seeking to advance an open and tolerant discussion to address how we as a society can provide better health care and social support to those who are uniquely vulnerable and suffering.

Acknowledgments

We gratefully acknowledge the contributions of several individuals who helped with the publication of this edited text. We are indebted to each of the authors, who patiently addressed the questions posed in reviewing their manuscripts and in formatting their chapters to reflect a coherent discussion of the physician-assisted suicide debate. We particularly thank Bette-Jane Crigger of the Hastings Center, for her editorial review of the text before it was submitted for publication; Yale Kamisar, who, in addition to contributing a chapter, read the entire manuscript and provided his legal expertise, encouragement, and enthusiasm for the project; and Bridget King, for her help in preparing the manuscript and researching references. Josephine Hendin, professor of English at New York University, helped with the writing and rewriting of the introduction and conclusion. We are grateful for help from colleagues at our respective institutions, but the views expressed in the book are those of the authors and do not necessarily reflect the opinions or policies of their institutions. Finally, we wish to thank Wendy Harris, our editor at the Johns Hopkins University Press, for her confidence in the project and her guidance in bringing it to fruition.

Contributors

Daniel Callahan, Ph.D., Director of International Programs and Co-founder, The Hastings Center, Garrison, New York

Harvey M. Chochinov, M.D., Ph.D., Professor of Psychiatry and Family Medicine, University of Manitoba, Winnipeg, Canada

Felicia Cohn, Ph.D., Program Officer, Institute of Medicine/National Research Council, Washington, D.C.

Diane Coleman, J.D., President, Not Dead Yet, Forest Park, Illinois

N. Gregory Hamilton, M.D., Clinical Professor, Department of Psychiatry, Oregon Health Sciences University; and President, Physicians for Compassionate Care, Portland, Oregon

Yale Kamisar, LL.B., LL.D. (hon.), Clarence Darrow Distinguished University Professor of Law, University of Michigan Law School, Ann Arbor, Michigan

Leon R. Kass, M.D., Ph.D., Addie Clark Harding Professor, the Committee on Social Thought and the College, University of Chicago, Chicago, Illinois

David W. Kissane, M.B., B.S., M.P.M., M.D., F.R.A.C.G.P., F.A.Ch.P.M., F.R.A.N.Z.C.P., Director of Palliative Medicine at

the University of Melbourne and the Center for Palliative
Care, St. Vincent's, Victoria, Australia

Joanne Lynn, M.D., M.A., M.S., Director, RAND Center to Improve
Care of the Dying, Arlington, Virginia

Edmund D. Pellegrino, M.D., John Carroll Professor of Medicine
and Medical Ethics and Director, Center for Clinical Bioethics,
Georgetown University, Washington, D.C.

Cicely Saunders, O.M., F.R.C.P., Founder and President,
St. Christopher's Hospice, London, United Kingdom

Leonard Schwartz, LL.B., LL.M., M.D., Department of Psychiatry,
University of Manitoba, Winnipeg, Canada

Zbigniew Zylicz, M.D., Fellow in Palliative Care, University of
Nijmegen; and Director, Hospice Rozenheuvel, Rozendaal,
the Netherlands

The Case against
Assisted Suicide

Introduction:
A Medical, Ethical, Legal, and Psychosocial Perspective

Kathleen Foley, M.D., and Herbert Hendin, M.D.

Should we legalize physician-assisted suicide and euthanasia? Few issues have the potential to divide society as much as this one. Polls show that opinion divides old against young and black against white and sets the disabled apart. In the spring of 1997 the U.S. Supreme Court rejected a federal constitutional right to assisted suicide, essentially returning the struggle over legalization to the states and to the court of public opinion. Assisted suicide is an issue about which the public needs to be informed, one whose importance will only increase with the increasing percentage of elderly people in the population.

The conditions peculiar to our age have made those who are dying in our culture profoundly vulnerable. The bonds of community are weak, and insistence on individual rights is strong. Advances in high-technology life-support systems, growing numbers of cancer and AIDS patients struggling with fatal diagnoses, the aging population, and increasing limitations on health care resources create an environment that particularly threatens patients with terminal illnesses. Such patients have multiple physical and psychosocial symptoms compounded by a substantial degree of existential distress.

Physicians have increasingly identified their own attitudinal, behavioral, educational, and economic barriers to providing humane, compassionate, appropriate care to such patients. Such barriers make us seriously concerned that physicians inadequately equipped to care for those who are dying would substitute physician-assisted suicide for rational, therapeutic, psychological, and social interventions that could enhance the quality of life for dying patients. Health care professionals need to take the lead in developing guidelines for good care of the dying in the management of pain, the treatment of psychosocial distress, and the provision of social support for caregivers.

Surveys of both the general public and health care professionals conclude that our society provides woefully inadequate care for those who are dying and that we need to improve the care of such patients. We endorse the World Health Organization recommendation that governments not consider the legalization of physician-assisted suicide and euthanasia until they have demonstrated the full availability and practice of palliative care for all citizens. In the United States, we have a long way to go to reach this goal.

Given public awareness of the inadequacies of care for those who are dying, it is not surprising that if asked "Are you in favor of euthanasia?" most people reply that they are. Further questioning reveals, however, that they mean little more than that they would rather die painlessly than painfully. When people are asked, "If terminally ill, would you rather be given treatment to make you comfortable or have your life ended by a physician?" their responses are quite different.

What most people do not know is that such treatment is now possible. Having experienced the painful death of a family member or friend, many assume it is not. When a knowledgeable physician addresses the desperation and suffering that underlie the request for assisted suicide and assures patients that he or she will continue to do so until the end of their lives, most patients change their minds, no longer want to hasten death, and are grateful for the time remaining to them. But at this time only a minority receive such care.

In the 1997 ruling upholding the constitutionality of state laws prohibiting assisted suicide, the U.S. Supreme Court declared that assisted suicide was not necessary for the plaintiffs in the New York and Washington State cases it was considering because modern medical methods of obtaining relief from suffering were available to the plaintiffs. Justice Sandra Day O'Connor summarized the opinion of the majority of the justices in saying that for terminally ill patients in great pain there were "no legal barriers to obtaining medication from qualified physicians to alleviate that suffering, even to the point of causing unconsciousness and hastening death."[1]

As important as what the Court rejected—a federal constitutional right to assisted suicide—was what the majority of the justices embraced: the right of terminally ill patients not to suffer. The Court's opinion was an implicit challenge to every state to prevent tragedies of neglect, care that only prolongs suffering, and abuses of assisted suicide by providing to all people the good palliative care now received by only a few.

For society, a more precise framing of the assisted suicide question would be, Does our need to care for people who are seriously or terminally ill and to reduce their suffering require us to permit physicians to end patients' lives? Our perspective in answering this question is largely medical and empirical, that is, it is derived from the practice and ethics of medicine and from the evidence of the medical and social consequences of legalization. We believe there is convincing evidence that legalization of assisted suicide and euthanasia undermines the care provided to patients at the end of life.

Many proponents of legalization maintain that opposition to legalization is fundamentally religious in nature and that secular objections are only a cloak for underlying moral convictions concerning the sanctity of life. As Thomas Preston, a prominent advocate, put it, "For many the question is: Does physician-assisted suicide represent compassionate relief of suffering or a violation of God's will?"[2] From our perspective, it represents neither. Although we understand and respect the position of those who oppose legalization of physician-assisted suicide and euthanasia on religious grounds, if we believed that legalization were necessary to relieve suffering at the end of life, our position would be different.

It is worth noting that such nonreligious organizations as the American Medical Association, the American Geriatrics Society, the American Hospital Association, and the National Hospice and Palliative Care Organization are strongly opposed to legalization for reasons that are obviously medical and social. Studies have shown that the less physicians know about palliative care, the more they favor legalization; the more they know, the less they favor legalization.[3]

Opposition to legalization is strongest among physicians who know most about caring for terminally ill patients (i.e., palliative care specialists, gerontologists, psychiatrists who treat patients who become suicidal in response to medical illness, hospice physicians, and oncologists). They know that patients requesting a physician's assistance in suicide are usually telling us as strongly as they know how that they desperately need relief from their suffering and that without such relief they would

rather die. They are making an anguished cry for help and a very ambivalent request to die. When they are treated by a physician who can
hear their ambivalence, understand their desperation, and relieve their
suffering, the wish to die usually disappears.

People responding to the knowledge of serious or terminal illness
with anxiety, depression, and a wish to die are similar to people who
react to other crises with a desire to end the crisis by ending their lives.
People vulnerable to suicide are particularly prone to setting absolute
conditions on life: "I won't live . . . without my husband" or "if I lose my
looks, power, prestige, or health" or "if I am going to die soon." They are
afflicted by the need to make demands on life that cannot be fulfilled.
Determining the time, place, and circumstances of their death is the most
dramatic expression of their need for control. Depression, often precipi-
tated by discovering that they have a serious illness, exaggerates their
tendency to see problems in black-and-white terms, overlooking solutions and alternative possibilities.[4]

Policy recommendations regarding assisted suicide made by those
who are not knowledgeable about the care of dying patients are often
removed from the realities these patients face. Writing for the Ninth Circuit Court of Appeals, which declared the State of Washington law banning assisted suicide to be unconstitutional, Judge Stephen Reinhardt
dismissed the danger of abuse were assisted suicide to be legalized:
"Should an error actually occur it is likely to benefit the individual by
permitting a victim of unmanageable pain and suffering to end his life
peacefully and with dignity at the time he deems most desirable."[5] The
assumption by this respected jurist that even a mistaken death would be
welcomed by any person who is terminally ill is somewhat frightening
in its removal from the experience of patients and their families in such
cases.

Removal from actual patient care permitted another distinguished
legal philosopher, Ronald Dworkin, to maintain that respect for the consistency and integrity of the way individuals live their lives, including
the way they wish to die, requires that we grant their requests for euthanasia.[6] Just what does this mean? Does the fact that individuals who
respond to every life crisis with depression, panic, and the desire to die
are facing a serious or terminal illness demand that we heed their request
to die because it is consistent with their character? For others, the panic
that accompanies serious or terminal illness is not in keeping with their
prior life or character. When the panic is addressed, it usually subsides

and the request for death disappears. When the panic is not addressed and the physician simply heeds the request, the patient often dies in a state of unrecognized terror.

The word *euthanasia* was coined from the Greek language (*eu* for "good" or "noble," and *thanatos* for "death") in the seventeenth century by Francis Bacon to refer to an easy, painless, happy death. In modern times it has come to mean the active causation of a patient's death by a physician, usually through the injection of a lethal dose of medication. In physician-assisted suicide, the patient self-administers the lethal dose that has been prescribed by a physician who knows the patient intends to use it to end his or her life. Both the terms "physician-assisted suicide" and "euthanasia" are often avoided by their advocates, who prefer the nonspecific euphemism "assistance in dying."

Although throughout history individual philosophers—from Plato and Seneca to Montaigne and Hume—justified suicide for those who were severely sick and suffering, the notion that physicians should assist in such suicides is relatively recent. The earliest literary references to assisted suicide involve help from comrades, and not because of illness. Some, like King Saul, who asked his armor bearer to hold the sword on which he impaled himself, wished to avoid the humiliation of capture in battle.

The mythological story of the death of Hercules provides a rare detailed account of an assisted suicide intended to put an end to pain and suffering.[7] Hercules has been unintentionally poisoned by his wife, Denira, who has been deceived into believing that a blood potion she has been given will cure him of his infatuation with another woman. Mistakenly believing the time has come to use the potion and unaware that it is lethal, Denira sprinkles a robe with it and has the robe sent to Hercules. The effect of the poisoned robe, which would have killed anyone else but Hercules, is to cause him unbearable pain from which there is no relief. In his first agony Hercules kills the messenger who brought the robe to him. Denira, in turn, kills herself when she realizes what she has done.

Hercules wants death but it will not come. He continues to live a tortured existence until he decides to arrange his own death. He orders a great pyre to be built on a mountain; he is carried there and lifted to the top of the pyre, where he lies down. He asks his youthful follower, Philoctetes, to set the wood on fire, first giving him the bow and arrows that Philoctetes later uses so effectively in the Trojan War. Before being engulfed in flames, he expresses his anticipated relief: "This is rest. This is the end."

Pain so great that even a Hercules cannot stand it, and a choice between continued suffering and a hastened death, is the prototype of the cases today that are said to warrant assisted suicide or euthanasia. That a terminally ill person should seek a physician to assist in suicide, however, was not seriously proposed until the eighteenth century, with the discovery of analgesics and anesthetics that, while having the potential to relieve suffering for dying patients, could even more easily and painlessly end life.

As medicine learned to control acute infectious disease, life expectancy gradually increased from a norm of forty in 1850 to almost double that figure today, and degenerative and late-onset diseases, of which cancer was the epitome, made the discussion of end-of-life care more urgent and made the role of the physician more important. The first articles advocating euthanasia in the context of modern medicine appeared in the United States and England in the 1870s. The first proposal for the legalization of euthanasia was made and defeated in Ohio in 1905. Following a similar defeat in Iowa, no further proposals were made in the United States for three decades.

The euthanasia movement revived in the United States and was even stronger in England in the 1930s. Euthanasia societies were formed in both countries, and there were accounts of suffering patients who desired euthanasia as well as accounts by physicians who had performed it surreptitiously.

Interest in euthanasia had coincided in the late nineteenth and early twentieth centuries with the development of the eugenics movement in both the United States and Europe. Stimulated by advances in genetics and a misguided attempt to hasten the process of natural selection that had been described by Charles Darwin shortly before, proponents of eugenics envisioned a perfection of the human race, initially through sterilization of the unfit or degenerate, variously defined as criminals, prostitutes, alcoholics, epileptics, and the mentally ill. Thirty states passed sterilization laws, eventually sixty thousand Americans were sterilized, and the movement was embraced by figures ranging from Teddy Roosevelt and Woodrow Wilson to Oliver Wendell Holmes. As late as the beginning of World War II, the most prominent euthanasia advocate in this country, Dr. Foster Kennedy, favored compulsory euthanasia for retarded children on eugenic grounds. He came to believe that the certainty of the diagnosis and prognosis in these cases justified such involuntary deaths more than those resulting from voluntary euthanasia in adults diagnosed as terminally ill, whose diagnosis and prognosis could turn out to be wrong and who might indeed recover.[8]

Although Germany was not the first country to embrace eugenics, it took hold there more deeply than elsewhere, led by Ernest Haeckel, a famed and respected biologist and social scientist. Haeckel advocated euthanasia for the "hundreds of thousands of incurables—lunatics, lepers, people with cancer etc. . . . artificially kept alive," whom he saw as a drain on the economy and a threat to the health of the Aryan race.[9] Alfred Hoche and Karl Binding, a psychiatrist and an attorney, respectively, built on Haeckel's work to write in 1920 *The Permission to Destroy Life Unworthy of Life,*[10] the influential book much admired by Adolf Hitler. Hoche and Binding proposed that those who were retarded, deformed, or terminally ill and those damaged by accident or disease should be put to death for racially hygienic purposes or because they were a burden to society, or both.

When the Nazis came to power, they first legalized voluntary euthanasia but eventually adopted the Haeckel/Hoche/Binding proposals on a scale that even the three of them could hardly have imagined. Euthanasia was used by German doctors first to end the lives of several hundred thousand mentally ill children and adults considered incurable and subsequently to eliminate Jews, gypsies, and others designated as racially or genetically undesirable.

The postwar revulsion to the Holocaust, and to the role of physicians in implementing it, discredited the euthanasia movement. A significant minority of advocates, however, while not emphasizing the eugenic aspects of euthanasia, continue to see it as a necessary social remedy for the increasing number of old people, the inadequacy of nursing homes, and the economic cost to families and society of caring for elderly persons. In the words of Eliot Slater, an English psychiatrist and advocate of euthanasia, "If a chronically sick man dies, he ceases to be a burden on himself, on his family, on the health services and on the community."[11] Derek Humphry, founder of the Hemlock Society, wrote in a recent book, "One must look at the realities of the increasing cost of health care in an aging society, because in the final analysis, economics, not the quest for broadened individual liberties or increased autonomy, will drive assisted suicide to the plateau of acceptable practice."[12] Pietr Admiraal, one of the foremost Dutch practitioners of euthanasia, believes that in twenty-five years Europe may resort to euthanasia to deal with a large population of elderly people. Admiraal says he is glad he will not be alive to see it, but he remains a strong advocate of euthanasia.[13]

The contemporary revival of interest in euthanasia in the 1970s and 1980s, however, was primarily centered on compassion for suffering patients. It was considered in part to have been a reaction to modern medical technology that permits us to maintain a pointless semblance of life and creates fear of painful and undignified death. The Netherlands became the first country to give legal sanction to physician-assisted suicide and euthanasia. Unrelievable pain and suffering were conditions that the Dutch stipulated must be met for euthanasia to be performed. When, in the mid-1990s, however, Oregon became the only state to pass a law permitting physician-assisted suicide, pain and suffering were not a requirement: a diagnosis of a terminal illness with a prognosis of six months to live was enough. The guiding principle was not pain and suffering but patient autonomy or choice.

In varying degrees, compassion for suffering patients, respect for patient autonomy, and the fact that suicide can be a rational act on the part of the patient now serve as the basis for the strongest arguments in favor of legalization and were the foundation for an amicus curiae brief filed with the Supreme Court in the 1997 case by a group of bioethicists supporting a constitutional right to assisted suicide. In the next section of this book we have asked three pioneers in the field of medical ethics, Leon Kass, Edmund Pellegrino, and Daniel Callahan, to address from their different perspectives the inadequacies of attempting to justify assisted suicide on these grounds.

Kass outlines the basic principles and values of the profession of medicine, explaining why ending the patient's life is not compatible with those values. He addresses the destructive impact of legalization of assisted suicide and euthanasia on the intrinsic trust that must underlie the relationship between doctor and patient. He points out that compassion and voluntariness are often contradictory guiding principles, since those suffering most are often unable to express their wishes. The result is likely to be decisions to end the lives of patients who have not requested death. He indicates how seldom the decisions made by dying patients are truly autonomous, how easily they are influenced or manipulated.

Pellegrino explores and explains how frequently compassion can be misdirected. A physician may confuse his or her own anguish at the patient's condition or the plight of the family with compassion for the patient. Nor is even genuine compassion a guarantee against doing harm. A physician who does not know how to relieve a patient's suffering may compassionately but inappropriately agree to end the patient's life.

Callahan analyzes the claim that if suffering makes life seem meaningless to patients, patient autonomy dictates that physicians should grant their requests for assisted suicide. He indicates that this comes close to saying that life can have meaning only if marked by self-determination, yet a "noble and heroic life can be achieved by those who have little or no control over the external conditions of their lives, but have the wisdom and dignity necessary to fashion a meaningful life without it." Only further confusion results when rationality is used as the basis for determining the rightness or wrongness of euthanasia in a particular case or as the basis for any social policy. Callahan points out how wrong decisions are made by rational people all the time. Medicine has neither the expertise nor the wisdom to relieve all the problems of human mortality, the most central of which is why we have to die at all or die in ways that seem pointless to us.

In law, autonomy is usually addressed as a matter of rights. The legal basis for the U.S. Supreme Court's rejection of the notion of a federal constitutional right to assisted suicide is explained and explored by Yale Kamisar, the dean of constitutional experts on the subject. He addresses why the Court drew a clear distinction between a patient's right to refuse or withdraw from any unwanted treatments, even if doing so would be fatal, and the request for physician-assisted suicide. He discusses why the justices did not see it as reasonable to recognize the right to physician-assisted suicide only for terminally ill patients and not for chronically ill patients who have longer to suffer or for those who have emotional pain not accompanied by physical disease. He analyzes why the Court did not consider it possible to realize such a right with assisted suicide, in which a patient takes a lethal dose of medication prescribed by a doctor, and yet forbid physicians to give lethal injection (euthanasia) to those patients who were unable to swallow drugs or otherwise effect their own death. In addition, he analyzes the impact of the Court's decision on the national debate.

What happens to autonomy, compassion, and rationality when assisted suicide and euthanasia are given legal sanction? Chapters in the next section look at the difference between theory and practice in three places where this occurred—the Netherlands, the state of Oregon, and the Northern Territory of Australia.

With twenty years' experience, the Netherlands, the only country in which assisted suicide and euthanasia have had legal sanction, provides the best laboratory to help us evaluate what they mean in actuality. Herbert Hendin was one of three foreign observers to have had the opportunity to study the situation in the Netherlands extensively, to discuss specific cases with leading Dutch practitioners, and to interview Dutch government-sponsored euthanasia researchers about their work. All three observers independently concluded that guidelines established by the Dutch for the practice of euthanasia—a competent patient who has unrelievable suffering makes a voluntary request to a physician, who before going forward must consult with another physician, and afterward must report the case to the authorities—were consistently violated and could not be enforced.[14]

Concern over charges of abuse led the Dutch government to undertake studies of the practices in 1990 and 1995.[15] Many violations of guidelines were evident from these two studies. For example, 60 percent of Dutch cases of assisted suicide and euthanasia are not reported, which by itself makes regulation impossible.

The most alarming finding of the Dutch studies is the fact that there are several thousand cases a year in which patients who have not given their consent have their lives ended by physicians. About a quarter of physicians stated that they had "terminated the lives of patients without an explicit request" from the patient to do so, and a third more of the physicians could conceive of doing so.

The evidence of the Dutch experience also indicates that, contrary to the expectations of euthanasia proponents, legal sanction empowers physicians, not patients. Physicians often suggest death, which compromises the voluntariness of the process; do not present obvious alternatives; ignore patient ambivalence; and even end the lives of patients who have not requested them to do so. Practicing euthanasia appears to encourage physicians to think they know best who should live and who should die, an attitude that leads them to make such decisions without consulting patients. Hendin will address the Dutch situation in a chapter in this section.

Given legal sanction, euthanasia, intended originally for the exceptional case, has become an accepted way of dealing with serious or terminal illness in the Netherlands. In the process, palliative care has become one of the casualties, while hospice care has lagged behind that of other countries. In testimony before the British House of Lords, Zbigniew Zylicz, a medical oncologist who specializes in palliative medicine and one of the few palliative care experts in the Netherlands, emphasized Dutch deficiencies in palliative care, attributing them to the easier alternative of euthanasia.

Zylicz has for over a decade been treating terminally ill patients at one of the few hospices in the Netherlands. He also makes more than a hundred house calls a year to such patients as a consultant to physicians responsible for their care, and he has been attempting to educate Dutch physicians regarding palliative care. His chapter describes what it is like for a palliative care physician to care for terminally ill patients in a country where euthanasia is considered a form of palliative care.

For anyone inclined to believe that assisted suicide can be implemented in this country in some way that avoids the problems seen in the Netherlands, careful study of the situation in Oregon—the one state that has legalized assisted suicide—provides contrary evidence. Under the Oregon law, when a terminally ill patient makes a request for assisted suicide, physicians are required to point out that palliative care and hospice care are feasible alternatives. They are not required, however, to be knowledgeable about how to relieve either physical or emotional suffering in terminally ill patients. Without such knowledge, the physician cannot present feasible alternatives. It would seem necessary to require physicians lacking such training to refer any patient requesting assisted suicide for consultation with a physician knowledgeable about palliative care. However, there is no such requirement in the Oregon law.

Our opportunity to learn from the Oregon experience is curtailed, since Oregon physicians participating in assisted suicide are not asked to provide significant medical information about their patients to the Oregon Health Division (OHD), which monitors the law. Physicians are merely asked to check off a list on an OHD form indicating that such statutory requirements as a written request for the lethal dose of medication, a fifteen-day waiting period, and consultation with another physician have been met. Only one line is provided for both diagnosis and prognosis, although a diagnosis of terminal illness and prognosis of death within six months are the essential requirements for assisted suicide in the state. The form does not even inquire as to patient's reasons for making the request for assisted suicide. The data collected by OHD do not make it possible to know what transpired in any particular case. What we know of the few individual cases in which the information has become public, combined with the inadequate monitoring by OHD, provides cause for concern. We participated in a detailed analysis of the Oregon law, and together we examined the reports OHD issued after each year of the law's operation. We also analyzed the few Oregon cases in which the details have become known. This analysis forms the basis for a chapter on the Oregon experience, which indicates how little the law's presumed safeguards actually protect patients.

Gregory Hamilton, an Oregon psychiatrist who heads Physicians for Compassionate Care, a group in Oregon advocating improved palliative care as an alternative to legalization of physician-assisted suicide, lives daily with the ramifications of the Oregon law. He describes how the culture of silence and secrecy that surrounds the law attempts to conceal and ignore violations of the law's guidelines. He helps make us aware of how the economics of medical care in Oregon encourage assisted suicide. He also discusses his personal experience with the operation of the Oregon law.

Finally, the Northern Territory of Australia has had experience, although brief, with legalized euthanasia. The parliament of the territory voted to legalize euthanasia in 1996, and the law was in operation for nine months before it was overturned by Australia's national parliament. The effort to overturn the Northern Territory act was stimulated in part by the fact that sick Australian Aborigines, who live for the most part in the Northern Territory, were not seeking medical care out of fear that physicians would now feel free to end patients' lives without their consent. That these fears of being killed, although exaggerated, had some basis in fact was evident in a study of physicians throughout Australia done before the passage of the Northern Territory act but published in this period. The study, by Helga Kuhse and Peter Singer, indicated that euthanasia and involuntary euthanasia were being secretly practiced in the country.[16] These findings were used by the authors and others to argue that legalization might reduce the number of cases in which decisions were made without consulting patients.

During the legalization period, one physician (Philip Nitschke) reported that he performed euthanasia in a number of cases. He agreed to be interviewed by and jointly published an outline of his cases with David Kissane, a leading palliative care expert in Australia.[17] In his chapter, Kissane presents his analysis of these cases, which is quite different from Nitschke's, as well as an analysis of the study of physicians' practices and the effect of legalization and its aftermath on the care of terminally ill patients in Australia.

The vulnerability experienced by the Australian Aborigines when faced with legalization is not unique or without substance. In its 1997 decision, the U.S. Supreme Court recognized the importance of the state's interest in protecting from abuse, neglect, and mistakes groups who would be at particular risk if assisted suicide were legalized—those who are poor, elderly, depressed, or coping with disabilities. Their special concerns are the subject of the next section of this book.

Some of the most powerfully moving opposition to assisted suicide has come from patients with disabilities. They are acutely aware of the dangers of misguided compassion. They have seen the tendency of the medical profession and society in general to undervalue their lives and mistakenly to assume that any depression they suffer is inevitable and untreatable. Diane Coleman, an attorney who is disabled and has been the organizer and articulate leader of Not Dead Yet, an advocacy group representing disabled persons, addresses the reality of the problems they already face and the dangers to them inherent in legalization of assisted suicide.

Vulnerable individuals, elderly patients, the uninsured, members of minority groups, and the disenfranchised have reason to be particularly apprehensive. It is no accident that while polls show younger people favoring legalization, it is opposed by most people over sixty. African Americans of all ages oppose it by two to one. Joanne Lynn, a distinguished gerontologist and director of the RAND Center to Improve Care of the Dying, and her colleague Felicia Cohn have written a chapter discussing the problems in care faced by seriously or terminally ill patients in these groups and why legalization is of particular concern to them. These authors have responded specifically to nine arguments commonly used to justify legalization, indicating why these arguments are misleading or mistaken.

People who become depressed in response to serious or terminal illness are particularly vulnerable. Unfortunately, depression is commonly underdiagnosed and inadequately treated. Although most people who kill themselves are under medical care at the time of death, their physicians often fail to recognize the symptoms of their depressive illness or fail to provide adequate treatment. Harvey Chochinov, a professor of psychiatry and family medicine in the Department of Psychiatry at the University of Manitoba and one of the leading authorities on this subject, and his colleague Leonard Schwartz, help us understand the impact of depression, anxiety, and existential factors on terminally ill patients' will to live as well as what can be done to relieve their psychological suffering and to help them find satisfaction and meaning in the time remaining to them.

The next section of the book addresses the question, If assisted suicide is not the answer, how can we improve the care and reduce the suffering of those who are seriously and terminally ill? Better hospice care and improved palliative care, including better psychiatric care, are some of the solutions. Hospice has been able to provide for many the relief from suffering and the humane treatment that make death with dignity a reality rather than a slogan. Dame Cicely Saunders, the founder of the modern hospice movement, discusses the evolution and development of hospice and its integration into medical practice.

Kathleen Foley defines palliative care and describes the major barriers—physician related, patient related, and institutional—that prevent patients and families from receiving appropriate humane care at the end of life. She examines the various components of suffering—physical, psychological, existential—in both patient and caregiver and discusses how palliative care approaches can be clearly distinguished from physician-assisted suicide. She points out that major initiatives to improve care are under way. Death is an issue the whole society faces, requiring a compassionate response. But we should not confuse compassion with competence in the care of terminally ill persons.

The conclusion outlines a policy that can address the needs of dying patients, their physicians, and society. The U.S. Supreme Court's challenge to the states to provide good-quality medical care at the end of life suggests that we begin with the role the states are, can be, or should be playing in meeting this challenge. Is there a role for the federal government? What can and should organized medicine do to improve the quality of care at the end of life? What role can and should psychiatry play? What can consumer advocacy groups do? What can we do to meet the needs of patients so that assisted suicide does not seem a needed option?

*Autonomy, Compassion,
and Rational Suicide*

1

"I Will Give No Deadly Drug":
Why Doctors Must Not Kill

Leon R. Kass, M.D., Ph.D.

That we die is certain. When and how we die is not. Because we want to live and not to die, we resort to medicine to delay the inevitable. Yet in some cases, medicine's success in preserving life has been purchased at a heavy price, paid in the coin of *how* we die: often in conditions of great pain and suffering, irreversible incompetence, and terminal loss of control. In these circumstances, many Americans increasingly seek greater control over the end of life, and some even wish to elect death to avoid the burdens of lingering on. Ironically, they also seek assistance in doing so from the death-defying art of medicine. People no longer talk only about refusing medical treatment. The demands of the day are for physician-assisted suicide and euthanasia. Voters in the state of Oregon have legalized physician-assisted suicide; a large segment of national public opinion approves the practice of doctor-induced death; and even many physicians appear ready to overturn the centuries-old taboo against medical killing. Euthanasia practiced by physicians seems to be an idea whose time has come.

But in my view, it remains a bad idea whose time must not come—not now, not ever. Powerful reasons, of both prudence and principle, have for centuries supported such a judgment, and, as I will argue, they do so still, despite our changed circumstances—indeed, all the more so because of them. The heart of the argument rests on understanding the special moral character of the medical profession and the ethical obligations that it entails. Accordingly, I will be considering these interrelated questions: What are the norms that all physicians, *as physicians,* should agree to observe, whatever their personal opinions and private morality? What is the basis of such a medical ethic? What does it say— and what should we think—about doctors intentionally killing?

Contemporary Ethical Approaches

The question about physicians killing appears, at first glance, to be just a special case of this general question: May or ought one kill people who ask to be killed? Those who answer this general question in the affirmative offer two reasons. First is freedom or autonomy: Each person has a right to control his or her body and his or her life, including the end of it. Some go as far as to assert a right to die, a strange claim in a liberal society founded on the need to secure and defend the inalienable right to life. But strange or not, for patients too weak to oppose potent life-prolonging technologies wielded by aggressive physicians, the claim based on choice, autonomy, and self-determination is certainly understandable. In this view, physicians (or others) are bound to acquiesce in demands not only for termination of treatment but also for intentional killing through poison, because the right to choose—freedom—must be respected, even more than life itself, and even when the physician would never recommend or concur with the choices made. Physicians, as keepers of the vials of life and death, are morally bound actively to dispatch the embodied person out of deference to autonomous personal choice.

The second reason for killing the patient who asks for death has little to do with choice. Instead, death is to be directly and swiftly given because the patient's life is deemed no longer worth living, according to some substantive or "objective" measure. Unusually great pain or a terminal condition or an irreversible coma or advanced senility or extreme degradation is the disqualifying quality of life that pleads—choice or no choice—for merciful termination. Choice may enter indirectly to confirm the judgment: if the patient does not speak up, the doctor (or a relative or some other proxy) may be asked to affirm that he would not himself choose—or that his patient, were he able to choose, would not choose— to remain alive with one or more of these stigmata. It is not his autonomy but rather the miserable and pitiable condition of his body or mind that justifies doing the patient in. Absent such substantial degradations, requests for assisted death would not be honored. Here the body itself offends and must be plucked out, from compassion or mercy, to be sure.

Not the autonomous will of the patient, but the doctor's benevolent and compassionate love for suffering humanity justifies the humane act of mercy killing.

These two reasons advanced to justify the killing of patients correspond to the two approaches to medical ethics most prominent in the field today: the school of autonomy and the school of general benevolence and compassion (or love). Despite their differences, they are united in their opposition to the belief that medicine is intrinsically a moral pro fession, with *its own* immanent principles and standards of conduct that set limits on what physicians may properly do. Each seeks to remedy the ethical defect of a profession seen to be in itself *a*moral, technically competent but morally neutral.

For the first ethical school, morally neutral technique is morally used only when it is used according to the wishes of the patient as client or consumer. The model of the doctor-patient relationship is one of contract: the physician—a highly competent hired syringe, as it were—sells his services on demand, restrained only by the law. Here's the deal: for the patient, autonomy and service; for the doctor, money, graced by the pleasure of giving the patient what he wants. If a patient wants to fix his nose or change his gender, determine the sex of unborn children, or take euphoriant drugs just for kicks, the physician can and will go to work—provided that the price is right.[1]

For the second ethical school, morally neutral technique is morally used only when it is used under the guidance of general benevolence or loving charity. Not the will of the patient, but the humane and compassionate motive of the physician—not as physician but as human being—makes the doctor's actions ethical. Here, too, there can be strange requests and even stranger deeds, but if they are done from love, nothing can be wrong—again, providing the law is silent. All acts—including killing the patient—done lovingly are licit, even praiseworthy. Good and humane intentions can sanctify any deed.

In my opinion, both of these approaches misunderstand the moral foundations of medical practice and therefore provide an inadequate basis for medical ethics. For one thing, neither of them can make sense of some specific duties and restraints long thought absolutely inviolate under the traditional medical ethic (e.g., the proscription against having sex with patients). Must we now say that sex with a patient is permissible if the patient wants it and the price is right, or, alternatively, if the doctor is gentle and loving and has a good bedside manner? Or do we glimpse in this absolute prohibition a deeper understanding of the medical vocation, which the prohibition both embodies and protects? Indeed, as I will now try to show, the medical profession has its own intrinsic ethic, which a physician true to the calling will not violate, either for love or for money.

Profession: Intrinsically Ethical

Let me propose a different way of thinking about medicine as a profession. Consider medicine not as a mixed marriage between its own value-neutral technique and some extrinsic moral principles, but as an inherently ethical activity, in which technique and conduct are both ordered in relation to an overarching good, the naturally given end of health. This once-traditional view of medicine I have defended at length in my book *Toward a More Natural Science*.[2] Here I will present the conclusions without the arguments. It will suffice, for present purposes, if I can render this view plausible.

A profession, as etymology suggests, is an activity or occupation to which its practitioner publicly professes—that is, confesses—devotion. Learning may, of course, be required of, and prestige may, of course, be granted to, the professional, but it is the profession's goal that calls, that learning serves, and that prestige honors. Each of the ways of life to which the various professionals profess their devotion must be a way of life worthy of such devotion—and so they all are. The teacher devotes himself to helping people learn, looking up to truth and wisdom; the lawyer (or judge) devotes himself to rectifying injustice for his client (or for the parties before the court), looking up to what is lawful and right; the clergyman devotes himself to tending the souls of his parishioners, looking up to the sacred and the divine; and the physician devotes himself to healing the sick, looking up to health and wholeness.

Being a professional is thus more than being a technician. It is rooted in our moral nature; it is a matter not only of the mind and hand but also of the heart, not only of intellect and skill but also of character. For it is only as a being willing and able to devote himself to others and to serve some high good that a person makes a public profession of his way of life. To profess is an ethical act, and it makes the professional qua professional a moral being who prospectively affirms the moral nature of his activity.

Professing oneself a professional is an ethical act for many reasons. It is an articulate public act, not merely a private and silent choice—a confession before others who are one's witnesses. It freely promises continuing devotion, not merely announces present preferences, to a way of life, not just a way to a livelihood, a life of action, not only of thought. It serves some high good, which calls forth devotion because it is both good and high, but which requires such devotion because its service is most demanding and difficult, and thereby engages one's character, not merely one's mind and hands.

The good to which the medical profession is chiefly devoted is health, a naturally given although precarious standard or norm, characterized by "wholeness" and "well-working," toward which the living body moves on its own. Even the modern physician, despite great technological prowess, is finally but an assistant to natural powers of self-healing. As the healing profession, medicine uses artful means to serve the human body's natural efforts to maintain its integrity and its native powers and activities.

But health, though a goal tacitly sought and explicitly desired, is difficult to attain and preserve. It can be ours only provisionally and temporarily, for we are finite and frail. Medicine thus finds itself in between: the physician is called to serve the high and universal goal of health while also ministering to the needs and relieving the sufferings of the frail and particular patient. Moreover, the physician must respond not only to illness but also to its meaning for each individual, who, in addition to symptoms, may suffer from self-concern—and often fear and shame—about weakness and vulnerability, neediness and dependence, loss of self-esteem, and the fragility of all that matters to him. Thus the inner meaning of the art of medicine is derived from the pursuit of health and the care for the ill and suffering, guided by the self-conscious awareness, shared (even if only tacitly) by physician and patient alike, of the delicate and dialectical tension between wholeness and necessary decay.

When the activity of healing the sick is thus understood, we can discern certain virtues requisite for practicing medicine—among them, moderation and self-restraint, gravity, patience, sympathy, discretion, and prudence. We can also discern specific positive duties, addressed mainly to the patient's vulnerability and self-concern—including the demands for truthfulness, patient instruction, and encouragement. And, arguably, we can infer the importance of certain negative duties, formulable as absolute and unexceptionable rules. Among these, I submit, is this rule: Doctors must not kill. The rest of this chapter attempts to defend this rule and to show its relation to the medical ethic, itself understood as growing out of the inner meaning of the medical vocation.

I confine my discussion solely to the question of direct, intentional killing of patients *by physicians*—so-called mercy killing. Though I confess myself opposed to such killing even by nonphysicians,[3] I am not arguing here against euthanasia per se. More importantly, I am not arguing against the cessation of medical treatment when such treatment merely prolongs painful or degraded dying; nor do I oppose the use of certain measures to relieve suffering that have, as an unavoidable consequence, an increased risk of death. Doctors may and must allow to die, even if they must not intentionally kill.

Bad Consequences

Although the heart of my argument will turn on my understanding of the special meaning of professing the art of healing, I begin with a more familiar mode of ethical analysis: assessing needs and benefits versus dangers and harms. Still the best discussion of this topic is a now-classic essay by Yale Kamisar, written more than forty years ago.[4] Kamisar makes vivid the difficulties in ensuring that the choice for death will be freely made and adequately informed, the problems of physician error and abuse, the troubles for human relationships within families and between doctors and patients, the difficulty of preserving the boundary between voluntary and involuntary euthanasia, and the risks to the whole social order from weakening the absolute prohibition against taking innocent life. These considerations alone are, in my view, sufficient to rebut any attempt to weaken the taboo against medical killing; their relative importance for determining public policy far exceeds their relative importance in this chapter. But here they serve also to point us to more profound reasons why doctors must not kill.

There is no question that fortune deals many people a very bad hand, not least at the end of life. All of us, I am sure, know or have known individuals whose last weeks, months, or even years were racked with pain and discomfort, degraded by dependency or loss of self-control, or characterized by such reduced humanity that it cast a deep shadow over their entire lives, especially as remembered by the survivors. All who love these suffering individuals would wish to spare them such an end, and there is no doubt that an earlier death could do it. Against such a clear benefit, attested to by many a poignant and heartrending true story, it is difficult to argue, especially when the arguments are necessarily general and seemingly abstract. Still, in the aggregate, the adverse consequences—including real suffering—of being governed solely by mercy and compassion may far outweigh the aggregate benefits of trying to relieve agonal or terminal distress by direct medical killing.

The first difficulty emerges when we try to gauge the so-called need or demand for medically assisted killing. This question, to be sure, is in part empirical. But evidence can be gathered only if the relevant categories of "euthanizable" people are clearly defined. Such definition is notoriously hard to accomplish—and it is not always honestly attempted. On careful inspection, we discover that if the category is precisely defined, the need for mercy killing seems greatly exaggerated, and if the category is loosely defined, the poisoners will be working overtime.

The category always mentioned first to justify mercy killing is the group of persons suffering from incurable and fatal illnesses, with intractable pain and with little time left to live but still fully aware, who freely request a release from their distress (e.g., people rapidly dying from disseminated cancer with bony metastases unresponsive to chemotherapy). But as experts in pain control tell us, the number of such people with truly untreatable pain is in fact rather low. Adequate analgesia is apparently possible in the vast majority of cases, provided that the physician and patient are willing to use strong enough medicines in adequate doses and with proper timing.[5]

But, it will be pointed out, full analgesia induces drowsiness and blunts or distorts awareness. How can that be a desired outcome of treatment? Fair enough. But then the rationale for requesting death begins to shift from relieving experienced suffering to ending a life no longer valued by its bearer or, let us be frank, by the onlookers. If this becomes a sufficient basis to warrant mercy killing, now the category of euthanizable people cannot be limited to individuals with incurable or fatal painful illnesses with little time to live. Now persons in all sorts of greatly reduced conditions—from persistent vegetative state to quadriplegia, from severe depression to the condition that now most horrifies, Alzheimer disease—might have equal claim to have their suffering mercifully halted. The trouble, of course, is that most of these people can no longer request for themselves the dose of poison. Moreover, it will be difficult—

if not impossible—to develop the requisite calculus of degradation or to define the threshold necessary for ending life.

In view of the obvious difficulty in describing precisely and "objectively" what categories and degrees of pain, suffering, or bodily or mental impairment could justify mercy killing, advocates repair (at least for the time being) to the principle of volition: the request for assistance in death is to be honored because it is freely made by the one whose life it is, and who, for one reason or another, cannot commit suicide alone. But this too is fraught with difficulty: How free or informed is a choice made under debilitated conditions? Can consent long in advance be sufficiently informed about all the particular circumstances that it is meant prospectively to cover? And in any case, are not such choices easily and subtly manipulated, especially in those who are vulnerable?

Truth to tell, the ideal of rational autonomy, so beloved of bioethicists and legal theorists, rarely obtains in actual medical practice. Illness invariably means dependence, and dependence means relying for advice on physician and family. This is especially true with those who are seriously or terminally ill, where there is frequently also depression or diminished mental capacity that clouds one's judgment or weakens one's resolve. With patients thus reduced—helpless in action and ambivalent about life—someone who might benefit from their death need not proceed by overt coercion. Rather, requests for assisted suicide can and will be subtly engineered.

To alter and influence choices, physicians and families need not be driven by base motives or even be consciously manipulative. Well-meaning and discreet suggestions, or even unconscious changes in expression, gesture, and tone of voice, can move a dependent and suggestible patient toward a choice for death. Simply by making euthanasia or assisted suicide an option available to gravely ill persons, will we not, as Kamisar wrote long ago, "sweep up, in the process, some who are not really tired of life, but think others are tired of them; some who do not really want to die, but who feel that they should not live on, because to do so when there looms the legal alternative of euthanasia is to do a selfish or cowardly act?"[6] Anyone who knows anything at all about the real life of elderly persons and those who are incurably ill knows that many of them will experience—and be helped to experience—their *freedom* or *right* to choose physician-assisted death as an *obligation* or *duty* to do so.

In the great majority of medical situations, the idealistic assumptions of doctor-patient equality and of patient autonomy are in fact false, even when the patient is in relatively good health and where there is an intimate doctor-patient relationship of long standing. But with those who are seriously ill, or hospitalized, and, even more, with the vast majority of patients who are treated by physicians who know them little or not at all, many choices for death by the so-called autonomous patient will not be truly free and fully informed. Physicians hold a monopoly on the necessary information: prognosis, alternative treatments, and their costs and burdens. Like many technical experts, they are masters at framing the options to guarantee a particular outcome. This they do already in presenting therapeutic options to the "autonomous patient" for decision, and there is no reason to think that will change should one of those options now become "assistance for death." When the physician presents a depressed or frightened patient with a horrible prognosis and includes among the options the offer of a "gentle, quick release," what will the patient likely choose, especially in the face of a spiraling hospital bill or edgy children? The acceptance of physician-assisted death, ostensibly a measure enhancing the freedom of dying patients, will thus in many cases become a deadly license for physicians to recommend and prescribe death, free from outside scrutiny and immune from possible prosecution.

Contrary to the foolish hopes of advocates for autonomy, the insistence on voluntariness as the justifying principle cannot be sustained. It is naive to think that one can draw and hold a line between, on the one hand, physician-assisted suicide or voluntary euthanasia (practiced by doctors on willing patients) and, on the other hand, *non*voluntary euthanasia (where physicians perform mercy killing without the patient's request). Just think through how the situation will develop in practice. Almost no physician will accede to a request for deadly drugs unless he himself believes there are good reasons to justify the patient's choice for death (too much pain, loss of dignity, lack of self-command, poor quality of life, etc.); otherwise, the physician will try to persuade the patient to accept some other course of treatment or palliation, including psychotherapy for suicidal wishes. Thus, *in actual practice* physician-assisted suicide and euthanasia will be performed by physicians not out of simple deference to patient choice, but for reasons of mercy: this is a "useless" or "degrading" or "dehumanized" life that pleads for active, merciful termination, and therefore deserves medical assistance.

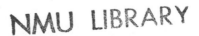

But once assisted suicide and euthanasia are deemed acceptable for reasons of "mercy," then delivering those whom illness or dependence have dehumanized will also be acceptable, whether such deliverance is chosen or not. Once legalized, physician-assisted death will not remain confined to those who freely and knowingly elect it—nor do the most energetic backers of "death with dignity" really want it thus restricted. They see the slippery slope and eagerly embrace the principle that will justify the entire downward slide. Why? Because the vast majority of candidates who "merit" an earlier death cannot request it for themselves. Persons in a so-called persistent vegetative state; those with severe depression, mental illness, or dementia; infants who are deformed; and retarded or dying children—all are incapable of requesting death but are equally deserving of the new, humane "aid in dying."

Lawyers and doctors, subtly encouraged by advocates of cost containment, will soon rectify this inequality. Invoking the rhetoric of equal protection, they will ask courts and ethics committees why those who are comatose or who have dementia should be denied a right just because they cannot claim it for themselves. With court-appointed proxy consenters, we will quickly erase the distinction between the right to choose one's own death and the right to request someone else's—as we already have done in the termination-of-treatment cases.

Doctors and relatives will not even need to wait for such changes in the law. Who will be around to notice when those who are elderly, poor, disabled, weak, powerless, retarded, depressed, uneducated, demented, or gullible are mercifully released from the lives that their doctors, nurses, and next of kin deem no longer worth living?

Precisely because most of the cases that are candidates for mercy killing are of this sort, the line between voluntary and involuntary euthanasia cannot hold, and will be effaced by the intermediate case of mentally impaired or comatose persons who are declared no longer willing to live because someone else wills that result for them. It is easy to see the trains of abuses that are likely to follow the most innocent cases, especially because the innocent cases cannot be precisely and neatly defined so that they are distinguished from the rest.

That the specter of unauthorized euthanasia is no mere scaremongering is confirmed by reports from Holland, where assisted suicide and voluntary euthanasia practiced by physicians have been encouraged for over twenty years, under guidelines established by the medical profession. Although the guidelines insist that the choosing of death must be informed and voluntary, a 1989 survey of 300 physicians disclosed that (already then) over 40 percent had performed *non*voluntary euthanasia and over 10 percent had done so five times or more.[7] Another survey, this one commissioned by the Dutch government, provides even more alarming data: in 1990, besides the 2,300 cases of voluntary euthanasia and 400 cases of physician-assisted suicide per year, there were over 1,000 cases of active *non*voluntary euthanasia performed without the patient's knowledge or consent, *including roughly 140 cases (14%) in which the patients were mentally totally competent.* (Comparable rates of nonvoluntary euthanasia for the United States would be roughly 20,000 cases per year.) In addition, there were 8,100 cases of morphine overdose with the intent to terminate life, of which 68 percent (5,508 cases) took place without the patient's knowledge or consent.[8] Responding to international criticism and concern, the Dutch government commissioned another survey in 1995, which, the researchers claim, shows that the practice of physician-assisted suicide and euthanasia is now well regulated.[9] But, as Dr. Herbert Hendin and colleagues have shown by careful scrutiny of the Dutch government's data, there remains high cause for concern. The incidence of physician-caused death increased (4.7% of all deaths in 1995, up from 3.7% in 1990); 59 percent of Dutch physicians, defying the requirement of notification, still do not report their death-dealing deeds; more than half feel free to suggest euthanasia to their patients, and about 25 percent admit to ending patients' lives without consent. In 1995, 948 patients were directly put to death without their consent; another 1,896 patients died (1.4% of all Dutch deaths that year) as a result of opiates given with the explicit intent to cause death (in over 80% of these cases, no request for death was made by the patient).[10]

And why are Dutch physicians performing nonvoluntary euthanasia? "Low quality of life," "relatives' inability to cope," and "no prospect for improvement" were reasons physicians gave for killing patients without request; pain or suffering was mentioned by only 30 percent.[11] Is there any reason to believe that Dutch physicians are less committed than their American counterparts to the equal dignity of every life under their care?

Actual abuses aside, the legalized practice of physician-assisted death will almost certainly damage the doctor-patient relationship. True, some may be relieved to know that their old family doctor will now provide

personal standards. One will choose to assist death over against moderate or impending dementia, another against paraplegia, a third against blindness or incurable incontinence or prolonged depression. Only those requests resonating with the physician's own private criteria of "intolerable" or "unworthy" lives will be honored. True, many people hold opinions and make judgments about which lives are worthier than others and even about which might be unworthy of continued existence. The danger comes when people *act* on these judgments, and especially when they do so under the cloak of professional prestige and compassion. Medical ethics, mindful that medicine wields formidable powers over life and death, has for centuries prevented physicians from acting professionally on the basis of any such personal judgment. Medical students, interns, and residents are taught—and acquire—a profound repugnance to medical killing as a major defense against committing, or even contemplating, the worst action to which their arrogance or their weakness, or both, might lead them.

Even the most humane and conscientious physicians psychologically need protection against themselves and their weaknesses and arrogance, if they are to care fully for those who entrust themselves to them. A physician-friend who worked many years in a hospice caring for dying patients explained it to me most convincingly: "Only because I knew that I could not and would not kill my patients was I able to enter most fully and intimately into caring for them as they lay dying." The psychological burden of the license to kill (not to speak of the brutalization of the physician-killers) could very well be an intolerably high price to pay for physician-assisted euthanasia.

The point, however, is not merely psychological; it is also moral and essential. My friend's horror at the thought that he might be tempted to kill his patients, were he not enjoined from doing so, embodies a deep understanding of the medical ethic and its intrinsic limits. Let us now move from assessing consequences to looking at medicine itself.

Medicine's Outer Limits

Every activity can be distinguished, more or less easily, from other activities. Sometimes the boundaries are indistinct: it is not always easy, especially today, to distinguish some music from noise or some art from smut or some teaching from indoctrination. Medicine and healing are no different: it is sometimes hard to determine the boundaries, with regard to both ends and means. Is all cosmetic surgery healing? Are placebos—or food and water—drugs?

There is, of course, a temptation to finesse these questions of definition or to deny the existence of boundaries altogether: medicine *is* whatever doctors *do,* and doctors do whatever doctors can. Technique and power alone define the art. Put this way, we see the need for limits: technique and power are ethically neutral, notoriously so, usable for both good and ill. The need for finding or setting limits to the use of powers is especially important when the powers are dangerous: it matters more that we know the proper limits on the use of medical power—or military power—than, say, the proper limits on the use of a paintbrush or violin.

The beginning of ethics regarding the use of power generally lies in nay-saying. The wise setting of limits on the use of power is based on discerning the excesses to which the power, unrestrained, is prone. Applied to the professions, this principle would establish strict outer boundaries—indeed, inviolable taboos—against those "occupational hazards" to which each profession is especially prone. Within these outer limits, no fixed rules of conduct apply; instead, prudence—the wise judgment of the person on the spot—finds and adopts the best course of action in the light of the circumstances. But the outer limits themselves are fixed, firm, and non-negotiable.

What are those limits for medicine? At least three are set forth in the venerable Hippocratic Oath: no breach of confidentiality; no sexual relations with patients; no dispensing of deadly drugs.[13] These unqualified, self-imposed restrictions are readily understood in terms of the temptations to which the physician is most vulnerable, temptations in each case regarding an area of vulnerability and exposure that the practice of medicine requires of patients. Patients necessarily divulge and reveal private and intimate details of their personal lives; patients necessarily expose their naked bodies to the physician's objectifying gaze and investigating hands; patients necessarily expose and entrust the care of their very lives to the physician's skill, technique, judgment, and character. The exposure is, in all cases, one-sided and asymmetric: the doctor does not reveal his intimacies, display his nakedness, or offer up his embodied life to the patient. Mindful of the meaning of such nonmutual exposure and vulnerability, and mindful too of their own penchant for error and mischief, Hippocratic physicians voluntarily set limits on their own conduct, pledging not to take advantage of or to violate the patient's intimacies, naked sexuality, or life itself.

The prohibition against killing patients, the first negative promise of self-restraint sworn to in the Hippocratic Oath, stands as medicine's first and most abiding taboo: "I will neither give a deadly drug to anybody if asked for it, nor will I make a suggestion to this effect. . . . In purity and holiness I will guard my life and my art." In forswearing the giving of poison, the physician recognizes and restrains a godlike power he wields over patients, mindful that drugs can both cure and kill. But in forswearing the giving of poison *when asked for it,* the Hippocratic physician rejects the view that the patient's choice for death can make killing the patient—or assisting the patient in suicide—right. For the physician, at least, human life in living bodies commands respect and reverence—by its very nature. As its respectability does not depend on human agreement or patient consent, revocation of one's consent to live does not deprive one's living being of respectability. The deepest ethical principle restraining the physician's power is neither the autonomy and freedom of the patient nor the physician's own compassion or good intention. Rather, it is the dignity and mysterious power of human life itself, and, therefore, also what the Oath calls the purity and holiness of the life and art to which the physician has sworn devotion. A person can choose to be a physician but cannot simply choose what physicianship means.[14]

The Central Core

The central meaning of physicianship derives not from medicine's powers but from its goal, not from its means but from its end: to benefit the sick by the activity of healing. The physician as physician serves only the sick. The physician does not serve the relatives or the hospital or the national debt inflated due to Medicare costs. Thus the true physician will never sacrifice the well-being of the sick to the convenience or pocketbook or feelings of the relatives or society. Moreover, the physician serves the sick not because they have rights or wants or claims, but because they are sick. The healer works with and for those who need to be healed, in order to help make them whole. Despite enormous changes in medical technique and institutional practice, despite enormous changes in nosology and therapeutics, the center of medicine has not changed: it is as true today as it was in the days of Hippocrates that the ill desire to be whole; that wholeness means a certain well-working of the enlivened body and its unimpaired powers to sense, think, feel, desire, move, and maintain itself; and that the relationship between the healer and the ill is constituted, essentially even if only tacitly, around the desire of both to promote the wholeness of the one who is ailing.

The wholeness and well-working of a human being is, of course, a rather complicated matter, much more so than for our animal friends and relations. Health and fitness seem to mean different things to different people, or even to the same person at different times of life. Yet not everything is relative and contextual; beneath the variable and cultural lies the constant and organic: the well-regulated, properly balanced, and fully empowered human being. Indeed, only the existence of this natural and universal subject makes possible the study of medicine.

But human wholeness goes beyond the kind of somatic wholeness abstractly and reductively studied by the modern medical sciences. Whether or not doctors are sufficiently prepared by their training to recognize it, those who seek medical help in search of wholeness are not *to themselves* just bodies or organic machines. Each person intuitively knows himself to be a center of thoughts and desires, deeds and speeches, loves and hates, pleasures and pains, but a center whose workings are none other than the workings of his enlivened and mindful body. The patient presents himself to the physician, tacitly to be sure, as a psychophysical unity, as a *one*, not just a body, but also not just as a separate disembodied person who simply *has* or *owns* a body. The person and the body are self-identical. True, sickness may be experienced largely as belonging to the body as something other, but the healing one wants is the wholeness of one's entire embodied being. Not the wholeness of just *soma*, not the wholeness of just *psyche*, but the wholeness of *anthropos* as a (puzzling) concretion of *soma-psyche* is the benefit sought by the sick. This human wholeness is what medicine is finally all about.

Can wholeness and healing, thus understood, ever be compatible with intentionally killing the patient? Can one benefit the patient *as a whole* by making him dead? There is, of course, a logical difficulty: how can any good exist for a being that is not? "Better off dead" is logical nonsense—unless, of course, death is not death indeed but instead a gateway to a new and better life beyond. Despite loose talk to the contrary, it is in fact impossible to compare the goodness or badness of one's existence with the goodness or badness of one's "nonexistence," because it nonsensically requires treating "nonexistence" as a condition one is nonetheless able to experience and enjoy. But the error is more than logical: in fact, to intend and to act for someone's good requires that person's continued existence for the benefit to be received.

To be sure, certain attempts to benefit may in fact turn out, unintentionally, to be lethal. Giving adequate morphine to control pain might induce respiratory depression leading to death. But the intent to relieve the pain of the living presupposes that the living still live to be relieved. This must be the starting point in discussing all medical benefits: no benefit without a beneficiary.

Against this view, someone will surely bring forth the hard cases: patients so ill-served by their bodies that they can no longer bear to live, bodies riddled with cancer and racked with pain, against which their "owners" protest in horror and from which they insist on being released. Cannot the person "in the body" speak up against the rest and request death for "personal" reasons?

However sympathetically we listen to such requests, we must see them as incoherent. Such person-body dualism cannot be sustained. "Personhood" is manifest on earth only in living bodies; our highest mental functions are held up by, and are inseparable from, lowly metabolism, respiration, circulation, and excretion. There may be blood without consciousness, but there is never consciousness without blood. Thus one who calls for death in the service of personhood is like a tree seeking to cut its roots for the sake of growing its highest fruit. No physician, devoted to the benefit of the sick, can serve the patient *as person* by denying and thwarting the patient's personal *embodiment*. The boundary condition, "No deadly drugs," flows directly from the center, "Make whole."

Against this defense of the venerable taboo against medical killing, a number of objections can be—indeed, have been—raised. Some will say that medicine has no central purpose, while others will protest that I have defined it too narrowly. For example, Franklin G. Miller and Howard Brody, criticizing an earlier version of this argument, complain that I am guilty of "essentialism"—believing that medicine serves only the goal of healing (despite the fact that I have always held that relief of suffering, along with promoting wholeness, is a necessary part of the medical task).[15] Instead, they propose that medicine serves a plurality of goals, "which includes healing, promoting health, and helping patients achieve a peaceful death." To achieve this last "important goal for medicine," they argue that in some circumstances "physician-assisted death may become, unfortunately, the best among the limited options."[16]

Where does this allegedly *medical* goal of "helping patients achieve a peaceful death" come from? Miller and Brody do not say. It surely lacks the support of medical tradition and standard medical ethics. In their discussion, it rather appears out of the blue, simply stipulated and asserted, without an attempt at reasoned justification. Yet even if we place the best construction on their assertion and admit that medicine has something to offer patients regarding the end of life, Miller and Brody are victims of imprecise thought. They have confused helping patients "experience peaceful *dying*" with helping them *"achieve* a peaceful *death."* As I will argue more fully in what follows, medicine surely owes patients assistance in their dying process—to relieve their pain, discomfort, and distress. This is simply part of what it means to seek to relieve suffering, always an essential part of caring *for the living*, including when they are in the process of their dying. But medicine has never, under anyone's interpretation, been charged with *producing or achieving death itself.* Physicians cannot be serving their art or helping their patients—whether regarded as human beings or as persons—by making them disappear.

Despite their errors, Miller and Brody are at least clear that the "achievement of a peaceful death" is a goal *distinct* from healing; they will not try to smuggle euthanasia ("a peaceful death") into medicine under a revisionist idea of healing or relief of suffering. But others are willing to play the sophist. For example, Dr. Else Borst-Eilers, former chair of the Dutch Health Council, has claimed that "there are situations in which the best way to heal the patient is to help him die peacefully and the doctor who in such a situation grants the patient's request acts as the healer *par excellence."*[17] This kind of euphemistic talk should produce chills for those who remember how a distinguished German jurist, Professor Karl Binding, and a distinguished German psychiatrist, Dr. Alfred Hoche, proposed in 1920 the destruction of "life unworthy of life," which they described as "purely a healing treatment" and as a "healing work."[18] Argue if you must that killing those who are infirm and those who are miserable should be acceptable. But, for goodness' sake, have the decency not to pretend that it is healing.

To say it plainly, to bring nothingness is incompatible with serving wholeness: one cannot heal—or comfort—by making nil. Healers cannot annihilate if they are truly to heal. The physician-euthanizer is a deadly self-contradiction.

When Medicine "Fails"

We must acknowledge a difficulty. The central goal of medicine—health—is, in each case, a perishable good: inevitably, patients get irreversibly sick, patients degenerate, patients die. Healing the sick is in principle a project that must at some point fail. And here is where all the trouble begins: how does one deal with "medical failure"? What does one seek when restoration of wholeness—or "much" wholeness—is by and large out of the question?

Contrary to what the euthanasia movement would have people believe, there is, in fact, much that can be done. Indeed, by recognizing finitude yet knowing that we will not kill, we are empowered to focus on easing and enhancing the lives of those who are dying. First of all, medicine can follow the lead of the hospice movement and—abandoning decades of shameful mismanagement—provide truly adequate (and now technically feasible) relief of pain and discomfort. Second, physicians (and patients and families) can continue to learn how to withhold or withdraw those technical interventions that are, in truth, merely burdensome or degrading medical additions to the unhappy end of a life—including, frequently, hospitalization itself. Ceasing treatment and allowing death to occur when (and if) it will seem to be quite compatible with the respect life commands for itself. For life can be revered not only in its preservation, but also in the manner in which we allow a given life to reach its terminus. Rightly understood, removing unwanted and burdensome medical interventions serves not a patient's choice for death but rather the patient's choice to continue to live as well as he can, even while he is dying. Doctors may and must allow to die, even if they must not intentionally kill.

Ceasing medical intervention, allowing nature to take its course, differs fundamentally from mercy killing. For one thing, death does not necessarily follow the discontinuance of treatment; Karen Ann Quinlan lived more than ten years after the courts allowed the "life-sustaining" respirator to be removed. Not her physician but the underlying fatal illness became the true cause of her death.[19]

What is most important *morally* is that the physician who ceases treatment does not intend the death of the patient. Even if death follows as a result of the physician's action or omission, his intention is to avoid useless and degrading medical additions to the already sad end of a life.

By contrast, in assisted suicide and all other forms of direct killing, the physician must necessarily and indubitably intend primarily that the patient be made dead. And he must knowingly and indubitably cast himself in the role of the agent of death. This remains true even if the physician is merely an assistant in suicide. Morally, a physician who provides the pills or lets the patient plunge the syringe after he leaves the room is no different from one who does the deed himself. "I will neither give a deadly drug to anybody if asked for it, nor will I make a suggestion to this effect."

The same prohibition against physician killing continues to operate in other areas of palliative care where some have sought to deny its importance. For example, physicians often and quite properly prescribe high doses of narcotics to patients with widespread cancer in an effort to relieve severe pain, even though such medication carries an increased risk of death. But it is wrong to say that the current use of intravenous morphine in advanced cancer patients already constitutes a practice of medical killing. The physician here intends only the relief of suffering, which presupposes that the patient will continue to live in order to be relieved. Death, should it occur, is unintended and regretted.

The well-established rule of medical ethics that governs this practice is known as the principle of double effect, a principle widely misunderstood. It is morally licit to embrace a course of action that intends and serves a worthy goal (like relieving suffering), employing means that may have, as an unintended and undesired consequence, some harm or evil for the patient. Such cases are distinguished from the morally illicit efforts that indirectly "relieve suffering" by deliberately providing a lethal dose of a drug and thus eliminating the sufferer.

True, it may not always be easy to distinguish the two cases from the outside. When death occurs from respiratory depression following administration of morphine, the outcome—a dead patient—is the same, and the proximate cause—morphine—is the same. Physical evidence alone, obtained after the fact, will often not be enough to tell whether the physician acted with intent to relieve pain or with intent to kill. But that is *exactly* why the principle of double effect is so important. Only an ethic opposing the intent to kill, reinforced by the law, keeps the physician from such deliberately deadly acts. Only such an ethic enables physicians to serve and care for our residual wholeness and humanity right to the very end.

Being Humane and Being Human

Once we refuse the technical fix, physicians and the rest of us can also rise to the occasion: we can learn to act humanly in the presence of finitude. Far more than adequate morphine and the removal of burdensome chemotherapy, those who are dying need our presence and our encouragement. Dying people are all too easily reduced ahead of time to "thinghood" by those who cannot bear to deal with the suffering or disability of those they love. Withdrawal of contact, affection, and care is the greatest single cause of the dehumanization of dying. Not the alleged humaneness of an elixir of death, but the humanness of connected living-while-dying is what physicians—and the rest of us—most owe someone who is dying. The treatment of choice is company and care.

The euthanasia movement would have us believe that the physician's refusal to assist in suicide or perform euthanasia constitutes an affront to human dignity. Yet one of euthanasia advocates' favorite arguments seems to me rather to prove the reverse. Why, it is argued, do we put animals out of their misery but insist on compelling fellow human beings to suffer to the bitter end? Why, if it is not a contradiction for the veterinarian, does the medical ethic absolutely rule out mercy killing? Is this not simply inhumane?

Perhaps inhumane, but not thereby inhuman. On the contrary, it is precisely because animals are not human that we must treat them (merely) humanely. We put dumb animals to sleep because they do not know that they are dying, because they can make nothing of their misery or mortality, and, therefore, because they cannot live deliberately (i.e., humanly) in the face of their own suffering or dying. They cannot live out a fitting end. Compassion for their weakness and dumbness is our only appropriate emotion, and given our responsibility for their care and well-being, we do the only humane thing we can. But when a conscious human being asks us for death, by that very action he displays the presence of something that precludes our regarding him as a dumb animal. Humanity is owed humanity, not humaneness. Humanity is owed the bolstering of the human, even or especially in its dying moments, in resistance to the temptation to ignore its presence in the sight of suffering.

What humanity needs most in the face of evils is courage, the ability to stand against fear and pain and thoughts of nothingness. The deaths we most admire are those of people who, knowing that they are dying, face the fact frontally and act accordingly: they set their affairs in order, they arrange what could be final meetings with their loved ones, and yet, with strength of soul and a small reservoir of hope, they continue to live and work and love as much as they can for as long as they can. Because such conclusions of life require courage, they call for our encouragement—and for the many small speeches and deeds that shore up the human spirit against despair and defeat.

Many doctors are in fact rather poor at this sort of encouragement. They tend to regard every dying or incurable patient as a failure, as if an earlier diagnosis or a more vigorous intervention might have avoided what is, in truth, an inevitable collapse. The enormous successes of medicine these past fifty years have made both doctors and laymen less prepared than ever to accept the fact of finitude. Physicians today are not likely to be agents of encouragement once their technique begins to fail.

It is, of course, partly for these reasons that doctors will be pressed to kill—and many of them will, alas, be willing. Having adopted a largely technical approach to healing, having medicalized so much of the end of life, doctors are being asked—often with thinly veiled anger—to provide a final technical solution for the evil of human finitude and for their own technical failure: If you cannot cure me, kill me. The last gasp of autonomy or cry for dignity is asserted against a medicalization and institutionalization of the end of life that robs those who are old and those who are incurably ill of most of their autonomy and dignity: intubated and electrified, with bizarre mechanical companions, once proud and independent people find themselves cast in the roles of passive, obedient, highly disciplined children. People who care for autonomy and dignity should try to reverse this dehumanization of the last stages of life, instead of giving dehumanization its final triumph by welcoming the desperate goodbye-to-all-that contained in one final plea for poison.

The present crisis that leads to the demand for assisted suicide and active euthanasia is thus an opportunity to learn the limits of the medicalization of life and death and to recover an appreciation of living with and against mortality. It is an opportunity for physicians to affirm the residual humanity—however precarious—that can be appreciated and cared for even in the face of incurable and terminal illness. Should doctors cave in, should we allow them to become technical dispensers of death, we will not only be abandoning our loved ones and our patients and our duty to care for them. We will also exacerbate the worst

tendencies of modern life, embracing technicism and so-called humaneness where humanity and encouragement are both required and
sorely lacking. On the other hand, should physicians hold fast, should
we all learn that finitude is no disgrace and that human wholeness can
be cared for to the very end, medicine may serve not only the good of its
patients, but also, by example, the moral health of modern times.

2

Compassion Is Not Enough

Edmund D. Pellegrino, M.D.

A certain Samaritan . . . had compassion on him.

Luke 10:33

Compassion and patient autonomy are the two commonest reasons advanced in favor of physician-assisted suicide and euthanasia. Of the two, compassion is the more universal and the more appealing. Few of us would consciously want to act noncompassionately. All of us would want to be treated compassionately when we need help. Without compassion, a society cannot be humane.

Compassion softens the realities of life. It succors the vulnerable, mollifies the wrath and power of the strong, and cushions the frailties to which, sooner or later, all must succumb. Without compassion, there would be no brake on selfish self-interest or hatred or all-out indifference to the plight of others. Few of us could—or would want to—live in a world devoid of compassion.

But even an emotion so powerful, necessary, and ubiquitous needs the restraint of reason. Like all our passions, compassion can be distorted, self-defeating, and even harmful. In the name of compassion, many have been deprived of their human dignity, condescended to, and even led unwillingly to their deaths. Reason and compassion need each other; one without the other can become self-justifying and tyrannize the human soul and psyche.

This is especially the case in the presence of human suffering, particularly when death is near and inevitable. In the presence of suffering and pain, most of us feel compassion and a desire to relieve the suffering. For the protagonists of assisted suicide or euthanasia, compassion is a sufficient moral reason to relieve human anguish—even an obligation. For the antagonists, compassion is a necessary attribute of beneficence but not, of itself, a sufficient moral justification for ending a human life. For them, compassion unrestrained by reason becomes dangerous.

This chapter examines the nature of compassion, the way it is used in moral arguments, its validity as the basis for an ethic of care, and its proper—and improper—place in the care of suffering human beings.

The Nature of Compassion

While it is a word in common parlance, *compassion* has many shades of meaning philosophically, psychologically, and theologically. At the outset, therefore, it is useful to disentangle some of the overlapping ideals subsumed in the word.

Etymologically, *compassion* derives from two Latin words: *cum,* meaning "with," and *patior,* meaning "I suffer." *Patior* comes from the Greek *pathos,* which means "feeling" or "emotion." Compassion literally means "to suffer with, or feel with, another person." In the presence of suffering or dying persons, compassion entails feeling something of that person's pain, suffering, and anguish.

Encompassed within this understanding of compassion are several other closely related emotions, like sympathy, pity, mercy, and empathy. Those terms are often used interchangeably, but there are some important nuances of difference among them.

Etymologically and phonetically, sympathy and empathy have a close relationship. They share the common root *pathos* (feeling or suffering). Nonetheless they have important differences in meaning. *Sympathy* connotes affinity of feeling, sentiment, or temperament with others. *Empathy* suggests a more intimate "getting inside" another person's experiences. *Pity* places emphasis on feeling sorry for another, sometimes tinged with a spirit of condescension or superiority. *Mercy,* on the other hand, connotes mitigation of punishment or kind treatment where severity might be expected.

For some philosophers, one or the other of these senses of compassion has been central to ethics.[1] In this chapter, I will take compassion in its common usage of co-suffering, co-feeling, a sense of "being in the other person's shoes," without trying to specify which of the possible mixtures of nuances is dominant in any particular instance.

The proponents of euthanasia and assisted suicide argue that we should feel compassion in the presence of another human being's suffering, that the existence of that emotion compels us to want to relieve suffering, and that it generates an obligation to relieve suffering. They propose what is in essence an ethic of compassion, one that gives normative moral force to a human emotion. This species of emotivist ethics dates as far back as Epicurus (371–341 B.C.E.). It was best enunciated in the eighteenth century by the English and Scottish school of "moral sense" theorists, of whom David Hume was the most articulate and influential representative.[2]

For Hume, moral sentiment, sympathy, and the emotions were the prime determinants of moral judgment. Hume held sympathy to be a virtue more reliable than reason, which should be sympathy's slave, not its master.[3] By itself, he argued, reason cannot move us to action; emotion does. Humans have a natural tendency to sympathize and to be benevolent, and this accounts for moral and virtuous acts.

In similar fashion, proponents of an ethic of compassion today treat the emotion of compassion or its cognates as moral imperatives. Margaret Battin,[4] for example, speaks of the "principle of mercy" in justifying intentionally hastening the death of suffering or dying persons whose suffering elicits compassion in us. In one way or another, this is the justification underlying tolerance for euthanasia or assisted suicide, whether it is the rare case in which all else has failed or the legal or social approbation of euthanasia on demand.[5]

There are understandable reasons why an emotivist ethic with compassion at its root is so appealing. For one thing, there is the growing disaffection with more traditional moral systems based in principles, duties, or rules that are deemed too abstract, too intellectual, and too distant from the concrete experience of moral choice to give adequate moral guidance. Emotions, it is said, put us into closer touch with our own humanity as well as that of others. Then there is the prevalent skepticism about the possibility that there exist any moral truths and the sense that reason is unable to grasp such truths if they do exist. All of this is accentuated by cultural differences, with their pluralism of moral judgment and their strong pull toward moral relativism.

Together, these factors give credence to emotions, feelings, and "values" as more reliable indicators of right and wrong than reasoned discourse. From this viewpoint, if reason has a place, it is secondary to emotion.

Its purpose is to adjust means and actions so that compassion is actual-
ized and empowered. Reason functions more as a rationalization or an
instrumental device than as a guide to the moral expression of the emotions. Some go further and excise philosophy from ethics altogether as
a distracting illusion, psychologizing the moral life completely.[6]

An Ethic of Compassion

In an interview on the subject of euthanasia and assisted suicide shortly
before his death, Hans Jonas, one of the most perceptive modern philosophers of biology and technology, took a different view: "We mustn't
let ourselves be governed by an ethic of compassion but only by a sense
of responsibility for the consequences arising from our attitudes, and our
willingness to consider, on occasion, taking life. We ought not, and must
not, let this be our starting point."[7] Jonas clearly questioned the propri-
ety of compassion as a self-justifying moral imperative. This is not the
place for a full critique of ethical systems based solely on compassion.
However, as Jonas suggested, a look at some of the logical consequences
of accepting and applying such an ethic to the intentional taking of
human life for humane reasons is in order.

To oppose a compassion-based ethic is not to deny the place of emotion in moral judgment. In fact, judgments that our own acts, or those
of others, are morally right or wrong are usually accompanied by feelings of approval or revulsion. But an emotive evaluation does not, in
itself, explain *why* these judgments are right or wrong. They are right or
wrong because they conform to or contravene a moral norm—some
virtue, duty, or principle. There must be some reasoned basis for moral
judgment, and that basis must be distinguishable from emotional evaluation. Without reason, there is no way to distinguish good emotional responses from bad ones.[8]

This is not to oppose reason and emotion in any absolute way. Rather,
it is to recognize their complex interrelationship without confusing one
with the other. The precise relationship of passion and reason is still a
subject of study even in as longstanding a moral system as that of Aristotle, who was the first to confront the consonance of action and feelings
in a formal way.

This relationship is especially relevant for compassion, which is an
emotion accompanied by a desire to act. The emotion, itself, is com-

mendable. Without compassion, human relationships would be brutish for the vulnerable among us. The emotion of compassion has engendered some of the most admirable and heroic acts of which humans are capable. But the fact that we experience the emotion of compassion does not per se give moral legitimacy to any action that compassion might motivate.[9]

After all, not all persons feel compassion in the same way, to the same degree, or with the same commitment to act. In a few, compassion is a negligible emotion or one that does not arise at all; in others, it may be suppressed or distorted by other emotions, like fear, anxiety, or self-interest. In such circumstances, compassion can become so diluted or altered that the acts it motivates are not at all benevolent.

Manifestly, it cannot be a duty to feel the emotion of compassion. We cannot command emotions to occur in others. Compassion is too personal, intimate, and internal to be mandated externally. Nor can the mere experience of a feeling of co-suffering justify any action it motivates as morally good. Rather, the duty of beneficence and the virtue of benevolence require us to act in such a way that we do, in fact, relieve suffering by means that are morally acceptable.

The key question in the euthanasia and assisted suicide debates, therefore, is not whether we are obliged to respond to the desire to relieve suffering. This is entailed by the duty of beneficence and the virtue of benevolence. Rather, we must ask ourselves, What constitutes an ethically appropriate way to act out the emotion of compassion? How are we to act compassionately in a *morally* justifiable way? How do we keep compassionate feelings from leading to maleficent acts?

The Argument from Compassion

Presumably, both those who favor and those who oppose euthanasia and assisted suicide aspire to act benevolently with respect to the relief of human suffering. Compassionate people are motivated by what they take to be the good of the person suffering. What is at issue is the definition of the good of that person. Protagonists of euthanasia and assisted suicide, for example, see suffering as an absolute evil to be relieved at any cost. From their viewpoint, we fail in compassion if we do not satisfy patients' wishes to end their own lives when they desire, and on their own terms—either by killing them on their request or by providing the means whereby they may kill themselves. If this is so, when we experience the emotion of compassion, relief of pain and suffering becomes a moral mandate irrespective of the means we use.

It follows from this line of reasoning that the means we use to end life should be as efficient as possible. But in fact, self-administered prescriptions may fail in a significant number of cases. As a result, the act of dying may be prolonged and unpleasant. The dose of the lethal medication may well have to be repeated or replaced by direct euthanasia. If this is so, it would require the physician to administer the dose, or to be present and ready to accelerate death more directly if the first effort fails. Assisted suicide quickly becomes direct and active euthanasia with the transfer of power from the patient to the physician—the antithesis of the expression of autonomy so many seek.

For some, voluntary euthanasia and assisted suicide may not satisfy the full extent of compassion and the obligation to relieve suffering. They might argue, for example, that it is unjust to allow persons who are physiologically unable to request termination of their lives to suffer because they lack decision-making capabilities. This is the case with persons in a permanent vegetative state, or with infants, children, or retarded persons. From this viewpoint, when quality of life is "poor" or lacking in future prospects, compassion requires involuntary or nonvoluntary euthanasia. To restrict hastening death only to those capable of making a voluntary decision is, in the minds of some, to narrow the obligation of compassion in unjust ways. For them, compassion should not wait on informed consent.

Likewise, should compassion be felt only for the person suffering? The continued existence of a dying or severely ill and handicapped person imposes suffering on those around the individual—families, physicians, and nurses, as well as society at large. Should we not save resources and reduce burdens on the whole health care system by hastening inevitable deaths? The resources thus saved could be used for other compassionate causes, like providing health care, food, housing, and education for the poor. To follow this line of reasoning, it would be compassionate to relieve the anguish, frustration, and emotional exhaustion of the caregiver by accelerating the death of a patient in a permanent vegetative state. It would also be a praiseworthy act of self-sacrifice on the patient's part to request acceleration of death to spare others the burdens of his or her care.

If compassion is absolutized in this way as a social value, it implies an obligation on the part of physicians to be the preferred instruments of hastening death.[10] Physicians know what drugs to use and in what combination and dosage. They know how to administer them. Laws give them exclusive control over the prescription of controlled substances. Physicians also know what to do if the patient's attempt at self-administration fails. On the rule of absolutized compassion, doctors should be society's delegated agents for release from suffering. Indeed, in this view, by virtue of the medical power they possess, physicians have a duty to terminate certain lives.[11]

Some even interpret the physician's refusal to participate in assisted suicide when requested as moral abandonment and a violation of the Hippocratic Oath. Today, the Hippocratic prohibition against administration of a lethal medication is under serious challenge. Many hold that the oath must no longer be interpreted "dogmatically," that is to say, strictly. Instead, it has been suggested that the benefit of death must be assessed by the patient, and only the patient. The patient should be allowed to choose intentional death. Physicians who comply would not violate their professional ethic.[12] Rather, they would replace an outmoded precept with commendable compassion.

To exalt compassion over traditional professional obligations or to make it one of such obligations is seductive but dangerous. Danger lurks behind the benign face of compassion so flexibly interpreted. An Auschwitz survivor put it bluntly: "The doctor ... if not living in a moral situation ... where moral limits are very clear ... is dangerous." This is not to argue against compassion, but to be reminded that without linking the emotion to a moral standard, evildoers can, and have, convinced themselves that they were acting "compassionately": To persuade good and moral people to do evil, then, it is not necessary to persuade them to become evil. It is necessary only to teach them that they are doing good.[13]

Another example of how compassion is misused as an argument for assisted suicide is the way some of its major advocates use it in treating intractable pain in dying patients.[14] They usually propose a process in which a series of steps are taken in cooperation with the patient to alleviate pain and suffering. If those fail, by joint agreement with the patient, the physician assists in suicide, presumably as a last resort, that is, presumably as the last step in a compassionate response to the patient's plight.

This process seems to have the attraction of an orderly decision-making event that the compassionate physician and the responsible patient will presumably not abuse. Superficially, the process appears to protect the patient's autonomy and evinces sympathy for the patient's plight: the driving force and the justifying argument is compassion for the sufferer. Several things are wrong with this reasoning.

First, it begs the central question, Is intentional hastening of death ever justified? It assumes an assisted death can be a "good" death. It presumes that taking life, even indirectly, is consistent with the ethics of medicine. It assumes a patient can resist the subtle coercion of others—doctors, nurses, family members, and friends who think the patient's life is not worth living or is one that they would not want to live.

Second, the patient autonomy that assisted suicide and euthanasia presume to protect and empower is illusory.[15] The physician decides when the patient is suffering intolerably enough to use the last resort. The physician controls the availability of the medication and its dose. The physician makes the judgment about the quality of the patient's life and suffering and what is good for the patient. The patient's autonomy is submerged in the observer's emotion of compassion. This form of paternalism is no less objectionable for its compassionate motivation. Indeed, the paternalism neutralizes the strong versions of the argument for autonomy as the moral basis for assisting suicide.[16]

Finally, the argument is often made from a "paradigm" case on the assumption that all compassionate persons would agree that a given life is not worth living. Extreme cases can elicit compassion, but to be normative morally, there must be some moral reason beyond the case itself. Lacking this, our capacity to elicit an emotion is erroneously transformed into a justification for imposing our values on the dying person, for doing what we would want for ourselves or our families.[17]

The fundamental error in any argument from compassion and any ethic based solely in compassion is the conversion of an emotion, with its multiple and various manifestations in different persons, into a moral obligation to act in any way that the emotion dictates. Emotion disengaged from moral reasons distorts compassion, just as reason without emotion distorts the reality of human moral experience.[18]

Compassion: What True Co-suffering Entails

Rejecting the argument from compassion used by the protagonists of euthanasia and assisted suicide is not the same as rejecting the role of compassion in the care of suffering persons. The proper role of the emotion of co-suffering is to compel us to act in such a way toward the sufferer that our effort to put ourselves in the sufferer's place is authentically compassionate. This is not simply to communicate pity or mercy, but genuinely to make some of the suffering person's burden our own. True compassion is an emotion accompanied by a desire to help, but to help in a way that communicates our solidarity with the sufferer without losing our ethical bearings in the process.

To be helpful, we do need to show our emotional solidarity with the one who is suffering. At appropriate times—through voice, touch, silence, or conversation—our feelings for the dying person can be made manifest to him or her. True compassion makes clear our attachment *to the person*, not to our own philosophy of dying or reasons for living.

Genuine compassion is indispensable in humane and loving care of suffering and dying persons. Without it, the suffering individual feels abandoned, ostracized from the world of human interaction and communal feeling, pitied, despised, devalued, and without dignity. Absence of compassion—or the perception of its absence—adds immeasurably to suffering and reinforces any incipient tendency to seek death in the face of suffering.

There are times, however, when some degree of detachment is appropriate. Patients need to know that our compassion does not undermine our professionalism, or our capacity to act with benign paternalism when the patient's response to illness is self-destructive. The traditional medical virtue of equanimity has been seriously misunderstood.[19] It is not a call to serene, uninterested detachment, but a call for calm appraisal of the clinical situation when emotions are threatening to engulf the doctor as well as the patient and the patient's family.

In my own clinical teaching, I often ask dying patients what message they want most to communicate to medical students and residents. Invariably, they say, "Please tell them to put themselves in my place." These words sum up our professional failings to show true compassion for those who are suffering or dying. These patients are speaking not only of the cruder aspects of the many impersonal ways in which we relate to them, the rudeness and uninterested detachment, but also of the subtler lapses as well: our overly hasty visits, our failure to touch the patient physically, our demeaning turns of phrase, our habit of belittling the patient's fear or of hearing without listening, the subtle imputations of loss of dignity, self-pity, and fear—all of which reinforce the patient's loss of self-worth.

Seriously ill, dying, or suffering patients have a heightened sensitivity to everything and everyone in their milieu. They tend to associate even the most minor occurrences with their own existential plight. They can sense indifference and insincerity as well as fear, anxiety, or the fascination-repulsion their physical appearance may induce in others. Much of the guilt, sense of worthlessness, and loss of dignity that suffering patients feel arises from how they perceive our responses to their predicament. By offering the possibility of an assisted suicide or leaving the lethal drugs at the bedside, we confirm the sufferer's devaluation of his or her own life. Our "compassion" contributes to the patient's suffering and reinforces the desperate plea for release by any means.

True compassion means we truly share the other's suffering. Saint Anselm puts it this way: "Compassion is our heart made wretched by the suffering of the wretched." Obviously, we cannot enter the world of another's suffering completely. But by our behavior we can communicate our concern, care, and feeling for the sufferer, our human identification with him or her. In this way, the sufferer can regain some sense of the worth and dignity the predicament of illness has taken away. True compassion is a response to a plea for help. It is a sign that we comprehend, to some extent, what is happening to suffering people even when we cannot relieve that suffering entirely. Patients know that we cannot enter their predicament fully, but they can recognize when we try to see ourselves in their "place."

True compassion requires that family members, friends, and physicians recognize their complicity in the patient's loss of dignity. We must recognize, too, that for those who assist in or approve of it, assisting in suicide may be an act of self-pity as much as compassion for another. The patient's death releases caregivers from frustration, fatigue, hostility, and guilt. A person who is debilitated, dying, and emaciated reminds us of our own finitude, of the fact that we, too, may someday suffer the same way. Our desire to rid ourselves of this reminder can be the unconscious motive for our "compassionate" act of euthanasia or assisted suicide.

It goes without saying that true compassion means relieving pain to the greatest extent possible. Pain per se is the reason for seeking death in a minority of cases, but it is a serious moral failure, and serious malpractice as well, not to use pain medication optimally. Compassion also means recognizing the futility of treatment when the burdens dispro-portionately outweigh the benefits. It means appreciating the fact that every person suffers differently and for different reasons. True compas-sion requires discernment of the unique constellation of causes that gen-erate suffering in *this* patient. It means directing our relief to those causes as they express themselves in the person of the patient.

Above all, compassionate participation in the other person's suffering means being present, available, and accessible, even in silence if we do not know what to say. Our presence assures the person that we will not let him or her die alone—a major source of fear and suffering in termi-nally ill patients. Assurance of our presence is more comforting than the availability of a lethal dose of medication on the bedside table, as the ad-vocates of suicide so confidently aver. That lethal dose only assures the patient that we, too, think his or her life is unworthy of living.

Compassionate caring permits the sufferer to continue as a valued member of the human community until death occurs. It confirms our solidarity with the sufferer and, paradoxically, allows for healing and even emotional and spiritual growth. It is neither compassionate nor car-ing to assuage our own emotion of co-suffering by hastening the death of the sufferer.

The Rightful Place of Compassion

Compassion is a universal emotion generated in all persons of goodwill in the face of another's suffering. It is accompanied by a desire to help the one who suffers and, as such, it can be a motive for beneficent acts that are essential to a good death. Compassion is not, however, a self-justifying reason for relieving pain or suffering at any cost, including taking the life of the sufferer. Compassion has its own serious limitations as a sole basis for professional or personal ethics.

Compassion that motivates true acts of co-suffering—and, by their performance, relieves the sufferer's anguish—is an essential component of a good death. To reject compassion as a justification for assisted sui-cide and euthanasia in no way vitiates the duty of beneficence that in fact does make compassionate behavior a moral obligation.

3

Reason, Self-determination,
and Physician-Assisted Suicide

Daniel Callahan, Ph.D.

Claiming the right to control our bodies and our lives is characteristically American. "Give me liberty or give me death" is a part of our history. It could thus well be said that the physician-assisted suicide movement represents the last, definitive step in gaining full individual self-determination: "Give me liberty and, if I want it, give me death." As a movement, physician-assisted suicide seeks to reassure us that we can die as we choose and, with a physician's expert help, be certain that we will die in the most technically expeditious fashion.

However mistaken in its direction and emphasis (as I will argue it is), a turn to physician-assisted suicide is a perfectly understandable response to the increased difficulty of dying a peaceful death, a dying ever more ensnared in technological and moral traps. First, there are all the cultural and medical obstacles now thrown in the way of simply allowing people to die from disease. Medicine tends to conflate the value of the sanctity of life and the technological imperative, rendering an acceptance of death morally suspect. Moreover, by increasingly judging all deaths to be events for which humans can and should take responsibility, we are blurring the distinction between killing and allowing to die; there is now every incentive to seek final and decisive control over the process of dying. Physician-assisted suicide seems to present the perfect way to do just that.

The physician-assisted suicide movement rests on two basic claims, secondarily supported by other considerations as well. Those claims are our right to self-determination and the obligation we all owe to each other to relieve suffering, but especially the obligation of the physician to do so. The movement's deepest point might simply be understood as this: If we cannot trust disease to take our lives quickly or peacefully, and we cannot rely on doctors to know with great precision how or when to stop treatment to allow that to happen, then we have a right to turn to more direct means. In the name of mercy, physicians should be allowed to end our lives at our voluntary request, or, alternatively, be permitted to put into our hands those means that will allow us to commit suicide. We will then be assured a peaceful death, one that we have fashioned for ourselves. For the peaceful death no longer (and never assuredly and perfectly) given us by nature, we must shape, by our choice, a death of our own making.

This is a dangerous direction to go in the search for a peaceful death. This path to peaceful dying rests on the illusion that a society can safely put in the hands of physicians the power directly and deliberately to take life, euthanasia, or to assist patients in taking their own life, physician-assisted suicide. (I see no moral difference between them—just as the law in most places would see no difference between my shooting someone and my giving a gun to another so he or she can do it.) It threatens to add still another sad chapter to an already sorry human history of giving one person the liberty to take the life of another. It perpetuates and pushes to an extreme the very ideology of control—the goal of mastering life and death—that created the problems of modern medicine in the first place. Instead of changing the medicine that generates the problem of an intolerable death (which, in almost all cases, good palliative medicine could do), allowing physicians to kill or provide the means to take one's own life simply treats the symptoms, all the while reinforcing, and driving us more deeply into, an ideology of control.

The suffering that leads people to embrace physician-assisted suicide can seem compelling: prolonged agony; a sense of utter futility; pain that can be relieved only at the price of oblivion; a desperate gasping for breath that, if relieved, will be followed again and again by the same gasping; or the prospect of months or years in a nursing home, or dependent on a trapped, overburdened family member. The possibilities of suffering, physical and psychological, should not be minimized, and I do not want to rest my resistance to physician-assisted suicide on any slighting of that kind. I can well imagine situations that could drive me to want such relief or feel driven to want it for others. The movement to euthanasia and assisted suicide is a strong and, seemingly, historically inevitable response to that fear. It draws part of its strength from the failure of modern medicine to reassure us that it can manage our dying with dignity and comfort. It draws another part from the desire to be masters of our fate. Why must we endure that which need not be endured? If medicine cannot always bring us the kind of death we might like through its technical skills, why can it not use them to give us a quick and merciful release?

The Relief of Suffering: Virtues and Duties

No moral impulse seems more deeply ingrained than the need to relieve human suffering. It is a basic tenet of the great religions of the world. It has become a foundation stone for the practice of medicine, and it is at the core of the social and welfare programs of all civilized nations. Unless we have been brutalized, our feelings numbed by cruelty or systematic indifference, we cannot stand to see another person suffer. The tears of another, even a total stranger, can bring tears to our own eyes. At the heart of the virtue of compassion is the capacity to feel with, and for, another. With those closest to us, that virtue often leads us to feel the pain of another as if it were our own. And sometimes it is stronger than that: it is a source of intensified anguish that we cannot lift from another the pain we would, if we could, make our own. A parent feels that way about the suffering of a child, and a spouse or friend about the suffering of a loved one who is trapped by pain that cannot be moved from one body to another.

Yet for all the depth of our common response to suffering, and our general agreement as a civilized society that it should be relieved, the scope and depth of that moral duty are not clear, especially for physicians. The problem of physician-assisted suicide forces us to answer a hard question: Ought the general duty of the physician to relieve suffering encompass the right to assist a patient to take his or her own life if that is desired and seems necessary? The question can be put from the patient's side as well: Is it a legitimate moral request for a patient to ask a doctor for assistance in committing suicide?

But there is an even more fundamental question that must be explored before turning to those questions: What should be done in response to such suffering? Is it simply a nice thing to relieve suffering if we can, a gesture of charity or kindness worthy of praise? We might say that our impulse of compassion is a good to be cultivated and expressed—that we will all be better off if we entertain that as an ideal in our lives together. Or is there more to it than that? Might it be that the relief of suffering is a moral duty, not just a noble ideal, to which we are obliged even if our sense of compassion is faint, even if what is asked of us might cause some suffering on our own part? How far and in what way, that is, does our duty extend in the relief of suffering, and just what kind of suffering is encompassed within such a duty?

One common answer to such questions is that we are, at the least, obliged to relieve the suffering of others when we can do so at no high cost to ourselves, and that we should do so when the suffering at stake is unnecessary. But that does not tell us much that is helpful, though it is surely important to repeatedly remind ourselves and others of such obligations. The hard cases are those in which the demands on us may be morally or psychologically stressful, and in which there is uncertainty about the significance of the suffering.

It is useful to distinguish two kinds of burdens. In one, the demand on us is to act, to do something specifically to relieve the suffering. That may mean giving our already overcrowded time just to be with someone in pain, someone whose first need is for companionship, for closeness; or providing otherwise needed money to improve the nursing care of a dying parent; or taking the trouble to find a better doctor, or hospital, for a spouse receiving poor care. Demands of that kind can be heavy, pressing our sense of duty to the limit; sometimes it can be unclear just where the limit is.

The other burden is subtler: the need to discern when suffering cannot, or should not, be wholly overcome, when our duty may be to accept the suffering of another, just as the person whose suffering it is must accept it. Many legitimate moral demands, for instance, will carry with them the possibility of suffering, and they should not for that reason be shirked. To take an unpopular position, to stand up for one's rights, to remain true to one's promises and commitments can all entail unavoidable suffering. A parent's commitment to the good of a child may require, and probably will at times require, that for the sake of the child's development the parent accept the need for the child to bear the penalties of his or her own choices and mistakes, and thereby to suffer as a parent in watching that happen. The same can be said of many other human relationships—those with friends, lovers, husbands, and wives. As bystanders to the suffering, we have to accept its unavoidability for the sufferer. We cannot relieve that suffering. The demand in some cases is to accept the suffering that another must endure, not run from it. Patience, loyalty, steadfastness, and fortitude are called for in accompanying the persons who must suffer, to help and allow them to do and be what they must, however heavy the burden on them and others. We are called on to suffer with the other, to be a supportive presence.

For just those reasons it cannot be fully correct to say that our highest moral duty to each other is the relief of suffering. More precisely, our duty is to enhance one another's good and welfare, and the relief of suffering will ordinarily be an important way to accomplish that. But not always. What we need to know is whether the suffering exists because without it some other human good cannot be attained; and that is exactly the case with the suffering caused by living out one's moral duties or ideals for a life.

Therein lies the ambiguity of the term "unnecessary suffering," frequently invoked as the kind of suffering physician-assisted suicide can obviate. Suffering will surely be "unnecessary" when it serves no purpose, when it is not an inextricable part of achieving important human goals. Unavoidable necessary suffering, by contrast, is that which is the essential means, or accompaniment, of valuable human ends, and not all suffering is. Yet the real problem here is in deciding on our goals, and the hardest choice will be in deciding whether, and how, to pursue goals that may entail suffering. If we make the avoidance or relief of suffering itself the highest goal, we run the severe risk of sacrificing, or minimizing, other human purposes. Life would then be focused on avoiding pain, minimizing risk, and craftily eying all possible life projects and goals in light of their likelihood of producing suffering.

If that is hardly desirable in the living of our individual lives, it is no less problematic in devising social policy. A society ought, so far as it can, to work for the relief of pain and suffering; and that is to state a simple moral principle. But a more complex principle is needed: A society should work to relieve only suffering that is not an unavoidable part of living out its other values and aspirations. That means it must ask, on the one hand, what those values are or should be and, on the other, what policies for the relief of suffering might subvert society's general values.

The most profound question we must then ask is this: If the suffering of illness and dying comes from the profound assault on our sense of integrity and self-direction, what is the best way we can—as those who give care, who want to do right by a person—honor that integrity? The claim of proponents of physician-assisted suicide is that the assault of terminal illness on the self is legitimately relieved, even mercifully and honorably so, by recognizing the right to self-determination to end that life.

Yet notice what we have accepted here. It is the idea that our integrity can be served only by the self-determination that brings death, by the direct implication of another in our death, and by accepting the implicit assumption that the suffering is "unnecessary"—meaningless, avoidable. To accept that comes close to declaiming that life can have meaning only if marked by self-determination, a strange notion indeed, flying directly in the face of human experience. That experience shows that a noble and heroic life can be achieved by those who have little or no control over the external conditions of their lives, but have the wisdom and dignity necessary to fashion a meaningful life without it. We would also be declaring that a life not marked by self-mastery, self-determination, is a meaningless one once burdened with unwanted suffering. It is not for nothing perhaps that modern medicine in its quest for cure has itself contributed to the harmful idea that all suffering is pointless, representing not life and its natural condition but the failure of medicine to overcome, or relieve, that suffering.

Is Self-empowerment Socially Neutral?

But might it not be said, in response, that permitting physician-assisted suicide would not involve taking a general position on the meaning of life, death, and suffering, but only empowering each individual and his or her physician-accomplice to make that determination? Would it not be, in that sense, socially neutral? Not at all. To establish physician-assisted suicide as social policy is, first, to side with those who say that some suffering is meaningless and unnecessary, to be relieved as decisively as possible, and that only individuals can determine what such suffering is; and, second, to say that such a highly variable, highly subjective matter is best left to the irrevocable judgment of doctor and patient. That is not a neutral policy at all, but one that makes a final judgment about what constitutes an appropriate, socially acceptable response to dying (the mutually agreed-on deliberate death of a person) and about social policy (the legitimation of physician-assisted suicide as a response to perceived threats of suffering and loss of self-integrity).

A great hazard of this approach is that it declares some forms of human suffering—but only those forms determined by private, variable responses—to be so beyond human help and caring that they are open only to death as a solution. It is, moreover, a striking break with both the medical and moral traditions of medicine to treat the desires and wishes of patients as if they alone legitimate a doctor's skills. It is to make doctors artisans in the fashioning of a patient's life (and in this case death), a role well beyond the traditional role of medicine, which has been to restore and maintain health.

There is little disagreement about the duty of the physician to relieve physical pain, even though there are some significant disputes about how far that effort should go. Of more pertinence to my concern here, however, is the extent of the duty of the physician to relieve suffering, that is, to try to relieve the psychological or spiritual condition of a person who as a result of illness suffers (whether in pain or not). I contend that the duty is important but limited.

Two levels of suffering can be distinguished. At one level, the principal problem is that of the fear, uncertainty, dread, or anguish of the sick person in coping with the illness and its meaning for the continuation of life and intact personhood—what might be called the psychological penumbra of illness. At a deeper level, the problem touches on the meaning of suffering for the meaning of life itself. The question here is more fundamental: What does my suffering tell me about the point or purpose or end of human existence, most notably my own? The questions here are no longer just psychological but encompass fundamental philosophical and religious matters.

The physician should do all in his or her power to respond, as physician, to the first level, but it is inappropriate, I contend, to attempt to solve by lethal means the problems that arise at the second level. What would that distinction mean in practice? It means that the doctor should, through counseling, pain relief, and cooperative efforts with family and friends, do everything possible to reduce the sense of dread and anxiety, of disintegration of self, in the face of a threatened death. The doctor should provide care, comfort, and compassion. But when the patient says to the doctor that life no longer has meaning, or that the suffering cannot be borne because of its perceived pointlessness, or that a loss of control is experienced as an intolerable insult to a patient's sense of self—at that point the doctor must draw a line. Those problems cannot properly be solved by medicine, and it is a mistake for medicine even to attempt to solve them.

The purpose of medicine is not to relieve all the problems of human mortality, the most central and difficult of which is why we have to die at all or die in ways that seem pointless to us. The purpose of medicine is not to give us control over our human destiny, or to help us devise a life to our private specifications—and especially the specification most desired these days, that of complete control of death and its circumstances. That is not the role of medicine because medicine has no competence to manage the meaning of life and death, only the physical and psychological manifestations of those problems.

Medicine's role must be limited to what it can appropriately do, and it has neither the expertise nor the wisdom necessary to respond to the deepest and oldest human questions. What it can do is relieve pain and bring comfort to those who psychologically suffer because of illness. That is all, and that is enough. When physicians would use medical knowledge, designed to help with that task, to directly cause death as a way of solving a patient's problems with life and mortality itself, they go too far, exceeding their own professional and moral rights. There has been a longstanding, historical resistance to giving physicians the power to assist in suicide precisely because of the skill they could bring to that task. Their technical power to help death along must not be matched by a moral or legal authority to engage in physician-assisted suicide; that would open the way for a corruption of their vocation.

I do not claim that a sharp and precise line can always be found between the two levels of suffering, but only that some limits can be feasibly set to enable us to say when the physician has strayed too far into the thickets of the second level. For ordinary purposes, it remains appropriate to speak of the duty of the physician to "relieve pain and suffering," but only as long as it is understood that this can be done to relieve only the problems of illness, not the problems of life itself. What life itself may give us, at its end, is a death that seems, in the suffering it brings, to make no sense. That is a terrible problem, but it is the patient's problem, not the doctor's. The doctor can, at that point, relieve pain, make the patient as comfortable as possible, and be another human presence. Beyond that, the patient must be on his or her own. Patients have no resource left but themselves at that point.

Suffering and Subjectivity

There is also another side to the issue. When physician-assisted suicide is requested, the doctor is being asked to act on the subjective suffering of another—variable from person to person, externally unverifiable, and always in principle reversible—with an action that will be objective and irreversible. As the human response to evil and suffering suggests, there is nothing in a particular burden of life, or in the nature of suffering itself, that necessarily and inevitably leads to a desire to be dead, much less a will to bring that about. That will and must always be a function of the patient's values and the way those values are either legitimated or rejected by the culture of which that patient is a part. Suffering in and of itself is not a good clinical predictor of a desire to be dead, which is why depression or a history of previous mental health problems is a far better predictor of a serious desire for suicide than illness, pain, or old age is. Thus we face a complex double challenge: to determine if, under those ambiguous circumstances, we should empower one person to help another to kill him- or herself; and if so, what the moral standard should be for the one who is to do the helping.

Physician-assisted suicide is mistakenly understood as only a personal matter of self-determination, the control of our own bodies, not to be forbidden since it is only a small step beyond our no longer forbidding suicide. But unlike unassisted suicide, an act carried out solely by the person, physician-assisted suicide should be understood as a social act. It requires the assistance of someone else. Legalizing physician-assisted suicide would also provide an important social sanction for suicide, tacitly legitimating it, and affecting many aspects of our society beyond the immediate relief of individual suffering. It would in effect say that suicide is a legitimate and reasonable way of coping with suffering, acceptable to the law and sanctioned by medicine. Suicide is now understood to be a tragic situation, no longer forbidden by the law but hardly anywhere understood as the ideal outcome of a life filled with suffering. That delicate balance would be lost and a new message delivered: Suicide is morally, medically, legally, and social acceptable.

All civilized societies have developed laws to reduce the number of situations in which one person is allowed to kill another. Most have resisted the notion that private agreements can be reached allowing one person to help another take his or her life. Traditionally, three circumstances have primarily been acceptable for the taking of life: killing in self-defense or to protect another life, killing in the course of a just war, and killing in the case of capital punishment. Killing in war and killing by capital punishment have been opposed by some, more successfully in the case of capital punishment, which is now banned in many countries, most notably in western Europe.

The proposal to legalize physician-assisted suicide is nothing less than a proposal to add a new category of acceptable killing to those already socially legitimated. To do so would be to reverse the long-developing trend to limit the occasions of legally sanctioned killing (most notable in the campaigns to abolish capital punishment and to limit access to handguns). Civilized societies have slowly come to understand how virtually impossible it is to control even legally sanctioned killing. Even with carefully fashioned safeguards, having legally sanctioned killing invites abuse and corruption.

Does it not make a difference that the absolute power is given, not to subjugate another (as in slavery), but as an act of mercy, to bring relief from suffering? No. Although the motive may be more benign than in the case of slavery as usually understood, that motive is beside the point. The aim in prohibiting physician-assisted suicide is to avoid introducing into society the inherent corruption of legitimated private killing. "All power corrupts," Lord Acton wrote, "and absolute power corrupts absolutely." It is that profound insight—a reflection on human despotism, usually justified initially out of good, empathetic motives—that should be kept in mind when we would give one person the right to kill another.

We come here to a striking pitfall of the common arguments for physician-assisted suicide. Once the key premises of that argument are accepted, there will remain no logical way in the future to (1) for long hold the line against euthanasia, to take care of those physically or psychologically unable to take their own lives; (2) deny euthanasia to any competent person who requests it for whatever reason, terminal illness or not; and (3) deny euthanasia and physician-assisted suicide to those who suffer but are incompetent, even if they do not request it. I am not saying that such a scenario will in fact take place, but only that the arguments given in favor of euthanasia logically entail the possibility. We can erect legal safeguards and specify required procedures to keep that scenario from coming to pass, but over time they will provide poor protection if the logic of the moral premises on which they are based is fatally flawed. The safeguards will appear arbitrary and flimsy and will invite covert evasion or outright rejection.

The Logic of the Arguments

Where are the flaws in these arguments? Recall that there are two classical arguments in favor of euthanasia and assisted suicide: our right of self-determination, and our claim on the mercy of others to relieve our suffering if they can do so, especially our claim on doctors. These two arguments are typically spliced together and presented as a single contention. Yet if they are considered independently—and there is no inherent reason they must be linked—they display serious problems. Consider, first, the argument for our right of self-determination. It is said that a competent adult ought to have a right to physician-assisted suicide for the relief of suffering. But why must the person be suffering? Does not that stipulation already compromise the right of self-determination? How can self-determination have any limits? Why are not the person's desires or motives, whatever they be, sufficient? How can we justify this arbitrary limitation of self-determination? The standard arguments for physician-assisted suicide offer no answers to those questions.

Consider next the person who is suffering but not competent, perhaps demented or mentally retarded. The standard argument would deny euthanasia and physician-assisted suicide to that person. But why? If a person is suffering but not competent, then it would seem grossly unfair to deny that person relief simply because he or she lacked competence. Are the incompetent less entitled to relief from suffering than the competent? Will it only be affluent, middle-class people, mentally fit and able, who can qualify? Will those who are incompetent but suffering be denied that which those who are intellectually and emotionally better off can have? Would that be fair? Do they suffer less for being incompetent? The standard argument about our duty to relieve suffering offers no response to those questions either.

Is it, however, fair to euthanasia advocates to do what I have done, to separate and treat individually the two customary arguments in favor of a legal right to euthanasia and physician-assisted suicide? The implicit reason for joining them is no doubt the desire to avoid abuse. By requiring a showing of suffering and terminal illness, the aim is to exclude perfectly healthy people from demanding that, in the name of self-determination and for their own private reasons, another person can be called on to kill them or assist them in suicide. By requiring a show of mental competence to effect self-determination, the aim is to exclude the nonvoluntary or involuntary killing of those who are depressed, retarded, or demented.

My contention is that the joining of those two requirements is perfectly arbitrary, a jerry-rigged combination if ever there was one. Each has its own logic, and each could be used to justify euthanasia and physician-assisted suicide. But that logic, it seems evident, offers little resistance to denying any competent person the right to be killed, sick or not, and little resistance to killing those who are not competent, so long as there is good reason to believe they are suffering. There is no principled reason to reject that logic, and no reason to think it could long remain suppressed by the expedient of an arbitrary legal stipulation that both features, suffering and competence, be present. In fact, in its statutes on physician-assisted suicide, the state of Oregon requires a terminal illness only, not a condition of suffering also. The result, of course, has been to remove a potential barrier to physician-assisted suicide.

There is a related problem worth considering. If the act of physician-assisted suicide, conventionally understood, requires the uncoerced request and consent of the patient, it no less requires that the person to do the assisting have his or her own independent moral standards for acceding to the request. The doctor must act with integrity. How can a doctor who voluntarily brings about, or is instrumental in, the death of another legitimately justify that act? Would the mere claim of self-determination on the part of someone be sufficient? "It is my body, doctor, and I request that you help me kill myself." There is historical resistance to that kind of claim, and doctors quite rightly have never been willing to do what patients want solely because they want it. To do so would reduce doctors to automatons, subordinating their integrity to patient wishes or demands. There is surely a legitimate fear, moreover, that if such claim were sanctioned, there would be no reason to forbid any two competent persons from entering into an agreement for one to kill the other, a form of consenting-adult killing. Perhaps the resistance also arises out of a reluctance to put doctors in the role of taking life simply as a means of advancing patient self-determination, quite apart from any medical reasons for doing so.

Physician Integrity

The most likely reason for resistance to a pure self-determination standard is that our culture has, traditionally, defined a physician as someone whose duty is to promote and restore health. It has thus been
customary, even among those pressing for euthanasia and physician-
assisted suicide, to hang on to some part of the physician's traditional
role. That is why a mere claim of self-determination, which requires no
reference to health at all, is not enough. A doctor will not cut off my
healthy arm simply because I decide my autonomy and well-being would
thereby be enhanced.

What may we conclude from these still-viable traditions? To justify
committing an act of physician-assisted suicide and still maintain
professional and personal integrity, the doctor must have his or her
own independent moral standards. What should those standards be?
The doctor will not be able to use a medical standard. A decision for
physician-assisted suicide is not a medical but a moral decision. Faced
with a patient reporting great suffering, a doctor cannot, therefore, justify physician-assisted suicide on purely medical grounds. The doctor
must believe that a life of subjectively experienced intense suffering is
not worth living in order to feel justified in taking the decisive and ultimate step of killing the patient. It must be *the doctor's* moral reason to act,
not the patient's reason (even though their reasons may coincide). But
if the doctor believes that a life of some form of suffering is not worth
living, then how can the doctor deny the same relief to a person who
cannot request it, or who requests it but whose competence is in
doubt? There is no self-evident reason why the supposed duty to
relieve suffering must be limited to competent patients claiming self-
determination—or why patients who claim death as their right under
self-determination must be either suffering or dying.

There is, moreover, the possibility that what begins as a right of doctors to engage in physician-assisted suicide under specified conditions will
soon become a duty to offer it up front to patients. On what grounds
could a doctor deny a request by a competent person for physician-
assisted suicide? It is not sufficient just to stipulate that no doctor should
be required to do that which violates his or her conscience. As commonly
articulated, the arguments about why a doctor has a right to assist in
suicide—the dual duty to respect patient self-determination and to re-

lieve suffering—are said to be central to the vocation of being a doctor. Why should duties as weighty as those be set aside on the grounds of "conscience" or "personal values"?

These puzzles make clear that the moral situation is radically changed once our self-determination requires the participation and assistance of a doctor. Executing our will is no longer a solitary act but a social act requiring two people. It is then that doctor's moral life, that doctor's integrity, that is also and no less encompassed in the act of physician-assisted suicide. What, we might then ask, should be the appropriate moral standards for a person asked to assist in a suicide? What are the appropriate virtues and sensitivities of such a person? How should that person think of his or her own life and find, within that life, a place for physician-assisted suicide?

Now I could imagine someone granting the weight of the considerations against euthanasia I have advanced and yet having this response: Is not our duty to relieve suffering sufficiently strong to justify running some risks? Why should we be intimidated by the dangers in decisive relief of suffering? Is not the present situation, where death can be slow, painful, and full of suffering, already a clear and present danger?

Our duty to relieve suffering—by no means unlimited in any case—cannot justify the introduction of new evils into society. The risk of doing just that in the legalization of physician-assisted suicide is too great, particularly since the number of people whose pain and suffering could not be otherwise relieved would never be large (as even most physician-assisted suicide advocates recognize). It is too great because it would take a disproportionate social change to bring it about, one whose implications extend far beyond those who are sick and dying, reaching into the practice of medicine and into the sphere of socially sanctioned killing. It is too great because, as the history of the twentieth century should demonstrate, killing is a contagious disease, not easy to stop once unleashed in society. It is too great a risk because it would offer medicine too convenient a way out of its hardest cases, those in which there is ample room for further, more benign reforms. We are far from exhausting the known remedies for the relief of pain (frequently, even routinely, underused) and a long way from providing decent psychological support for those who, not necessarily in pain, nonetheless suffer because of despair and a sense of futility in continuing life.

Reason, Rationality, and Physician-Assisted Suicide

Could it not be said, however, in those cases in which physicians cannot relieve the suffering of a patient, that suicide would be a rational act for that patient? "Rational suicide," as it has sometimes been called, surely has a kind of initial plausibility. Death is a definitive way to rid oneself of suffering and, if life with the suffering seems not worth living, then it would seem rational to be rid of that life.

In trying to evaluate this line of thought, some distinctions are necessary. The first is the need to distinguish between the rational and the reasonable. In its most minimal sense, an act can be said to be "rational" if it is consistent with the premises behind it. It does not matter what the premises are as long as the conclusion logically follows. In that sense, if it is believed that life is not worth living, then it is rational to end that life. It was no less rational for the Nazis, operating on the premise that inferior groups stood in the way of some imagined superior race, to conclude that it would be best to eliminate them. This form of rationality might be called instrumental rationality: it is indifferent to the quality of the premises and is interested only in coming up with deductions or conclusions consistent with them. Given consistent deductions or conclusions, the criterion of "rational" has been met.

The notion of what is "reasonable," however, is meant to deal with the failings of instrumental rationality. Good, reasonable premises can stand up to careful scrutiny. Being "rational" in the sense specified above is the easy part. Knowing what is a justifiable premise is the hard part. The history of moral and political debates has shown that rational errors, displaying bad and inconsistent reasoning, are possible but that far more common is disagreement about premises.

Hence, the important question is not whether suicide can be rational—it surely can be in the narrow instrumental sense—but whether it is a reasonable way for human beings to deal with suffering. There are good reasons to doubt this. One of them is the simple fact, which any physician (or even layperson) can readily verify, that there seems to be no correlation whatever between the suffering a person may undergo and a decision to commit suicide. Put another way, if suicide is seen as a rational way to handle suffering, why is suffering a poor predictor of suicide (and thus—one might speculate in the absence of any clear data on this point—of physician-assisted suicide as well)? Both the Dutch experience and the early evidence from Oregon suggest that suicide is most attractive to those who fear a loss of control—and that, as a general rule, the majority of people who commit suicide have some history of mental illness. That history hardly proves suicide to be irrational in any and all cases, but it does give credence to the view that suffering at the end of life is rarely a predictor of suicide—and one test of rationality is whether there is some general and observable consistency between the fact of suffering and the choice of suicide. There simply is no such consistency.

Why is that? I surmise that since life in general—and not just the end of life—can be filled with tragedy and suffering, it is generally judged unreasonable to use suicide as a way of coping with tragedy and suffering. On the contrary, whether it is death from cancer, or the loss of a beloved spouse, or a broken romance, or an economic failure, in almost every culture suicide has not been considered an appropriate response.

There are two likely reasons for this. One of them is that since suffering is likely to be part of every life at one or more stages, life should not end when it occurs. The other reason (and here I speculate) is that there is a kind of perceived or felt duty to bear suffering as a form of mutual human support. The kind of despair that suicide represents is a temptation for all of us when life is miserable. But my ability to put up with it, to show it can be endured, is helpful to my neighbor when he or she is miserable. We all suffer at one point or other, and we all need the witness of each other that we can get through it. If we are essentially social creatures, not simply isolated individuals, then our life with other people will affect the way we look at life; we will learn from them just as they will learn from us. Suicide is, in that sense, not a private act at all. Families have to live with its aftermath, even as do those who only collect the bodies of those who have committed suicide. We are all models for each other's lives, even if we are not aware of it. A society that accepted suicide as a way of life would be creating a set of models: those who chose to reject the earlier tradition of solidarity in favor of a more contemporary tradition of self-determination and the evasion of suffering.

It is probably some such insight that lies behind the traditional religious rejection of suicide and not, as more commonly thought, the belief that God is the author of life and thus has the final say over its disposal. In any event, I judge it to be reasonable to resist suicide as a way to manage suffering and unreasonable to think about it solely in instrumental terms, that is, that it ends our lives and thus releases us from misery.

Curing One Evil with Another

Physical pain and psychological suffering among those who are critically ill and dying are great evils. The attempt to relieve them by the introduction of euthanasia and assisted suicide is an even greater evil. Those practices threaten the future security of the living. They no less threaten the dying themselves. Once a society allows one person to take the life of another based on their mutual private standards of a life worth living, there can be no safe or sure way to contain the deadly virus thus introduced. It will go where it will thereafter. The belief that physician-assisted suicide can be safely regulated is a myth—the confidentiality of the doctor-patient relationship makes it impossible to provide adequate oversight. Since we cannot know what goes on in the privacy of the doctor-patient encounter, we can never know whether, and to what extent, laws regulating physician-assisted suicide (and euthanasia as well) will be violated or ignored. The lack of any correlation between suffering and a desire for suicide means, of necessity, that physicians will have enormous discretion in assisting in suicide—but no way of knowing how to make a definitive evaluation of the extent of, or the legitimacy of, the suffering the patient reports.

The Rise and Fall of the "Right" to Assisted Suicide

Yale Kamisar, LL.B., LL.D. (hon.)

W hen, more than forty years ago, I first wrote about the law and policy governing death and dying,[1] I never thought that someday it would be seriously argued that there is (or ought to be) a constitutional right to assisted suicide or active voluntary euthanasia, or both. Some would say I lacked the foresight or imagination to contemplate such a development. But I believe my attitude was understandable. As my colleague Carl Schneider recently observed, "Throughout most of American history no one would have supposed biomedical policy could or should be made through constitutional adjudication. No one would have thought that the Constitution spoke to biomedical issues, that those issues were questions of federal policy, or that judges were competent to handle them."[2] However, *Roe v. Wade*[3] and *Cruzan v. Director, Missouri Department of Health*[4] were to change all that.

The Significance of *Roe* and *Cruzan*

In *Roe* the Court informed us that a "right of privacy," which had earlier been invoked to invalidate restrictions on the use and distribution of contraceptives,[5] "is broad enough to encompass a woman's decision whether or not to terminate her pregnancy."[6]

The *Roe* Court cleared the way for its ultimate holding by rejecting the state's argument that "a fetus is a person" within the meaning of the Constitution—"the word 'person,' as used in the Fourteenth Amendment," it told us, "does not include the unborn."[7] However, the fact that *Roe* did not involve the termination of a human life (so far as the Court was concerned) did not prevent proponents of physician-assisted suicide from reading the case and its progeny very broadly to support a "right" or "liberty," under certain circumstances, to enlist the assistance of others in committing suicide.[8]

Proponents of physician-assisted suicide also found much solace in the capacious language appearing in a more recent abortion case, *Planned Parenthood v. Casey*.[9] In the course of reaffirming *Roe*, the *Casey* Court spoke at one point about "the right to define one's own concept of existence" and one's concept of "the mystery of human life" as being "at the heart of liberty." The language appears in the last two sentences of a long paragraph. The *entire* paragraph reads as follows:

> Our law affords constitutional protection to personal decisions relating to marriage, procreation, contraception, family relationships, child rearing, and education. Our cases recognize "the right of the *individual*, married or single, to be free from unwarranted governmental intrusion into matters so fundamentally affecting a person as the decision whether to bear or beget a child." Our precedents "have respected the private realm of family life which the state cannot enter." *These matters*, involving the most intimate and personal choices a person may make in a lifetime, choices central to personal dignity and autonomy, are central to the liberty protected by the Fourteenth Amendment. At the heart of liberty is the right to define one's own concept of existence, of meaning, of the universe, and of the mystery of human life. Beliefs about these matters could not define the attributes of personhood were they formed under compulsion of the State.[10]

Proponents of physician-assisted suicide seized on this language, maintaining that it strengthened the main argument for assisted suicide—respect for "personal autonomy" or "self-determination." As one proponent expressed it, paraphrasing the language in *Casey*, the right to assisted suicide stems from "the right to define one's concept of existence and to make the most basic decisions about bodily integrity."[11] But if one believes that respect for "personal autonomy" or "self-determination" entitles a person to decide whether, when, and how he or she wishes to end his or her life, is there any principled way to limit this right or liberty to the terminally ill?

The paragraph from *Casey* quoted above does contain some sweeping language that greatly encouraged proponents of physician-assisted suicide. But such language can plausibly be read (as the Supreme Court was eventually to read it) as explaining why "these matters"—"personal decisions relating to marriage, procreation, contraception, [and] family relationships" or, more summarily, "the private realm of family life"— have been given constitutional protection.

Viewed in isolation, the language about "defin[ing] one's own concept of existence" and "of the mystery of human life" does seem breathtaking. Literally, it would cover the right of terminally ill people to enlist the assistance of others in committing suicide. But literally it would also cover the right of at least *every sane adult*—terminally ill or not, indeed, physically ill or not—to enlist the aid of another in suicide.

Either the language quoted above refers only to personal decisions relating to marriage, procreation, contraception, child rearing, and the like, or it refers to all that plus personal decisions relating to suicide and suicide assistance. If the latter, why don't *all people* have the right to define their own concept of existence or their own concept of the mystery of life?

Why are these awesome rights, if they do exist, denied to the great majority of us because our lives are not about to end but are of indefinite duration? Why, if people so desire, can't they change that? Is the choice *whether* to end one's life and *how* to do so, "central to the liberty protected by the Fourteenth Amendment," or is it not?

If a *competent* person comes to the sad but firm conclusion that his or her existence is unbearable and voluntarily, clearly, and repeatedly requests assisted suicide and there *is* a constitutional right to some form of assisted suicide, why should this person be prevented from obtaining the assistance of another to end his or her life because he or she does not "qualify" under *somebody else's* standards? As Daniel Callahan has observed, "How can self-determination have any limits? [Assuming a person is competent and determined to commit suicide with the assistance of another,] why are not the person's desires or motives, whatever they may be, sufficient?"[12]

Although proponents of physician-assisted suicide have long found much support for their views in *Roe* and its progeny, the meaning of *Roe* has undergone a significant change. A growing number of commentators have maintained that the best argument for the right to abortion is based on principles of "sex equality," not "due process" or "privacy." As then-Judge Ruth Bader Ginsburg noted (shortly before her appointment to the U.S. Supreme Court) in *Casey,* which reaffirmed *Roe,* the majority "added an important strand to the Court's opinion on abortion": It "acknowledged the intimate connection between a woman's 'ability to control [her] reproductive li[fe]' and her 'ability [to] participate equally in the economic and social life of the Nation.'"[13]

"Laws restricting abortion so dramatically shape the lives of women, and only of women," Professor Laurence Tribe has observed, "that their denial of equality hardly needs elaboration."[14] Continues Tribe: "While men retain the right to sexual and reproductive autonomy, restrictions on abortion deny that autonomy to women. Laws restricting access to abortion thereby place a real and substantial burden on women's ability to participate in society as equals." The more the right to abortion is grounded on sexual equality, or the more *Roe* is justified on that ground, the less support that right offers proponents of a constitutional right to assisted suicide.

Proponents of physician-assisted suicide also relied heavily on *Cruzan,* the first Supreme Court case on death, dying, and the right of privacy ever decided and the only Supreme Court case on the subject until the 1997 physician-assisted suicide cases, *Washington v. Glucksberg*[15] and *Vacco v. Quill.*[16] The *Cruzan* Court did not need to, and did not, discuss the right or liberty interest in determining the time and manner of one's death, hastening one's death, or obtaining the active intervention of a physician to help bring about one's suicide. The only assumption that the *Cruzan* Court made for purposes of that case was that a competent person had a constitutionally protected interest in refusing unwanted life-sustaining medical treatment (even artificially delivered food and water).

Although the right to terminate artificial life-support systems and the right to enlist the assistance of another in committing suicide can be, and have been, lumped together under the rubric of "right to die," the two "rights" are different in important respects. As the New York State Task Force on Life and the Law noted, the so-called right to die should mean only, and until recently meant only, "a right against intrusion," a right to resist "a direct invasion of bodily integrity, and in some cases, the use of physical restraints, both of which are flatly inconsistent with society's basic conception of personal dignity."[17] To be sure, a total prohibition against assisted suicide does close an "avenue of escape," but, unlike a refusal to honor a competent patient's request to terminate life-sustaining treatment, it does not force one into "a particular, all-consuming, totally dependant, and indeed rigidly standardized life: the life of one confined to a hospital bed, attached to medical machinery, and tended to by medical professionals."[18]

Not only would a prohibition against rejecting life-sustaining treatment impose a more onerous burden on persons affected than does a ban against assisted suicide (indeed, in some cases a ban against forgoing or terminating life support could lead to the almost total "occupation" of a person's life by medical machinery and the "expropriation" of a person's body from his or her own will), it also would impair the autonomy of a great many more people. As Justice William Brennan pointed out in his dissenting opinion in *Cruzan,* more than three-fourths of the two million people who die in this country every year do so in hospitals and long-term care institutions, and most of these individuals die "after a decision to forgo life-sustaining treatment has been made."[19] If life-sustaining treatment could not be rejected, vast numbers of patients would be "at the mercy of every technological advance."[20] Moreover, if patients could refuse potentially lifesaving treatment at the outset but not discontinue the treatment once it went into effect, many patients probably would not seek such treatment in the first place. In short, allowing a patient to die at some point is a practical condition on the successful operation of medicine.

The same can hardly be said of physician-assisted suicide or physician-administered active voluntary euthanasia. Moreover, as Professor John Arras observed, "the practice of forgoing treatment is by now so deeply embedded in our social and medical practices that a reversal of policy on this point would throw most of our major medical instructions into a state approaching chaos."[21] Again, the same can hardly be said of a refusal to comply with requests for physician-assisted suicide or physician-administered active voluntary euthanasia.

However, the U.S. Court of Appeals for the Ninth and Second Circuits read *Roe* and *Cruzan* very differently from the way I and many other commentators have. As a result, in 1996, within the span of a single month, both the Ninth Circuit in *Compassion in Dying v. Washington* (renamed, when the case reached the U.S. Supreme Court, *Washington v. Glucksberg*) and the Second Circuit in *Quill v. Vacco* held that there was a constitutional right to physician-assisted suicide under certain circumstances. Until these decisions were handed down, no state or federal appellate court in this country had ever held that there was a constitutional right to assisted suicide no matter how narrow the circumstances or stringent the conditions.

The Ninth Circuit and Second Circuit decisions shattered a general consensus that withholding or withdrawing lifesaving treatment constitutes neither suicide nor assisted suicide nor homicide. Starting with the landmark *Quinlan* case,[22] various state supreme courts had explicitly recognized the significance of the distinction between refusal of medical treatment and active intervention to end life. To be sure, "the moral significance of the distinction has been subjected to periodic philosophical challenge," but the distinction "has remained a basic tenet of health care law and mainstream medical ethics."[23] As Alexander Morgan Capron has pointed out,[24] the Ninth Circuit viewed the right to forgo unwanted medical treatment and the right to enlist the assistance of a physician in committing suicide as nothing more than *sub*categories of *the same* broad right or liberty interest: "controlling the time and manner of one's death" or "hastening one's death."[25] The Ninth Circuit did not merely smudge the distinction between "letting die" and actively intervening to promote or to bring about death—it disparaged the distinction: "We see no ethical or constitutionally cognizable difference between a doctor's pulling the plug on a respirator and his prescribing drugs which will permit a terminally ill patient to end his own life. In fact, some might argue that pulling the plug is a more culpable and aggressive act on the doctor's part and provides more reason for the criminal prosecution. To us, what matters most is that the death of the patient is the intended result as surely in one case as in the other."[26]

If the Ninth Circuit belittled the distinction between letting die and actively intervening to help bring about death, it did not treat more kindly another distinction long relied on by opponents of physician-assisted suicide: the distinction between giving a patient a drug for the purpose of killing the patient and administering drugs for the purpose of relieving pain, with the knowledge that it may have a "double effect"—hastening the patient's death as well as reducing the patient's pain. The Ninth Circuit could "see little, if any, difference for constitutional or ethical purposes between providing medication with a double effect and providing medication with a single effect, as long as one of the known effects in each case is to hasten the end of the patient's life."[27]

Although the Second Circuit summarily rejected the Ninth Circuit's due process analysis, it was no more impressed than the other federal court of appeals with the distinction between "allowing nature to take its course" and "intentionally using an artificial death-producing device."[28] Indeed, the *Quill* court went a step further. What it considered to be "the moral and legal identity of those two modes of hastening death [became] the crux of [its] argument for prohibiting laws banning assisted suicide."[29] The Second Circuit maintained that New York had not treated terminally ill people facing similar circumstances alike: terminally ill persons on life support systems "are allowed to hasten their death by directing the removal of such systems," but persons off life support who are "similarly situated" except for being attached to life-sustaining equipment "are not allowed to hasten death by self-administering prescribed drugs."[30] The Second Circuit would have us believe that much like a person who has been speaking prose throughout life without being aware of it, many physicians and other health professionals have been helping people commit suicide almost every day of their professional lives without realizing it: "Withdrawal of life support requires physicians or those acting on their direction physically to remove equipment and, often, to administer palliative drugs which may themselves contribute to death. The ending of life by these means is nothing more nor less than assisted suicide. It simply cannot be said that those mentally competent, terminally-ill persons who seek to hasten death but whose treatment does not include life support are treated equally."

The 1996 decisions by the two federal courts of appeals generated a good deal of momentum in favor of physician-assisted suicide. The fact that the rulings came so close together, that there was no dissent in the Second Circuit case, and that the decision of the Ninth Circuit was supported by a lopsided majority all contributed to this momentum. So did the forcefulness of the language in the two majority opinions. But then the U.S. Supreme Court entered the fray—and brought the momentum to a screeching halt.

Chief Justice Rehnquist's Opinions in *Glucksberg* and *Quill*

Chief Justice Rehnquist wrote the opinion of the Court in both *Washington v. Glucksberg* (the Ninth Circuit case) and *Vacco v. Quill* (the Second Circuit case). The chief justice disagreed with the two lower federal courts virtually point by point, and he in effect eradicated all the lower courts' stirring language in favor of a constitutional right to physician-assisted suicide. It may be useful to summarize briefly the main arguments the *Glucksberg* and *Quill* plaintiffs made in assailing a *total* prohibition against physician-assisted suicide and the reasons Chief Justice Rehnquist gave for rejecting each of these arguments (using the chief justice's own language wherever possible).

Argument: Withdrawal of life support is nothing more or less than assisted suicide; there is no significant moral or legal distinction between the two practices. The right to forgo unwanted life-sustaining medical treatment and the right to enlist a physician's assistance in dying by suicide are merely *sub*categories of *the same* broad right or liberty interest—controlling the time and manner of one's death or hastening one's death.

Response: The distinction between assisting suicide and terminating lifesaving treatment is "widely recognized and endorsed in the medical profession and in our legal traditions [and] is both important and logical."[31] The decision to commit suicide with a physician's assistance "may be just as personal and profound as the decision to refuse unwanted medical treatment, but it has never enjoyed similar legal protection. Indeed, the two acts are widely and reasonably regarded as quite distinct."[32]

Argument: There is no significant difference between administering palliative drugs with the knowledge that it is likely to hasten the patient's death and prescribing a lethal dose of drugs for the very purpose of killing the patient. As the Ninth Circuit put it, there is no real distinction between providing medication with a double effect and providing it with a single effect "as long as one of the known effects in each case is to hasten the end of the patient's life."

Response: In some cases, to be sure, "painkilling drugs may hasten a patient's death, but the physician's purpose and intent is, or may be, only to ease his patient's pain. . . . The law has long used actors' intent or purpose to distinguish between two acts that may have the same result. . . . The law distinguishes actions taken 'because of' a given end [dispensing drugs in order to bring about death] from actions taken 'in spite of' their unintended but foreseen consequences [providing aggressive palliative care that may hasten death, or increase its risk]."[33]

Argument: The 1990 *Cruzan* case is not simply a case about the right to forgo unwanted medical treatment. Considering the facts, it is really a case about personal autonomy and the right to control the time and manner of one's death. *Cruzan's* extension of the right to refuse medical treatment to include the right to forgo life-sustaining nutrition and hydration was "influenced by the profound indignity that would be wrought upon an unconscious patient by the slow atrophy and disintegration of her body [and] can only be understood as a recognition of the liberty, at least in some circumstances, to physician assistance in ending one's life."[34]

Response: Cruzan is *not* a suicide or an assisted suicide case. The Court's assumption in that case was not based, as the Second Circuit supposed, "on the proposition that patients have a general and abstract 'right to hasten death,' but on well established, traditional rights to bodily integrity and freedom from unwanted touching."[35] Indeed, "in *Cruzan* itself, we recognized that most States outlawed assisted suicide—and even more do today—and we certainly gave no intimation that the right to refuse unwanted medical treatment could be somehow transmuted into a right to assistance in committing suicide."[36]

Argument: Fourteenth Amendment Due Process protects one's right to make intimate and personal choices, such as those relating to marriage, procreation, and child rearing—as well as the time and manner of one's death. As the Ninth Circuit observed, quoting language from *Planned Parenthood v. Casey:* "Like the decision of whether or not to have an abortion, the decision how and when to die is one of 'the most intimate and personal choices a person may make in a lifetime,' a choice 'central to personal dignity and autonomy.'"[37]

Response: The capacious, one might even say majestic, language in *Casey* simply "described, in a general way and in light of our prior cases, those personal activities and decisions that this Court has identified as so deeply rooted in our history and traditions, or so fundamental to our concept of constitutionally ordered liberty, that they are protected by the Fourteenth Amendment."[38] However, the fact that many of the rights and liberties protected by due process "sound in personal autonomy does not warrant the sweeping conclusion that any and all important, intimate, and personal decisions are so protected, and *Casey* did not suggest otherwise."[39]

Justice O'Connor's Concurring Opinion

I am well aware that in both *Glucksberg* and *Quill* Justice O'Connor provided the fifth vote (along with Justices Scalia, Kennedy, and Thomas) to make the chief justice's opinions the opinions of the Court—by stating that she joined Chief Justice Rehnquist's opinion, yet writing separately. I am aware, too, that in large measure two other members of the Court, Justices Ginsburg and Breyer, joined O'Connor's opinion.

However, there is no indication in Justice O'Connor's brief concurring opinion that she found any of the principal arguments made by physician-assisted suicide proponents any more persuasive than the chief justice did. There is no suggestion, for example, that she reads the *Cruzan* opinion any more broadly than does the chief justice or that she interprets the stirring language in *Casey* any more expansively. Nor is there

encompass an interest on the part of terminally ill, mentally competent adults in obtaining relief from the kind of suffering experienced by the plaintiffs in this case." Not only is a liberty interest implicated when a state inflicts severe pain or suffering on someone, continued the solicitor general, but also when a state "compels a person" to suffer severe pain caused by an illness by "prohibiting access to medication that would alleviate the condition." During the oral arguments General Dellinger maintained:

> A person states a cognizable liberty interest when he or she alleges that the state is imposing severe pain and suffering *or has adopted a rule which prevents someone from the only means of relieving that pain and suffering*. . . .
> If one alleges the kind of severe pain and agony that is being suffered here and that *the state is the cause of standing between you and the only method of relieving that*, you have stated a constitutionally cognizable liberty interest.[44]

Kathryn Tucker, the lead lawyer for the plaintiffs in the *Glucksberg* case, addressed the Court immediately after Solicitor General Dellinger. She was not pleased with the solicitor general's description of the liberty interest at stake: "The Solicitor General's comment that what we're dealing with here is simply a liberty interest in avoiding pain and suffering . . . absolutely trivializes the claim. We have a constellation of interests [including decisional autonomy and the interest in bodily integrity], each of great Constitutional dimension."[45] It may well be that a liberty interest in obtaining pain relief or not being denied access to such relief is only a "trivialized" version of the liberty interest really at stake. But Justices O'Connor and Breyer focused heavily, perhaps exclusively, on that trivialized or downsized version.

Since Justices Stevens and Souter, who also concurred in the judgments, seem even more receptive than O'Connor, Ginsburg, and Breyer to arguments in favor of a right to physician-assisted suicide, at least in compelling cases,[46] there is reason to think that at least five members of the Court are likely to resist state legislative efforts to reject or to modify the principle of double effect if such action would force some dying people to endure severe pain. Thus, although "Rehnquist's opinions did not endorse a constitutional right to adequate palliative care but simply rejected the conclusion of the Ninth and Second Circuit Courts of Appeals,"[47] it may well be that "[a] Court majority" (the five concurring Justices in *Glucksberg* and *Quill*) did effectively endorse such a right.[48]

In a sense, the Court's support for the principle of double effect is a victory for everybody. For whatever position they may take on assisted suicide or euthanasia, surely most people want those who are dying and severely ill to suffer as little physical pain as possible. And as Howard Brody observed, "Clinicians need to believe to some degree in some form of the principle of double effect in order to provide optimal symptom relief at the end of life. . . . A serious assault on the logic of the principle of double effect could do major violence to the (already reluctant and ill-informed) commitment of the mass of physicians to the goals of palliative care and hospice."[49]

In a way, however, the showing of support for the principle of double effect by the highest court in the land was a special victory for opponents of assisted suicide and euthanasia. For they have long defended the principle. And they did so again in the *Glucksberg* and *Quill* cases.

For example, in an amicus brief supporting the states of New York and Washington, the American Medical Association (AMA), the American Nurses Association, the American Psychiatric Association, and some forty other medical and health care organizations emphasized that a physician's obligation to relieve pain and suffering and to promote the dignity of dying patients "'includes providing palliative treatment even though it may foreseeably hasten death.'"[50] The AMA (and the many other medical organizations that joined it) told the Supreme Court: "[The] recognition that physicians should provide pain medication sufficient to ease [patients'] pain, even where that may serve to hasten death, is *vital* to ensuring that no patient suffer from physical pain" [emphasis added].

A good number of those favoring the legalization (or constitutionalization) of physician-assisted suicide have sharply criticized the principle of double effect. They have condemned the supposed hypocrisy in both permitting the use of analgesics that hasten death and banning euthanasia. They have further maintained that killing to relieve suffering has already been sanctioned in the context of "risky pain relief."[51] Moreover, it is worth recalling that it was the 8-3 majority of the U.S. Court of Appeals for the Ninth Circuit that disparaged the double effect principle—as Brody puts it, dismissing the principle as "moral hypocrisy."[52] A robust version of the principle of double effect—the view that even when the level of medication is likely to cause death, the principle may be constitutionally required—helps *opponents* of physician-assisted suicide, *not* proponents of the practice. For one of the main arguments against the legalization of physician-assisted suicide is that "properly trained health care professionals can effectively meet their patients' needs for compassionate end-of-life care without acceding to requests for suicide."[53] The principle of double effect eases the task of health care professionals—and eases the plight of their patients—and thus weakens the case for physician-assisted suicide.

Some Final Thoughts on Justice O'Connor's Concurring Opinion

Up to now, I have taken the position that if Justice O'Connor left the door open for future litigation in this area, she left it open only a crack. But I must say that I find the reason she gave for joining the chief justice's opinions quite baffling. At the outset of her concurring opinion she states that she is joining the Rehnquist opinions because she "agree[s] that there is no generalized right to 'commit suicide.'"[54] But nobody claimed that there *was* a "generalized right to commit suicide" or a general right to obtain a physician's assistance in doing so. *Nobody.* In their Supreme Court brief, the lawyers for the plaintiffs in the Washington case formulated the question presented as "whether the Fourteenth Amendment's guarantee of liberty protects the decision of a mentally competent, *terminally ill* adult to bring about impending death in a certain, humane, and dignified manner."[55] Furthermore, Tucker *began* her oral argument for the plaintiffs in the *Washington* case by telling the Supreme Court that "this case presents the question whether *dying citizens* in full possession of their mental faculties *at the threshold of death due to terminal illness* have the liberty to choose to cross the threshold in a humane and dignified manner."[56] It is hard to see how anyone could emphasize death, dying, and terminal illness any more than that.

Since one of the principal arguments made by opponents of physician-assisted suicide is that once established for terminally ill patients assisted suicide would not remain so limited for very long, it was not surprising that several justices voiced doubts about whether the claimed right or liberty interest would or could or should be limited to those on the threshold of death.[57] But Tucker stood her ground.

She told the Court that "we do draw the line at a patient who is confronting death" because, unlike other individuals who wish to die by suicide, one on the threshold of death *no longer* has a choice between living and dying, but "only the choice of *how* to die."[58] She also recognized that a state may prevent a *non*–terminally ill person from choosing suicide because one day that person might "rejoice in that," but the same could not be said for the person who is terminally ill—for his or her life is about to end anyhow.

Moreover, when asked to define the liberty interest Timothy Quill and other plaintiffs in the New York case were claiming, Tucker's co-counsel, Professor Laurence Tribe, told the Court that it "is the liberty, *when facing imminent and inevitable death,* not to be forced by the government to endure . . . pain and suffering"; "the freedom, *at this threshold at the end of life,* not to be a creature of the state but to have some voice in the question of how much pain one is really going through" [emphasis added]. This caused Justice Scalia to respond, "Why does the voice just [arise] when death is imminent?"

From the outset of the litigation, the lawyers for the plaintiffs in the Washington and New York cases insisted that the right or liberty interest they claimed was limited to those who are terminally ill because, among other reasons, I think they knew there was no appreciable chance that the courts would establish a general right to assisted suicide. Or, to put it somewhat differently, I think they knew that *the only chance they had of* prevailing in the courts was to ask for a narrowly limited right to physician-assisted suicide, one confined to terminally ill individuals. They were well aware that such a narrowly limited right would cause less alarm and command more support than a general right to assisted suicide.

In short, if all that the Supreme Court decided is that there is no general right to commit suicide, the Court decided virtually nothing—because everybody agreed that there was no such right.

Justice O'Connor observes that "the Court frames the issue in this case as whether the Due Process Clause . . . protects a 'right to commit suicide which itself includes a right to assistance in doing so,' and concludes that our [history and legal traditions] do not support the existence of such a right."[59] But this description of what "the Court" (or Chief Justice Rehnquist) did is incomplete.

In describing the claim at issue in *Glucksberg,* the Ninth Circuit had used such language as "a constitutionally recognized 'right to die'," "a due process liberty interest in controlling the time and manner of one's death," "a liberty interest in hastening one's own death," "a strong liberty interest in choosing a dignified and humane death," and an issue "deeply affect[ing] individuals' right to determine their own destiny."

Seemingly annoyed at what he apparently considered the Ninth Circuit's sloppy and emotive language, and perhaps displeased that in all its various descriptions of the claim at issue the Ninth Circuit had avoided the term "suicide" (a term that carries strongly negative connotations), the chief justice maintained that a more careful statement of the question presented would be "whether the 'liberty' specially protected by the Due Process Clause includes a right to commit suicide which itself includes a right to assistance in doing so."[60]

I readily admit that this passage caused a certain amount of confusion. But it should not be forgotten that the chief justice pointed out *at least three times* that the Ninth Circuit had held that the challenged law "was unconstitutional '*as applied to terminally ill* competent adults who wish to hasten their death with medication prescribed by their physicians.'" And in the penultimate paragraph of his opinion, the chief justice concluded, "We therefore hold that [the Washington law] does not violate the Fourteenth Amendment, either on its face or '*as applied* to competent, terminally ill adults who wish to hasten their deaths by obtaining medication prescribed by their doctors'" [emphasis added]. The Washington statute was challenged by three terminally ill patients and four physicians who periodically treat terminally ill patients and who wished to help such patients die by suicide. Although the patients died during the pendency of the case, the physicians remained.

Justice O'Connor did not argue that the physician-plaintiffs "lacked standing" to challenge the constitutionality of the ban against physician-assisted suicide insofar as it applied to competent, terminally ill patients. In contrast, Justice Stevens, who wrote a separate concurring opinion, came close to saying just that. Although the Ninth Circuit considered the Washington law *as applied* to terminally ill, competent adult patients who wished to hasten their deaths, observed Stevens, all the patient-plaintiffs had died by then and therefore the court of appeals' holding "was not limited to a particular set of plaintiffs before it." But Stevens's statement is incomplete.

To be sure, the physician-plaintiffs were not threatened with prosecution for assisting in the suicide of *a particular* patient. As the Ninth Circuit pointed out, however, "they ran a severe risk of prosecution under the Washington statute, which proscribes the very conduct in which they seek to engage."[61] Moreover, although Justice Stevens did not discuss this aspect of the case, both the district court and the court of appeals proceeded on the basis that the physician-plaintiffs had standing to sue on behalf of their terminally ill patients as well as on their own behalf. This is hardly surprising; the U.S. Supreme Court has frequently permitted physicians to assert their patients' rights in challenging abortion restrictions.[62] Moreover, it might be said that the Washington statute is aimed more directly at physicians than at their patients. It does not make *committing suicide* with the assistance of another a felony. It makes *aiding another* to commit suicide a felony.

If physicians lacked standing to challenge laws prohibiting assisted suicide, how could appellate courts *ever* consider an "as applied to terminally ill patients" challenge? All terminally ill patients *necessarily* will die before completion of the litigation. In fact, in the *Glucksberg* case all but one of the patient-plaintiffs had died by the time the district court issued its decision.

As Professor Sonia Suter noted, although the chief justice did not fully address Justice Stevens's argument, concurring Justice Souter did.[63] Souter saw the challenge to the Washington statute "not as facial but as applied"[64] and "conclude[d] that 'the statute's *application to the doctors* has not been shown to be unconstitutional'" [emphasis added]. Justice Souter pointed out that "although the terminally ill original parties have died during the pendency of this case, the four physicians who remain as respondents here continue to request declaratory and injunctive relief for their own benefit in discharging their obligations to other dying patients who request their help."

What is the most plausible explanation for Justice O'Connor's odd statement that she is joining the chief justice's opinions in *Glucksberg* and *Quill* because she "agree[s] that there is no generalized right to 'commit suicide'?" Although this is a conclusion that I am not eager to reach, I think the reason for Justice O'Connor's statement is a reluctance to rule out the possibility of a right to physician-assisted suicide in every set of circumstances and a desire to "proceed with special caution" in this area.[65]

The Future of the "Right" to Physician-Assisted Suicide in the Supreme Court

I have to agree with the many Court watchers (especially those who were unhappy with the result in the assisted suicide cases) who say that *Glucksberg* and *Quill* will not be the Court's last word on the subject. But it hardly follows that the next time the Court confronts the issue it will establish a right to assisted suicide in some limited form. There were a number of factors at work when the Supreme Court decided the 1997 physician-assisted suicide cases, and most of them will still be operating when the Court addresses the issue a second time.

The issue has recently been the subject of intense discussion and vigorous debate, and there is no indication this agitation will subside in the foreseeable future. As the chief justice observed (and concurring Justice O'Connor agreed), "public concern and democratic action are . . . sharply focused on how best to protect dignity and independence at the end of life, with the result that there have been many significant changes in state laws and in the attitudes these laws reflect."[66] Moreover, the rights of a politically vulnerable group are not at stake—as had been the situation when the Court intervened in prior cases. After all, "dying people are clearly not a discrete and insular minority in the same, sure way as are black people subject to race discrimination laws [or] women subject to abortion restrictions."[67] And when the issue is close and "there is no democratic defect in the underlying political process," courts "should not strike down reasonable legislative judgments."[68]

I think Justice O'Connor put it well when, reiterating a point she made during the oral arguments, she commented, "Every one of us at some point may be affected by our own or a family member's terminal illness. There is no reason to think the democratic process will not strike the proper balance between the interests of terminally ill, mentally competent individuals who would seek to end their suffering and the State's interests in protecting those who might seek to end life mistakenly or under pressure."[69]

Another reason, quite likely, for the Court's reluctance to establish a constitutionally protected right to or liberty interest in assisted suicide, and one that will apply the next time around as well, is capsuled in the solicitor general's amicus brief: once an exception to the general prohibition against physician-assisted suicide is mandated by the Court, however heavily circumscribed it might be at first, "there is no obvious stopping point."

For example, the Ninth Circuit invalidated the state's assisted suicide ban "only 'as applied to competent, terminally ill adults who wish to hasten their deaths by obtaining medication prescribed by their doctors.'" After noting Washington State's insistence that the impact of the

Ninth Circuit's decision "will not and cannot be so limited," the chief justice observed:

> The [Ninth Circuit's] decision, and its expansive reasoning, provide
> ample support for the State's concerns. The court noted, for example,
> that the "decision of a duly appointed surrogate decision maker is for
> all legal purposes the decision of the patient himself," that "in some in-
> stances, the patient may be unable to self-administer the drugs and . . .
> administration by the physician . . . may be the only way the patient may
> be able to receive them," and that not only physicians, but also family
> members and loved ones, will inevitably participate in assisting suicide.
> Thus, it turns out that what is couched as a limited right to "physician-
> assisted suicide" is likely, in effect, a much broader license, which could
> prove extremely difficult to solve and contain.[70]

Although concurring Justice Ginsburg neither joined the chief justice's opinion nor wrote an opinion of her own, during the oral arguments she voiced skepticism that any right to physician-assisted suicide,
no matter how narrowly limited initially, could or would be confined
to the terminally ill or could or would stop short of active voluntary
euthanasia. When Tucker urged the Court to recognize, or to establish,
a constitutionally protected liberty interest "that involves bodily integrity, decisional autonomy, and the right to be free of unwanted pain
and suffering,"[71] Justice Ginsburg retorted that "a lot of people would fit
[this] category," not just the terminally ill. How, she wondered, do you
"leave out the rest of the world who would fit the same standards?" At
another point, Justice Ginsburg suggested that the patient who is so
helpless or in so much agony that she "is not able to assist in her own
suicide," but must have a health professional administer a lethal injection, is "in a more sympathetic situation" than one who is able to commit suicide with the preliminary assistance of a physician.

Still another factor that must have had some impact on at least some
members of the Court, and is bound to influence at least some of the
justices in future cases, is the strong opposition of the AMA and other
medical groups to the constitutionalization or legalization of physician-
assisted suicide, regardless of how narrowly limited the constitutional
right or the statutory authorization might be. As Linda Greenhouse has
pointed out, the amicus brief filed by the AMA in *Glucksberg* and *Quill*
sharply contrasted with the one the same organization had filed seven
years earlier in the *Cruzan* case.[72] In *Cruzan*, the AMA told the Court that
under the circumstances, terminating life support was in keeping with

"respecting the patient's autonomy and dignity."[73] In *Glucksberg* and *Quill*, however, the AMA (and more than forty other national and state medical and health care organizations) told the Court that "the ethical prohibition against physician-assisted suicide is a cornerstone of medical ethics"; that the AMA had repeatedly "reexamined and reaffirmed" that ethical prohibition, as recently as the summer of 1996; and that "physician-assisted suicide remains 'fundamentally incompatible with the physician's role as healer, would be difficult or impossible to control, and would pose serious societal risks.'"[74]

Recent and continuing trends in medical practice may only heighten the AMA's resistance to physician-assisted suicide. The next time the issue is presented, the AMA and other medical groups might well tell the Court, as Leon Kass and Nelson Lund recently argued, that new trends and developments make the need to maintain the absolute prohibition against physician-assisted suicide "more important than ever."[75] As they put it, it would not be surprising if the next time around the AMA and other medical groups were to tell the Court something like this: "Given the great pressures threatening medical ethics today—including, among other factors, a more impersonal practice of medicine, the absence of a lifelong relationship with a physician, the push toward managed care, and the financially-based limitation of services—a bright line rule regarding medically-assisted death is a bulwark against disaster."[76]

Finally, another factor at work in the assisted suicide cases, and one that will operate as well the next time the Court confronts the issue, is the justices' realization that if they were to establish a right to assisted suicide, however limited, the need to enact legislation implementing and regulating any such right would generate many problems—which inevitably would find their way back to the Court.

Whether a regulatory mechanism would be seen as providing patients and physicians with much-needed protection or as unduly burdening the underlying right would be largely in the eye of the beholder. Thus it is not surprising that proponents of physician-assisted suicide even disagree among themselves as to how a particular procedural requirement should be regarded. For example, three of the nation's most respected proponents of physician-assisted suicide, Franklin Miller, Howard Brody, and Timothy Quill, have questioned the desirability of the fifteen-day waiting period required by the Oregon Death with Dignity Act, a provision designed to ensure that a patient's decision to elect assisted suicide is resolute.[77] According to Miller, Brody, and Quill, such an "arbitrary time period . . . may be highly burdensome for patients who are suffering intolerably and may preclude access to assisted death for those who request it at the point when they are imminently dying." The same three commentators also criticize a provision of a model state act requiring that the discussion between physician and patient concerning a request for assisted suicide be witnessed by two adults, calling it "unduly intrusive and unlikely to be effective." On the other hand, Miller, Brody, and Quill maintain that an Oregon provision requiring a second medical opinion on the assisted suicide decision is "not a reliable safeguard" because it "does not mandate that the consulting physician be genuinely independent."

Perhaps the most rigorous condition on physician-assisted suicide to be found is the requirement of Compassion in Dying (an organization that counsels people considering physician-assisted suicide and one of the plaintiffs in the *Glucksberg* case) that the approval of all of the would-be suicide's immediate family members be obtained.[78] It is hard to believe that any group favoring physician-assisted suicide would retain such a requirement if the Court were to establish a constitutional right to assisted suicide. But one can be fairly sure that if the Court were to establish such a right, opponents of physician-assisted suicide would fight hard to include a "family approval" provision in any legislation regulating assisted suicide—along with mandatory waiting periods, specified information, procedures to ensure that the decision to choose physician-assisted suicide is "truly informed," and all sorts of notification requirements and bans on the use of public facilities, public employees, and public funds.

Although not insubstantial, the differences among proponents of physician-assisted suicide over the requisite conditions and procedures for carrying out the practice pale compared to the differences likely to exist among those who disagree about legalizing physician-assisted suicide in the first place. In short, in many respects the legislative response to a Supreme Court decision establishing a right to assisted suicide is likely to be a replay of the response to *Roe v. Wade,* a specter that did not escape the attention of the justices.

At one point in the oral arguments, the chief justice told the lead lawyer for the *Glucksberg* plaintiffs:

> You're not asking that [this Court engage in legislation] now. But surely that's what the next couple of generations are going to have to deal with, what regulations are permissible and what not if we uphold your

position here. . . . You're going to find the same thing . . . that perhaps has happened with the abortion cases. There are people who are just totally opposed and people who are totally in favor of them. So you're going to have those factions fighting it out in every session of the legislature, how far can we go in regulating this. And that will be a constitutional decision in every case.[79]

Roe ignited what has aptly been called a "domestic war,"[80] one that, after a quarter-century of tumult, seems finally to have come to an end in the courts. The Court that decided the assisted suicide cases in 1997 was not eager to set off a new domestic war. Neither, I venture to say, will the Court be the next time around.

The Future of the "Right" to Physician-Assisted Suicide in the Political Arena

When the U.S. Supreme Court handed down its decisions in the *Glucksberg* and *Quill* cases, Barbara Coombs Lee, executive director of Compassion in Dying, purported to be quite pleased. The press reported that she was "really thrilled" that the Supreme Court had given her organization and her allies "a green light" to seek legislation authorizing physician-assisted suicide.[81] But proponents of physician-assisted suicide have *always had* the "green light" to persuade state legislatures to legalize the practice. The issue presented by *Glucksberg* and *Quill* was whether the U.S. Constitution *required* or *compelled* the states to legalize physician-assisted suicide under certain circumstances, not whether the states were *permitted* to do so.

Early in the oral arguments before the Supreme Court, Justice Stevens asked the attorney representing Washington State whether it was his view that a legislature had "the constitutional authority to authorize assisted suicide," and the answer was an unequivocal "yes."[82] A short time later, Justice Ginsburg asked the attorney representing New York whether he agreed that a legislature was free to legalize physician-assisted suicide, and he, too, left no doubt that he believed a legislature was so entitled. Nor did lawyers representing the plaintiffs in these cases deny that they had always had the green light to seek legislation authorizing physician-assisted suicide. But they made it clear that they were *not* thrilled about pursuing such a course. Thus when asked by Justice Breyer why a legislature was not "far more suited" to deal with end-of-life problems than a court interpreting a constitutional provision,

Tribe, the attorney for the proponents of assisted suicide in *Quill*, responded that although "in a sense there are 50 laboratories out there," they "are now operating largely with the lights out." And when asked a similar question by Justice O'Connor, Tucker, the attorney for the proponents of assisted suicide in *Glucksberg*, replied that because "ours is a culture of denial of death," she had "some concerns that the political process would not be expected to work in a usual fashion."

That the lawyers for the states, not the lawyers for the plaintiffs, urged the Court to let the state legislatures resolve the difficult issues involved in the physician-assisted suicide cases is hardly surprising. Proponents of physician-assisted suicide have not fared well in the political arena. They did achieve success in 1994 when Oregon voters passed a "death with dignity" act (a vote Oregon reaffirmed three years later), but so far Oregon has been a striking exception.

Washington and California ballot initiatives for "aid in dying" both failed in the early 1990s. Moreover, in the last decade bills to legalize physician-assisted suicide have been introduced in more than twenty states, and none has passed.[83] Indeed, in 1997 alone seven state legislative attempts to legalize physician-assisted suicide "died outright or . . . languished in committee."[84] On the other hand, bills expressly prohibiting assisted suicide have fared much better. Since 1989, sixteen such bills have been enacted into law.[85]

Some have made much of the fact that five months after the Supreme Court handed down its decisions in the physician-assisted suicide cases, Oregon voters reaffirmed their support for assisted suicide by a much larger margin than the initial 1994 vote. The state legislature had put the initiative (which had initially passed by a 51% to 49% vote) back on the ballot for an unprecedented second vote. This time the initiative was reaffirmed overwhelmingly, 60% to 40%. Barbara Coombs Lee hailed the event as "a turning point for the death with dignity movement."[86] David Garrow called the landslide vote "a good indicator of where America may be headed."[87] Still another commentator viewed the lopsided vote as a demonstration of "how far, and how fast, public opinion is moving on this issue."[88]

I think not. I think the most plausible explanation for the large margin by which Oregon voters rebuffed efforts to repeal the initiative in favor of physician-assisted suicide was their resentment and anger over the fact that the state legislature had forced them to vote on the issue again—the first time in state history that the legislature had tried to re-

peal a voter-passed initiative.[89] Those running advertisements in favor
of physician-assisted suicide, we are told by the press, "play[ed] on the
perceived anger" generated by the repeal effort itself.

The overwhelming defeat of a Michigan initiative to legalize physician-
assisted suicide (known as Proposal B) in the fall of 1998[90] underscores
the fact that the Oregon experience is the exception, not the rule. Several
months before the Michigan vote, polls indicated that Proposal B would
pass by a comfortable margin. (The prevote polls indicated the same
thing in Washington and California.) What changed the tide of public
opinion? Why did Proposal B lose by more than 40 percentage points?

The Michigan experience shows that it is much easier to sell the basic
notion of assisted suicide than to sell a complex statute making the idea
law. The wrenching case in which a dying person is suffering excruciating and unavoidable pain is the main reason there is so much support
for *the concept* of assisted suicide in this country (as opposed to support
for specific laws). All too often, a reporter thinks that the way to treat the
issue in depth is to present a detailed account of someone who is beg-
ging for help in committing suicide. But such compelling cases—which
are quite rare—blot out what might be called societal or public policy
considerations, such as how to tell if the patient actually has treatable
but hard-to-detect depression.

When pollsters ask about the issue, most people focus on the poignant
case. But when people are asked to approve a complex, 12,000-word
initiative, as in Michigan, the focus shifts. At this point, people start wor-
rying about whether the measure provides too few procedural safeguards or too many. They worry about whether the specific proposal
would impose too many burdensome requirements on dying patients
and their loved ones, as well as whether it provides too few safeguards.

For example, many Michigan voters seemed upset that the proposal
had no requirement that family members be notified of a patient's decision to seek assisted suicide. Critics of the proposal argued that one
might go to visit her father in a nursing home only to discover that a doctor had helped him commit suicide the previous day. But if the proposal
had required that all members of the family be informed, that provision,
too, would have been criticized as hindering a person's right to assisted
suicide.

Anecdotes about individual cases and stirring rhetoric about personal
autonomy and self-determination are one thing; concrete and detailed

proposals designed to cover thousands of cases are something else. As the eminent ethicist Sissela Bok recently observed, "No society has yet worked out the hardest questions of how to help those patients who desire to die, without endangering others who do not."[91] This is not the only problem confronting proponents of physician-assisted suicide. The Supreme Court not only reversed the Ninth and Second Circuit physician-assisted suicide decisions, it disagreed with the lower federal courts virtually point by point. As noted earlier, the Supreme Court in effect wiped out all the lower courts' very strong and very quotable language in favor of physician-assisted suicide.

Now that the Supreme Court has rejected their main constitutional arguments, I believe proponents of physician-assisted suicide are in a much weaker position then they were before these lawsuits were ever brought. For the constitutional arguments they made without success in the Supreme Court and the policy arguments they have been making, and will continue to make, in the state legislatures or state courts or on the op-ed pages of hundreds of newspapers greatly overlap. To be sure, despite the fact that the highest court in the land did not recognize (or is not yet ready to recognize) a constitutional right to physician-assisted suicide, even under narrow circumstances, one may still argue that there is a common law or state constitutional right or a "moral" or "political" right to physician-assisted suicide. Nevertheless, it will be a good deal more difficult to engage in any kind of "rights talk" after the Supreme Court decisions in *Glucksberg* and *Quill* than before.

There are only so many arguments one can make in favor of a "right" to physician-assisted suicide—and almost all of them were addressed by the Supreme Court in *Glucksberg* and *Quill*. I think it fair to say the Court did not find any of them convincing. Thus these arguments have lost a considerable amount of credibility and will be easier to rebuff when made again, albeit in a different setting.

Practice versus Theory

5

The Dutch Experience

Herbert Hendin, M.D.

In the spring of 2001 the Dutch Parliament passed a statute that formally legalized euthanasia and physician-assisted suicide in the Netherlands. Although the world media treated the passage as a major event,
both practices had long been legally sanctioned as the result of a series
of case decisions going back to the early 1970s that had made the Netherlands the only country where euthanasia and physician-assisted suicide
were widely practiced.

Those in the Netherlands who seek an explanation for the Dutch embrace of assisted suicide and euthanasia usually emphasize the country's
historical tradition of tolerance. The Dutch had fought to secure their religious freedom in the sixteenth and seventeenth centuries, and the
Netherlands became a refuge for Jews, Catholics, and free thinkers like
Spinoza and Descartes who fled there from religious oppression. Dutch
secular society in the same period was marked by the Netherlands becoming a major maritime power whose merchants had to learn to accept
different cultures, traditions, and practices.[1] In modern times the Dutch
point to the presence of fifty different religions—most due to schisms
in the Protestant church—and approximately twenty-five political parties. So much diversity in such a small country is seen as a sign of Dutch
tolerance.[2]

Tolerance does not imply integration. Splitting up into so many
autonomous groups has been seen as reflecting an inability to tolerate
the conflict that differences bring. Derek Phillips, professor of sociology
at the University of Amsterdam, sees the division into so many parties and
religious denominations as coming from a difficulty in accepting the ambiguity and tension that result when people of different viewpoints are

interacting in the same group. Dutch academic journals, for example, do not tend to reflect a diversity of viewpoints; more characteristically, different opinions find expression in separate journals.[3] Comparably, when the Royal Dutch Medical Association (KNMG) supported physician-assisted suicide and euthanasia, religious physicians formed a separate medical group opposed to euthanasia. The Dutch medical establishment believes that all opposition to euthanasia is fundamentally religious in nature but is far less tolerant of nonreligious physicians who oppose euthanasia on medical grounds and try to do so within the framework of organized medicine.[4] Compartmentalizing differences is seen as avoiding direct engagement and maintaining consensus within respective autonomous groups.

Most scholars point to Dutch Calvinism as an essential starting point in understanding the origins of contemporary Dutch attitudes toward euthanasia. Calvinism in the Netherlands had a puritanical self-righteous intensity in its faith in the virtue and guidance of the elect, its discouragement of pleasure, its belief that the endurance of suffering was admirable as well as redemptive, and its dedication to work, attitudes that once diffused throughout the society. These attitudes found expression in both the Roman Catholic Church and the Dutch Reformed Church. Protestantism and Catholicism were considered to be two of the three pillars on which Dutch society rested; the third was secularism. All three columns had a remarkable degree of autonomy, and each had its own schools, hospitals, and social organizations.[5]

As social revolution swept through the Western world in the 1960s, the influence of the Dutch Reformed Church and the Roman Catholic Church was eroded in the Netherlands, but the power of secularism remained. A new consensus emerged that held that individual autonomy should prevail whenever possible in seeking pleasure and avoiding pain. Such liberalization is viewed as a welcome shift away from an austere Puritanism toward a broad tolerance of diverse behavior. However, the emphasis on autonomy reflected the tendency to split along lines of difference that was now being defined in terms of autonomous individual behavior. The consensus that developed around euthanasia and other social changes was seen by Dutch observers as Calvinist in its intensity and self-righteousness but organized around the values of a secular culture. Dutch acceptance of drug use, dramatized by the crowds of young people who fill major public squares using drugs openly; acceptance of public displays of prostitution; and embrace of euthanasia have been seen as related evidence of antipuritanical changes that flowed from the social revolution. The view of Dutch tolerance of drug use, pornography, prostitution, and euthanasia as simply a reaction against an earlier set of religious values is not the whole story and will be explored from a contemporary perspective later in this chapter. Before the 1960s, however, there was not the interest in euthanasia in the Netherlands that had been present for some time in England and the United States and led to the formation of voluntary euthanasia societies in both countries in the 1930s—thirty-five years before such a society was organized in the Netherlands.

In 1973, against a background of social ferment, a euthanasia case first received widespread public attention in the Netherlands: a physician ended the life of her ailing seventy-eight-year-old mother at her mother's request. Popular support grew for the physician and for the Dutch court in Leeuwarden that found her guilty but refused to punish her. The court relied on an expert witness, a medical inspector for the national health service, who stated that it was no longer considered right for physicians to keep patients alive to the bitter end under certain conditions. These conditions were spelled out in detail in a subsequent case when, in 1981, a Rotterdam court, in finding a layperson guilty of assisting in a suicide, volunteered the opinion that a physician doing so might be exempt from punishment under the Dutch penal code if there had been a voluntary request from a person suffering unbearably with no reasonable alternatives for relief and if the physician had consulted with another physician in making the decision.[6]

In 1984, a case reached the Dutch Supreme Court. A physician who had assisted in the suicide of a ninety-five-year-old woman had been acquitted, but the decision for acquittal was reversed by an appellate court. The Supreme Court overturned the conviction, arguing that the appellate court had failed to consider whether the physician was placed in an intolerable position because of what it called a "conflict of duties." Was the patient's suffering such that the physician was forced to act in a situation "beyond [his or her] control?" The court referred the case back to an appellate court in The Hague with the instruction to consider the case with one dominant consideration from an objective medical perspective: could the euthanasia practiced by the physician be regarded as an action justified in a situation of medical necessity?[7]

This ruling invited and obliged the prosecutor in The Hague to rely heavily on the opinion of the Royal Dutch Medical Association (KNMG) as to the acceptability of euthanasia from the professions' standpoint. Critics of the Supreme Court's ruling were unhappy at what they perceived as the court's abdication of moral and legal authority to the medical profession. The statement given by the KNMG to the appellate court paraphrased the Supreme Court's language to declare that in a situation of necessity (force majeure) a physician could be justified in honoring a request for euthanasia.[8]

Even before the decision was issued in The Hague dismissing the charges against the physician, the KNMG had sent a letter to the Minister of Justice asking for a change in the law to permit euthanasia. Although there was public sympathy for the physicians involved in the euthanasia cases and support for the practice of euthanasia, there was not then support for changing the statute. Physicians were able to practice euthanasia with only the protection of case law. Prosecutions, however, were rare, and punishment, even in cases of conviction, was virtually nonexistent.

Eventually, a consensus on guidelines for practicing euthanasia was reached by the courts, the KNMG, the Ministry of Justice, and the Dutch Health Council. When patients experiencing intolerable suffering that could not be relieved in any other way made a voluntary, well-considered, and persistent request to a physician for euthanasia, the physician, if supported in the decision by another physician, would be justified in performing euthanasia. The doctor should not certify the death as due to natural causes and should notify the medical examiner, who would file a report with the local prosecutor, who could investigate further or allow the deceased to be buried. If these guidelines were followed the physician would not be prosecuted under Dutch law that, at the time, treated euthanasia as a criminal offense. In 1993, a statute was enacted that gave further protection to physicians by explicitly stipulating that a physician following the guidelines would not be prosecuted.

In response to domestic and international concern about reports of abuse, the Dutch government sponsored a study of physician-assisted suicide and euthanasia in 1990.[9] That study, which was largely replicated in a 1995 study, was supported by the KNMG with the promise that physicians who participated would receive immunity from prosecution for anything they revealed.

In 1996 the investigators published a report of their new findings in Dutch[10] and summarized their work in two articles in the *New England Journal of Medicine,*[11] which were supported by an editorial in that journal.[12] These reports concluded that, since matters had not grown worse during the five years between the two studies, there was no evidence that "physicians in the Netherlands are moving down a slippery slope."[13] That conclusion was misleading.

In this context, the "slippery slope" is the gradual extension of assisted suicide to widening groups of patients after it is legally permitted for patients designated as terminally ill. In the past three decades, the Netherlands has moved from considering assisted suicide (preferred over euthanasia by the Dutch Voluntary Euthanasia Society) to giving legal sanction to both physician-assisted suicide and euthanasia, from euthanasia for terminally ill patients to euthanasia for those who are chronically ill, from euthanasia for physical illness to euthanasia for psychological distress, and from voluntary euthanasia to nonvoluntary and involuntary euthanasia. ("Nonvoluntary" is used to describe euthanasia with patients not capable of requesting it; "involuntary" is used to describe euthanasia with patients who did not request it but were capable of doing so.)

According to the KNMG, it did not seem reasonable medically, legally, or morally to sanction only assisted suicide, thereby denying more active medical help in the form of euthanasia to those who could not effect their own death.[14] Most patients and physicians prefer euthanasia because they see it is less subject to complications and failure. Nor could the Dutch deny assisted suicide or euthanasia to chronically ill patients who have longer to suffer than those who are terminally ill, or to those who have psychological pain not associated with physical disease. To do so would be a form of discrimination. Nonvoluntary and involuntary euthanasia are not legally sanctioned by the Dutch, but they are increasingly excused as necessary to end the suffering of patients who, for a variety of reasons, are not able or willing to choose to hasten death.[15] Except for the legal sanction of euthanasia for mental suffering without physical illness, all of these other expansions of the practice of euthanasia had taken place by 1990 and were documented by the 1990 study.

Comparing the data for the 1990 and 1995 studies is revealing. From 1990 to 1995, the death rate from euthanasia increased from 1.9 percent to 2.2 percent of all deaths, when based on interviews with 405 Dutch physicians selected from a stratified random sample. The rate increased from 1.7 percent to 2.4 percent when based on responses to a question-naire completed by more than 4,600 physicians in both years (table 1). The increase in euthanasia deaths, ranging from 16 percent to 41 percent (from 573 to 1,064 deaths), would seem significant, but the *Dutch* inves-tigators do not regard it as such even though they give "generational and cultural changes in patients' attitudes" as a possible explanation for the increase.[16] The investigators describe the rates of physician-assisted sui-cide as remaining constant and low although, based on the interview study, the actual number increased from 380 to 542.

Table 1.
Estimated Incidence of Specific Medical Decisions at the End of Life

Medical Decision	1990 Study		1995 Study	
	Questionnaire Portion[a]	Interview Portion[b]	Questionnaire Portion[a]	Interview Portion[b]
Euthanasia	2,189 (1.7)	2,445 (1.9)	3,253 (2.4)	3,018 (2.2)
Physician-assisted suicide	244 (0.2)	380 (0.3)	271 (0.2)	542 (0.4)
Ending life without request[c]	1,030 (0.8)		948 (0.7)	
Opioids given with explicit intention of ending life[d]		1,350 (1.0)		1,896 (1.4)
Estimated total deaths caused by active inter-vention by physicians[e]	4,813 (3.7)		6,368 (4.7)	

Note: Values are the number of deaths with percentages of all deaths in parentheses, based on 128,786 deaths in the Netherlands in 1990 and 135,546 deaths in 1995.

[a] Figures based on questionnaire portions of the study. A total of 6,942 questionnaires mailed in 1991; 76 percent were returned. A total of 6,060 mailed in 1995; 77 percent were returned. Sample stratified to include a high percentage of cases where a decision at the end of life was likely to be made.

[b] Figures were from the interview portions of the study. A total of 405 physicians were in-terviewed in 1991 and another 405 in 1995. They were selected from stratified random sam-ple of 599 in 1991 and 559 in 1995. Only 9 percent refused to participate in 1991 and 11 percent in 1995. Others were not traceable, had chronic illness, or did not meet other criteria. Sample was stratified to include physicians likely to have participated in end-of-life decisions.

[c] Comparative figures available for only questionnaire portion of the study.

[d] Comparative figures available for only interview portion of the study.

[e] Total death estimates are based on projections from both the questionnaire and inter-view samples.

Guidelines Have Failed

The extension of euthanasia to more patients has been associated with the inability to regulate the process within established rules. Virtually every guideline set up by the Dutch—a voluntary, well-considered, persistent request; intolerable suffering that cannot be relieved; formal consultation with a colleague; and reporting of cases—has failed to protect patients or has been modified or violated.[17]

Many of the violations are evident from the officially sanctioned studies. For example, the studies reveal that more than 50 percent of physicians considered it appropriate to suggest euthanasia to patients.[18] Neither the physicians nor the study's investigators seem to acknowledge how much the voluntariness of the process may be compromised by such a suggestion.

Intolerable suffering that cannot be relieved has always been regarded as a necessary criterion for euthanasia in the Netherlands. In 74 percent of cases, physicians reported that such suffering was the major reason for patients requesting euthanasia. In a quarter of cases, however, fear of future suffering or loss of dignity was more important; neither of these reasons by itself would seem to satisfy the criterion of unrelievable suffering.

What if patients do not want treatments that will relieve their suffering? That is their right in the Netherlands as elsewhere, but then they do not meet the criterion for euthanasia. The Dutch Supreme Court affirmed that with regard to mental suffering, euthanasia is not permissible if palliative treatment is possible, even if it is refused by the patient. The KNMG stated that this should be true for somatically based suffering as well. In 17 percent of cases in 1995, however, physicians admitted that even though treatment alternatives had been available, euthanasia was performed.

Consultation takes place in about 80 percent of the reported cases, but interviews with physicians revealed that in only 11 percent of the unreported cases was there consultation with another physician.[19] Taken together, these figures indicate that there is consultation in about half of Dutch euthanasia cases. When life was terminated without request, there was no consultation in 97 percent of cases.

Of the physicians who had been a consultant more than once, 50 percent had previously been consulted by the same physician; 24 percent had themselves previously consulted the attending physician in euthanasia cases of their own.[20] Recognizing that such "pairs" may compromise the independence of consultants, the Dutch investigators subsequently recommended that independent consultants be chosen. In the overwhelming majority of cases, the physician's mind had been made up before consulting; not surprisingly, the consulting doctor disagreed in only 7 percent of cases. In 12 percent of cases the consulting physician did not actually see the patient. Convenience of location and agreement on life-ending decisions were the major reasons given for consulting a particular physician; knowledge of palliative care was hardly mentioned.

Under-reporting has been a serious problem. In only 18 percent of cases in 1990 had physicians reported their euthanasia cases to the authorities as required by Dutch guidelines. To encourage more reporting of cases, a simplified notification procedure was enacted. It ensured that physicians would not be prosecuted if guidelines were followed. The investigators credit this procedural change with contributing to an increase in the cases reported to 41 percent by 1995, while acknowledging that a 59 percent rate of unreported cases is still disturbingly high.

The Dutch studies reveal that half of the physicians who had not reported their most recent case of euthanasia gave as a reason their wish or that of their family to avoid a judicial inquiry, 20 percent the fear of prosecution, 16 percent the failure to fulfill the requirements for accepted procedures, and 14 percent the belief that euthanasia should be a private matter. Between 15 percent and 20 percent of doctors say they will not report their cases under any circumstances. Twenty percent of the physicians' most recent unreported cases involved ending a life without the patient's consent.[21] Such cases, both the 1990 and 1995 studies revealed, were virtually never reported.

Death without Consent

The most alarming concern to arise from the Dutch studies has been the documentation of cases in which patients who have not given their consent have had their lives ended by physicians. The 1990 study revealed that in 0.8 percent of the deaths (more than 1,000 cases) in the Netherlands each year, physicians admitted they actively caused death without the explicit consent of the patient. The 1995 figure is 0.7 percent (fewer than 1,000 cases), but the researchers, while pointing to the decline, concede that differences in the way this particular information was obtained make its significance uncertain. In both studies, however, about a quarter of physicians stated that they had "terminated the lives of patients without explicit request" from the patient to do so, and a third more of the physicians could conceive of doing so. The use of the word *explicit* is somewhat inaccurate, since in 48 percent of these cases there was no request of any kind[22] and in the others there were mainly references to patients' earlier statements of not wanting to suffer.[23]

The 1990 study documented, and the 1995 study confirmed, that cases classified as "termination of the patient without explicit request" were a fraction of the nonvoluntary and involuntary euthanasia cases. International attention had centered on the 1,350 cases (1% of all Dutch deaths) in 1990 in which physicians gave pain medication with the explicit intention of ending the patient's life.[24] The investigators minimized the number of patients put to death who had not requested it by not including these 1,350 patients in that category.

By 1995 there had been an increase in the number of deaths in which physicians gave pain medication with the explicit intention of ending the patient's life from 1,350 cases to 1,896 (1.4% of all Dutch deaths).[25] These are comparisons that the Dutch investigators do not make. As reported by the physicians in the 1995 study, in more than 80 percent of these cases (1,537 deaths), no request for death was made by the patient.[26] Since these are cases of nonvoluntary, and involuntary (if the patient was competent), euthanasia, this is a striking increase in the number of lives terminated without request and a refutation of the investigators' claim that there has been perhaps a slight decrease in the number of such cases.

If one totals all the deaths that resulted from euthanasia, assisted suicide, ending the life of a patient without consent, and giving opioids with the explicit intention of ending life, the estimated number of deaths caused by active intervention by physicians increased from 4,813 (3.7% of all deaths) in 1990 to 6,368 (4.7% of all deaths) in 1995 (table 1). Based on data from the questionnaire study, this is an increase of 27 percent in cases in which physicians actively intervened to cause death. Of the more than 6,000 deaths in which physicians admit to having actively and intentionally intervened to cause death, 40 percent involved no explicit request from the patient for them to do so.

The Dutch investigators minimize the significance of the number of deaths without consent by explaining that the patients were incompetent.[27] But in the 1995 study, 21 percent of the individuals classified as "patients whose lives were ended without explicit request" were competent; in the 1990 study, 37 percent were competent.[28] We are not told what percentage of those patients who were given pain medication intended to end their lives without discussing it with them were competent, but analysis of the data for opioid administration indicated that it is likely to be at least 20 percent.

More than 4,000 additional competent patients were given pain medication in amounts likely to end their lives by physicians who did not discuss the decision with them, but whose primary intention was not to end their lives.[29] Whether the intention was to end life or whether death was simply likely, physicians usually gave as the reason for not discussing the decisions with the patients that they had previously had some discussion of the subject with the patients.[30] Apparently they thought that was sufficient justification for ending a life or putting it at risk without determining the patient's current wishes.

The practice of involuntary euthanasia is often defended on the grounds of compassion. An illustration given me by the attorney for the Dutch Voluntary Euthanasia Society of why it was sometimes necessary for physicians to end the lives of competent patients without their consent was the case of a nun whose physician ended her life a few days before she would have died because she was in excruciating pain but her religious convictions did not permit her to ask for death.[31] Compassion is not the only motive in such cases. A Dutch woman with disseminated breast cancer who had said she did not want euthanasia had her life ended because, in the physician's words, "It could have taken another week before she died. I just needed this bed."[32]

The Limitations of the Dutch Studies

Political considerations have admittedly influenced the Dutch studies and their conclusions. I asked the Dutch investigators why physicians were not challenged when they offered implausible explanations for ending fully competent patients' lives without consulting them. The investigators explained that securing and retaining the cooperation of the KNMG and the participating physicians demanded that the physicians and policies not be challenged.[33]

The reasons given by physicians for failure to report their cases, such as the families' fear of judicial inquiry or the physician's fear of prosecution, also seem to require further questioning. The investigators state that the doctors' violations were not substantive but procedural, by which they mean failure to obtain written request from the patient, to write a written report, or to obtain a consultation. Failure to obtain a consultation is procedural only if the investigators have accepted the attitude of so many Dutch physicians that consultation is not for the benefit and protection of the patient but only to meet a legal requirement. In addition, the "procedural" explanation ignores the large number of unreported cases that involve the death of a patient who has not requested it, a matter that under any definition is not merely "procedural."

In addition, the researchers draw conclusions that exceed their evidence.[34] The 1990 and 1995 studies accepted physicians' assertions that their patients had received the best possible care and that there was no alternative to euthanasia. These statements are not supported by any objective data. Indeed, studies have demonstrated the inadequacy of physicians' training in palliative care in the Netherlands.[35] Since the statements of the responding physicians were accepted by the investigators without challenge, there was no exploration of possible alternatives to euthanasia.[36] Since neither the attending doctors, nor the consultants, nor the physician-interviewers in the government-sponsored studies were trained in palliative care, they were not in a position to ask the right questions.

The Dutch investigators, the KNMG, and the Dutch government are most sensitive to the charge of "involuntary euthanasia," a term they avoid by referring to such cases as "termination of the patient without explicit request." After the first report on the Dutch findings was published, the project investigators wrote an article and one of them published a thesis, trying in both publications to justify the involuntary cases (the patients did not have long to live; the same thing was happening in other countries but secretly), while admitting it would be preferable if such cases were kept to a minimum.[37] At some point the investigators seem to have realized that "termination of the patient without explicit request" had an Orwellian sound to the English-speaking world that was even worse than "involuntary euthanasia," and they now use the acronym LAWER, "life-ending acts without the explicit request of the patient," an acronym that vaguely suggests legality.

I asked Paul van der Maas, the principal Dutch investigator, why patients who had consented to be given pain medication by physicians with the explicit intention of ending their lives were not counted as euthanasia cases. He agreed that such cases could have been counted as euthanasia cases, thereby increasing that total. The only difference was that in ordinary euthanasia cases, since a drug to stop respiration was also administered, death took place almost immediately, while in patients given only overdoses of pain medication, death could take a number of hours. I then asked why patients who had not consented and were given pain medication by physicians with the explicit intention of ending their lives were not counted as cases whose lives had been terminated without explicit request. He not only was reluctant to do so, but also could not give me a reason. Of course, counting these cases would have made evident that their number had more than doubled since 1990, which would have aroused worldwide concern and criticism. The true number of cases in which patients' lives are terminated without their explicit request is being concealed by the way such deaths are labeled.

Both the 1990 and 1995 studies are flawed for all of the above-mentioned reasons. When cases are classified and counted so as to minimize disturbing findings, when implausible explanations are accepted without challenge, and when conclusions that might offend are not stated, there is a need for more objective and inclusive exploration and analysis. That exploration and analysis will have to include a realization that notification by physicians of all euthanasia cases would not by itself diminish abuse of euthanasia in the Netherlands. Nor could better case counting and classification do the job without exploring the interactive decision-making process that is at the heart of euthanasia and is not addressed in the Dutch research.

Despite the limitations of the government-sanctioned studies, on the basis of those studies alone it has been possible for investigators to conclude "that the so-called strict safeguards laid down by the courts and the Royal Dutch Medical Association . . . had largely failed."[38] When, as the 1990 and 1995 studies document, 59 percent of Dutch physicians do not report their cases of assisted suicide and euthanasia, when more than 50 percent feel free to suggest euthanasia to their patients, and when 25 percent admit to ending patients' lives without the patient's consent, it is clear that terminally ill patients are not adequately protected.

All of these problems were evident in the 1990 study, but it took a long time for them to be realized and understood. A brief article in the British journal the *Lancet*[39] followed by several equally brief articles hardly did justice to the findings. The study was published in a 1991 book that was translated and published in English a year later. The book is difficult to read in either Dutch or English, and much of the key information must

be found in tables. The few observations made in the book tend to minimize problems in ways that are misleading. For example, the book points
out that a large majority of the patients whose lives were ended without request were incompetent; the table reveals that 37 percent *were* competent, which means that hundreds of competent patients had their lives
ended without their consent.

The Dutch findings were accepted uncritically both in the Netherlands
and abroad by observers who, I have been surprised to find, had invariably not read the full report. The 1995 study was also published in
full in Dutch and in two articles in the *New England Journal of Medicine*,
but there are currently no plans to translate the full report into English.
It has taken years and a thorough comparison of the two studies by
scholars in the Netherlands, England, and the United States to begin finally to make the educated public fully aware of the extent of the problems in the Dutch system.

More Than Figures

Since the government-sanctioned Dutch studies in 1990 and 1995 are primarily numerical and categorical, they do not give a picture of what
these violations of guidelines mean in actual practice with patients. Nor
do the studies examine the interactions among physicians, patients, and
families that determine the decision for euthanasia. We need to look elsewhere for a fuller picture. Other studies conducted in the Netherlands
have indicated how voluntariness is compromised, alternatives are not
presented, and the criterion of unrelievable suffering is bypassed.[40] Some
examples may be helpful.[41]

A wife who no longer wished to care for her sick, elderly husband
gave him a choice between euthanasia and admission to a home for the
chronically ill. The man, afraid of being left to the mercy of strangers in
an unfamiliar place, chose to have his life ended; the doctor, although
aware of the coercion, ended the man's life. In a study done in Dutch hospitals, doctors and nurses reported that more requests for euthanasia
came from families than from patients themselves. The investigator concluded that the families, the doctors, and the nurses were involved in
pressuring patients to request euthanasia.[42]

A physically healthy fifty-year-old woman who had recently lost her
son to cancer refused all psychiatric treatment and said she would accept help only in dying. Her case contributed to extending the criteria

for euthanasia to include mental suffering without physical illness. It also provides some insight into the Dutch legal system.

The woman was assisted in suicide by a psychiatrist, Boudewijn Chabot, within four months of her son's death. Chabot had told her that he could not make such a decision until he knew her better, implying that if after time he considered her decision appropriate he would assist her. The woman saw him for a number of sessions over a two-month period, eventually telling him she would leave if he did not help her, at which point he did.

During the course of our interviews Chabot told me that his patient suffered from incurable grief. Her refusal of treatment was considered by him to make her suffering unrelievable. The woman had told Chabot that if he did not help her she would kill herself without him. He seemed on the one hand to be succumbing to emotional blackmail and on the other to be ignoring the fact that even without treatment, experience has shown that time alone was likely to have affected her wish to die. Before assisting in the suicide, Chabot had sent a written account of the case to a number of consultants, requesting their opinion and asking one of them to see the patient. The majority felt he should go forward, but none, including the one asked, felt it was necessary to see the patient. Since Chabot, as required, filed a report with the local coroner, and since the case was breaking new ground in being the first involving purely mental suffering to come to public attention, it was taken to court by a reluctant public prosecutor, who asked for a verdict of a year's suspended sentence. The prosecutor's own witness agreed that the assisted suicide was justified. Chabot was acquitted and that acquittal sustained on appeal.[43]

To American eyes accustomed to a legal system in which each side tries to win, the trial seems strange. In the Netherlands, however, the legal system is consensual, that is, it aims at a decision that tries to meet the needs of all concerned, including the community at large, rather than adversarial, where one side wins and the other loses. And the consensus shared by doctors, patients, lawyers, and judges in the Netherlands is strongly supportive of physicians in assisted suicide or euthanasia cases.

In reviewing this case, however, the Dutch Supreme Court, while affirming that mental suffering alone could be reason for performing euthanasia, found Chabot guilty of not having had a consultant see the patient, which it said was necessary in a case in which no physical illness was involved. No punishment was imposed because the court felt that in all other respects Chabot had behaved correctly. The KNMG felt even this mild reprimand was unfair, since in previous cases involving physical illness, courts had not been willing to convict simply because a consultant was not called, and Chabot had no reason to assume the situation in this case would be different. I felt that all of the consultants shared responsibility for not having asked to see the patient, whether required to or not, but this was not a view shared by those in the association with whom I spoke.

Wilfrid van Oijen, a Dutch physician who was filmed ending the life of a patient recently diagnosed with amyotrophic lateral sclerosis, said of the patient, "I can give him the finest wheelchair there is, but in the end it is only a stopgap. He is going to die and he knows it." That death may be years away, but a physician with this attitude may not be able to present alternatives to this patient. The patient in this case was clearly ambivalent about proceeding and wanted to put off the date for his death. This ambivalence was ignored by the doctor, who was supporting the desire of the patient's wife to move forward quickly. Van Oijen never saw the patient alone, permitted the wife to answer all questions for the patient about whether he wanted to die, and presented an exaggerated picture of the death that awaited him without euthanasia.[44]

In *Appointment with Death,* a documentary film by the Dutch Voluntary Euthanasia Society that was intended to promote euthanasia, a forty-one-year-old artist was diagnosed as HIV positive. He had no physical symptoms but had seen others suffer with them and wanted his physician's assistance in dying. The doctor compassionately explained to him that he might live for some years symptom free. Despite this, over time the patient repeated his request for euthanasia. Although the doctor thought his patient was acting unwisely and prematurely, he did not know how to deal with his patient's terror. He rationalized that respect for the patient's autonomy required that he grant the patient's request.

Consultation in the case was pro forma; a colleague of the doctor saw the patient briefly to confirm his wishes. And while the primary doctor kept establishing that the patient was persistent in his request and competent to make the decision, thus formally meeting those criteria, the doctor did not address the terror that underlay the patient's request.

This patient had clearly been depressed and overwhelmed by the news of his situation. Had his physician been able to deal with more than formal criteria regarding a request to die—more likely in a culture not so accepting of assisted suicide and euthanasia—this man would probably not have been assisted in suicide.[45]

A Cure for Suicide

This last case appeared to cry out for psychiatric consultation, but one was never considered. Even though a desire for suicide is considered a primary indication for psychiatric evaluation, such consultation is not likely in the Netherlands. This is true despite the fact that terminally ill patients with a desire to hasten death are, like other suicidal patients, likely to have a depression that will respond to treatment. A survey of Dutch psychiatrists indicated that only 3 percent of Dutch patients requesting assisted suicide or euthanasia are referred for psychiatric consultation. In cases where there is physical illness, only 19 percent of Dutch psychiatrists thought a psychiatric consultation should always be requested.[46] They were perhaps unfamiliar with the substantial evidence that general physicians are not able to evaluate when patients have psychiatric disorders that may be interfering with their judgment. The Dutch psychiatrists and the government-sponsored investigators make a fairly rigid distinction between physical and mental suffering. Yet in most cases, as in the case of the young man discussed above, both physical and psychological suffering are apt to be present, and the psychological is often the more important. That physical/psychological dichotomy, pervasive in the Netherlands, has had an important impact on the treatment of medical patients who become suicidally depressed.

Since the early 1980s, as assisted suicide and euthanasia have become increasingly available in the Netherlands, the suicide rate among those over fifty has fallen by a third.[47] This is the age group containing the greatest number of euthanasia cases (86% of the men and 78% of the women) and the greatest number of suicides. The remarkable decline in suicide in this older age group appears to be due to the fact that older suicidal patients are now asking to receive euthanasia instead. The likelihood that patients would end their own lives if euthanasia was not available to them was one of the justifications given by Dutch doctors for providing such help. If any significant percentage of these cases had been counted as suicides, the suicide rate would actually have risen.

Of course, proponents of euthanasia can maintain that making suicide "unnecessary" for those over fifty who are physically ill is a benefit of legalization rather than a sign of abuse. Such an attitude depends, of course, on whether one believes that there are alternatives to assisted suicide or euthanasia for dealing with the problems of older people who become ill.

Among an older population, physical illness of all types is common, and many who have trouble coping with physical illness become suicidal. In a culture accepting of euthanasia, their distress is accepted as a legitimate reason for dying.

Procedure, Not Substance

Consistent with its view that any Dutch problems with euthanasia are basically procedural, the KNMG has made various recommendations to improve the procedures for dealing with euthanasia cases without addressing the basic substantive problems. In 1995 the organization refined its guidelines: assisted suicide rather than euthanasia should be performed whenever possible; a second physician who has no professional or personal ties to the first should actually see the patient; physicians need not participate in euthanasia but must refer the patient to doctors who will; and physicians must report all cases of euthanasia to the authorities.

The protection of the patient is usually cited as the reason for preferring assisted suicide to euthanasia, but the strain on the doctor was given by the KNMG as the reason for this suggested change. A KNMG spokesperson explained that "many doctors find euthanasia a difficult and burdensome action and the patient's participation diminishes the burden slightly."[48] Physicians who perform euthanasia infrequently may follow the KNMG suggestion, and the guideline seems intended to encourage reluctant doctors to participate. Physicians who perform euthanasia more often are not likely to be deterred, since they see assisted suicide as more open to complications and failure.

The KNMG does not see a contradiction between saying that doctors need not participate in euthanasia and demanding that they make a referral that is against their conscience. The KNMG spokesperson explained that a doctor cannot "leave a patient in the cold at the last moment. He should help find alternatives." But no alternatives other than suffering or euthanasia are envisioned.

The reasonable recommendation by the KNMG that independent consultants should actually see the patients is, unfortunately, not likely to make much of a difference. Practitioners of euthanasia are known by reputation to every doctor, but they are not expert in palliative care; their seeing the patient or their not being a friend of the referring physician is not apt to change the result.

The Dutch investigators have recommended that some physicians specialize as euthanasia consultants, building up experience in the "medico-technical aspects of assisted suicide and euthanasia and the possibilities of palliative care."[49] Acting as a consultant in euthanasia cases, however, does not somehow make a physician knowledgeable about palliative care. My own experience with a few physicians in the Netherlands who had performed or been consultants in dozens of euthanasia cases was that they were surprisingly uninvolved in palliative care. Nor did they show sensitivity to the ambivalence that accompanies most requests to die, which was clearly evident in some of the cases we discussed.[50] They seemed to be facilitators of the process rather than independent evaluators of the patient's situation who might be able to relieve suffering so that euthanasia seemed less necessary to the patient. One prominent consultant described his role as easing the doubts of physicians who were uncertain as to whether to go forward with euthanasia. He and the other consultants were certainly knowledgeable in the "medico-technical" aspects of euthanasia (i.e., they could end life quickly and efficiently).

Wilfrid van Oijen, the Dutch physician mentioned earlier who was filmed performing euthanasia on a patient with amyotrophic lateral sclerosis, is a case in point. Although the film seems to minimize van Oijen's role as a euthanasia consultant, showing him in his family practice attending to pregnant women and small children, he tells us, "I perform euthanasia three or four times a year. It's not like I plan to go out with my Uzi and mow down crowds of people." In the Dutch version of the film he indicates that he is the consulting physician in three or four euthanasia cases a year in addition to the three or four he "believes" he performs himself. The average Dutch doctor in a general practice, however, is not involved in six to eight cases a year and is likely to have performed euthanasia only a relatively few times in a career. The Dutch Voluntary Euthanasia Society was sufficiently familiar with van Oijen's work as a specialist in euthanasia that when approached by a filmmaker who wished to film an actual case the society referred him to van Oijen. And while the physician is certainly not a terrorist or mass murderer mowing down people with an Uzi, he is more of a professional hired for a special skill than he is willing to admit. His dismissive attitude toward a wheelchair for his patient makes clear that while he is a euthanasia consultant it is not because of any interest in or knowledge he has of palliative care.[51]

It is worth noting that in 2001, van Oijen was found guilty by a Dutch court of ending the life of an eighty-four-year-old woman at her daughters' request—not the woman's own. The woman had heart problems and was increasingly bedridden. She was not in pain and said she did not want to die but could not care for herself. She had indicated a desire to be with her daughters, who cared for her at home, but her care had evidently become burdensome to them. Van Oijen gave her a medication that paralyzed her breathing but claimed he was not intending to end her life, only to speed up the process of dying. The case turned on the opinion of expert witnesses that the medication as given could not be considered part of palliative care. Although declaring van Oijen legally guilty of murder, the court imposed no punishment since it felt that while he made an "error of judgment" he had acted "honorably and according to his conscience" in what he considered the interests of his patient. Van Oijen had not asked for a second opinion in the case; he had also falsely reported the death as due to natural causes, and for this he was found guilty and fined 5,000 guilders ($2,140). The KNMG defended van Oijen's actions, claiming that he acted with "complete integrity."[52]

Neither the opinion of the KNMG nor that of the Dutch Supreme Court is likely to prevent euthanasia in cases in which a patient has refused a viable treatment alternative. Patients in the Netherlands, like patients elsewhere, have a right to refuse unwanted treatment. The physician may in good faith wrongly believe there are no treatment options available, and there is no requirement that anyone with expertise be consulted. Moreover, the Dutch Minister of Justice explicitly stated and instructed the attorneys general that refusal by the patient of treatment alternatives does not render euthanasia illegal.[53] Some in the Netherlands see a shift away from justifying euthanasia on the basis of unrelievable suffering and the possibility of relieving it toward justifying euthanasia based on patient choice as the natural progression of a liberal society's increasing emphasis on autonomy.[54] Such a shift would remove one of the bedrock safeguards on which the Dutch system was built. It also ignores the reality of what actually happens when a suffering patient is confronted with a physician who does not know how to relieve that suffering except by euthanasia. If the only alternatives are continued suffering or an early death, patients are not likely to feel they have a choice.

To encourage more reporting of cases, in 1998 the Dutch government adopted a procedure whereby cases are reported to nongovernmental regional groups of three people who evaluate the case—a lawyer, a physician, and an ethicist—as well as to the coroner and the local prosecutor. The prosecutor was to be guided by the group's opinion in deciding whether the case required investigation. This procedure was incorporated into subsequent legislation with a significant modification stipulating that only if the three-person group considered that the physician violated the Dutch guidelines for assisted suicide or euthanasia would the case be reported to the coroner and the prosecutorial authorities. Since the physician in the group is not required or likely to have training in palliative care, and since the group members will know only what the physician reporting the case chooses to tell them, it is hard to see how the group will be able to evaluate such cases. Of course, if patient interests and protection were part of the Dutch agenda, the case reviews would be done while the patients were still alive.

The KNMG has also supported having cases in which physicians end the lives of patients who have not requested death treated in the same way by these regional groups. There has not so far been public or governmental support for this proposal. The new legislation did not include original language that would have permitted children over twelve to request and receive euthanasia even if their parents were opposed, while they could previously do so only if they were sixteen. Opposition to this provision caused the government to modify this proposal to permit child euthanasia in the twelve to sixteen age group, but not over parental objection. Dutch physicians have pointed out that young children and parents will seldom be in conflict in such a situation. That misses the essential point. There is more danger that the parents will become discouraged or exhausted by a child's illness and that the child will respond to a sense that the family would feel relieved if he or she were not there. What is needed are physicians who recognize this and can intercede to help the child by easing the burden on the family.

The original bill considered permitting physicians to perform euthanasia on persons with dementia if they made a request for euthanasia while they were still competent. The request would have been dispositive even if the individual later seemed content with a reduced mental status and did not want to die. And for individuals who develop dementia without having made such a request, their families would be empowered to request it for them. The bill as passed did not clearly address this question. The Health Ministry stated that it believes that only early-stage dementia patients in intolerable pain are eligible for euthanasia.

It is worth noting that the Dutch authors of the 1995 study concluded their report by saying that it would be desirable to reduce the number of cases in which life is terminated without the patient's request, but this must be the common responsibility of the doctor and the patient. The person who does not wish to have his or her life terminated should declare this clearly, in advance, orally and in writing, preferably in the form of a living will. In a press conference, one of the investigators went even further in stating that the person responsible for avoiding involuntary termination of life is the patient. That remark is both a harbinger of the direction in which Dutch euthanasia policies are heading and a summation of much that is wrong with them.

As we will see, Dutch efforts at regulating assisted suicide and euthanasia have served as a model for proposed statutes in the United States and other countries.[55] Yet the Dutch experience has indicated that these practices defy adequate regulation. Given legal sanction, euthanasia, intended originally for the exceptional case, has become an accepted way of dealing with serious or terminal illness in the Netherlands. In the process, palliative care is one of the casualties, while hospice care lags behind that of other countries.[56]

In recent testimony before the British House of Lords, Zbigniew Zylicz, one of the few palliative care experts practicing in the Netherlands, emphasized Dutch deficiencies in palliative care and the lack of hospice care in the Netherlands, attributing them to the availability of the easier alternative of euthanasia.[57] (His personal experience is described in the next chapter.) In its 1997 ruling denying a constitutional right to assisted suicide, the U.S. Supreme Court cited these deficiencies in particular and the Dutch experience in general as evidence that it is dangerous to give legal sanction to assisted suicide.

Conclusion: Culture, Character, and Change

The Dutch medical authorities view euthanasia as a form of healing that is an integral part of palliative care. In the words of the Dutch Minister of Health, the doctor who grants the patient's request for euthanasia "acts as the healer par excellence."[58] Given this attitude, it is understandable that many Dutch physicians feel comfortable suggesting euthanasia to their patients. So regarded, euthanasia can be seen as simply another option for patients, and failure to suggest it could be considered malpractice. Those, including some Dutch physicians, who believed euthanasia was to be a last resort in desperate situations are alarmed because frightened and suffering patients are inclined to listen to suggestions by doctors even when the doctors are telling them their lives are not worth living.

The casualness with which Dutch physicians treat the need for a second opinion in euthanasia cases reflects the view they frequently expressed to me that such consultations were for the purpose of meeting legal requirements. When I asked one of the leading Dutch practitioners of euthanasia whether consultation did not provide some protection for patients, he explained that the concept of patient protection, so accepted in the United States, was foreign to the Dutch. His view was supported by the official spokesperson for the KNMG.

Although these physicians are wrong in assuming that Dutch patients do not need protection, they are correct in assuming that the vast majority of the Dutch do not consider that they do. The Dutch accept the authority of physicians in ways that would seem foreign in the United States. Malpractice suits are rare in the Netherlands. Even when physicians end the lives of patients who have not requested it, the Dutch are inclined to be forgiving on the grounds that the physicians' intentions were benevolent. Seeing their choice when confronted with painful illness as between prolonged suffering and a quick death, a large proportion of people in the country are also unaware that there may be better alternatives.

The embrace by the Dutch medical establishment of euthanasia and the Dutch population's willingness to follow them in doing so can be understood in part by what we know of Dutch culture and character—particularly the uniquely ambivalent Dutch attitude toward authority. Although Calvinism was born in opposition to papal authority, magistrates were seen as "ministers of Divine Justice, vice regents of God."[59] In modern times the Dutch impulse seems to be to resist formal authority—the Catholic Church in the Netherlands is uniquely resistant to papal authority[60]—and to replace it with authority that is less direct and obvious; doctors and judges fall into this category.

Writing decades before euthanasia became a preoccupation in the Netherlands, the eminent Dutch social historian Johan Huizinga was concerned with a weakening of judgment and morality in the country. It was not crime, prostitution, or drunkenness that worried him (although the rise of fascism in Europe did) but a "betrayal of the spirit." He feared that his fellow citizens liked tranquility to the point of passivity and found them lacking in passion, insensitive to myth, self-satisfied, and obstinate.[61]

Huizinga and other historians have seen the virtues of Dutch character (sobriety, domesticity, commercial spirit, honesty, cleanliness, and respectability) as originating in the bourgeois nature of the society that developed in the seventeenth century.[62] Although Calvinist piety and faith played an important role in the culture, it was urban society that was mainly responsible for the miraculous Dutch achievements when, for a period of at least fifty years, this small country—still establishing its freedom from Spain—became the pre-eminent commercial and artistic center of the world.[63]

Political liberation, mercantile achievement, and the growth of Calvinism were matched by the simultaneous liberation from the sea of an enormous part of the land that forms the Netherlands today.[64] Mercantile success, Calvinism, and the triumph in claiming land from the sea shaped the Dutch as powerfully as the conquest of the Western frontier shaped the American experience.

If the seventeenth century shaped Dutch character, so too did dealing with the decline that followed it. In the first half of the eighteenth century, England and France were able to use their military power to end the pre-eminent position of the Dutch as world traders. To this period social historians attribute the origin of what are described as the Dutch middle-class vices—being unromantic, unemotional, unimaginative, and stubborn.[65]

What is seen as unimaginativeness and insensitivity is perhaps reflected in a concreteness illustrated by the way so many Dutch doctors did not hear the ambivalence expressed in patients' requests for euthanasia. Such deficiencies concerned a Dutch colleague who supported euthanasia. She told me a story about her mother, who had dementia and was in a nursing home. Her mother told her not to throw away some violets in her room because you "don't throw away living things." She feared that the doctors in the home would not understand her mother's expression of a desire to live even with diminished capacities.

From a different perspective, Derek Phillips, who although American born has lived and worked as a sociologist in the Netherlands for thirty years, shares Huizinga's concern about Dutch moral and social attitudes. He sees the Dutch as relatively uninterested in moral philosophy and as lacking in moral passion. The Dutch, he points out, tend to equate morality with religion, and most see themselves as nonreligious. He considers the single most important social fact regarding morality in the Netherlands to be that "indifference masquerades as tolerance."[66]

His observations resonated with one personal aspect of my own experience in the Netherlands. I was troubled, as were other foreign observers, by what we regarded as Dutch indifference to their system's failure to protect patients and their physicians' failure to follow their own euthanasia guidelines.[67] I found that while some physicians supportive of euthanasia were willing to admit abuses in general, and even to concede that in a particular case euthanasia should not have been performed or that a wrongful death had taken place, they did not express anger or indignation that a life had been taken unnecessarily. The common attitude was that the doctor may have been mistaken but was entitled to his or her judgment of the matter. This casualness, often rationalized by the Dutch as tolerance, appears to a foreign observer to border on a callousness that seems consistent with Huizinga's and Phillips's observations about the Dutch lack of moral passion and unwillingness to assign individual responsibility. Huizinga notes that "tolerance is a virtue that can become a vice. Respect for the rights of others too often leads to respect for their wrongs."[68] In an even stronger sentence that could become an epigram for euthanasia in the Netherlands, he states, "the belief that what is evil becomes good if only enough people want it is one of the most terrifying aberrations of the age."[69]

The Dutch government, acknowledging the country's deficiencies in palliative care, has taken steps to improve the care of dying patients. As part of a five-year program begun in 1996, the Dutch Health Research and Development Council designated six medical institutions as centers for palliative care and provided aid that made possible an increase in the number of palliative care units in nursing homes from three to thirty.[70] (A palliative care unit in these nursing homes usually consists of three to four beds set aside for this purpose.) The nursing home palliative care units are not staffed by palliative care specialists, but the physicians who do staff them are being trained in palliative care.[71]

Probably the greatest hope for change lies in the grassroots efforts of a small number of palliative care physicians to educate Dutch physicians in the care of terminally ill patients and in the response of the physicians to these efforts. Ten times a year since 1994 three palliative care physicians, including Zylicz, have conducted a one-day course in palliative care for twenty physicians. The course is booked a year in advance. The palliative care specialists make an additional effort to reach nursing home physicians by holding yearly a three-day basic course for fifty of them and an advanced course that can accommodate thirty-five.[72]

Similar local initiatives have been responsible for an increase in the number of hospices in the country from six to ten. In the traditional middle-class virtues of industriousness, initiative, and a desire for improvement expressed by these Dutch doctors lies the best opportunity to improve the care given to dying patients. Although the Dutch experience suggests that engaging physicians in palliative care is much harder when the easier option of euthanasia is available, for a significant number such training has become a welcome option. If education of Dutch doctors by their palliative care instructors is successful, a reduction in the number of cases of assisted suicide and euthanasia will be one measure of that success.

6

Palliative Care and Euthanasia in the Netherlands:
Observations of a Dutch Physician

Zbigniew Zylicz, M.D.

The Netherlands is one of the most secular European countries and one of the wealthiest, most modern, and best-structured Western democracies. The health care system is well developed, and per capita spending on health care is among the highest in Europe. During the past two decades, euthanasia and assisted suicide have become increasingly accepted. The Dutch believe that by regulation the door to legally sanctioned euthanasia and assisted suicide can be opened slightly, that the law can control entry, and that doing so will prevent or diminish illegal, uncontrolled euthanasia. Although originally based on compassion for suffering patients, the current justification for euthanasia and assisted suicide (the latter is relatively infrequent in the Netherlands) is increasingly the right of self-determination.[1]

The Dutch population, which comprises 15.7 million people (1999), is aging. Over the next twenty years, the number of people aged 65 or older will increase by 48 percent, while the number of people most able to care for those who need it (i.e., those aged 20–64) will increase by only 3 percent.[2] We are facing the daunting prospect of future generations of doctors and nurses who will need to care for large numbers of elderly and frail patients while there will probably be fewer financial resources available to them to do this. Right now there are not enough people to provide such care, even though we still can afford it. So there will be increasing pressure on those who are sick and frail, chronically ill, or dying to consume less care and fewer societal resources. It is thus improbable that the problem of euthanasia will decrease.

There are over 135,000 deaths in the Netherlands each year. Thirty per-cent of these cases involve end-of-life decisions that may hasten death, ranging from patient refusal of invasive or painful treatments to eutha-nasia. Of these more than 6,300 (4.7% of all deaths) are caused by active intervention by physicians: euthanasia (2.2%), assisted suicide (0.4%), ending life without a patient's explicit request (0.7%), and symptom treatment with the explicit intention of ending a patient's life (1.4%).[3] (See chapter 5 and table 1 [p. 102] for fuller treatment of this subject.)

General Practice and Nursing Homes in the Netherlands

General practitioners in the Netherlands are well trained in most aspects of family medicine. More than half of their time is spent visiting disabled or chronically or terminally ill patients and tending at home to sick chil-dren with infectious diseases. But these physicians are generalists with only a superficial knowledge of palliative medicine. Their formal train-ing and education in this field lasted no more than several hours. The average practice in the Netherlands has a patient list of around 2,100.[4] This means that the practice will see approximately ten new cases of can-cer annually. Half of these patients will be cured, and half will die. Two patients will die in a hospital or nursing home, out of the sight of the gen-eral practitioner, and only three at home. Among them, according to our observation, only one patient every two years will have complex prob-lems and need the support of a multidisciplinary palliative care team. Until now, this type of support was provided by either acute hospitals or nursing homes.

Nursing homes in the Netherlands (370 beds per 100,000) are com-parable to sophisticated geriatric hospitals, being fully staffed with well-trained nursing home physicians and providing round-the-clock specialized nursing care. They are able to provide complex care, includ-ing psychogeriatrics, for chronically ill patients for long periods of time.

In general, a given nursing home bed will have a turnover of no more than one patient per year. So the nursing home physicians will see only a limited number of terminally ill cancer patients in their facilities. It is understandable, therefore, that many nursing home physicians as well as many general practitioners feel that they lack sufficient expertise to manage these patients alone, although it took decades for them to begin to admit this. The majority of patients with end-stage cancer, however, want to be cared for at home by the general practitioner rather than

general practitioner will continue to care for the rest of the family. Mistakes and near-mistakes may have an impact on decades of care afterward.

Therefore, my role is to help the general practitioner, as discreetly as possible, while ensuring that I do not jeopardize the patient-doctor relationship. My advice can be taken or ignored by the physician, and there is little I can do about this. I must also be prepared for situations in which even the best advice will not alleviate all suffering and sedation may be indicated or the patient may choose euthanasia.

An eighty-year-old woman was diagnosed with disseminated breast cancer. She had become increasingly blind over the preceding fifteen years and had used a hearing aid for the past ten years. After having a mastectomy, she refused treatment with chemotherapy and radiotherapy. She moved in with one of her three daughters, who worked in a small business with her husband. The patient had increasing pain in her back, and her mobility rapidly declined to the extent that she was not able to move her legs. She lay in bed in one supine position and developed sacral bedsores. Her general practitioner treated her with increasing doses of oral morphine, but despite this the pain worsened. The clinical picture was further complicated by symptoms of severe constipation. The patient repeatedly requested euthanasia, but her general practitioner refused on principle. Instead, he asked me for a bedside consultation.

The patient was very happy to see me and felt that I was her and her daughter's only hope. Clinically, there was clear spinal cord compression due to vertebral metastases, and she was prescribed high doses of steroids and an analgesic for nerve injury. She improved within twenty-four hours and was pain free on rest, although not on movement. She was able to change her position, and I expected her to improve further.

Initially, she was happy that her pain had decreased but soon she began to feel that life in bed, paralyzed, had no meaning. She asked her general physician again for euthanasia. Her general practitioner, an older physician, asked a younger female colleague to take over the case in keeping with existing rules for physicians who refuse to perform euthanasia. The young colleague came and asked both the general practitioner and me not to visit again. She did not want to be one of two captains on the ship. I withdrew completely, but for my colleague it was more difficult because he came regularly to see the patient's daughter, who remained his patient.

One month after her mother's death, the daughter and her husband came to see me in the hospice. They asked where I had been while their mother was dying. The subcutaneous morphine pump initiated by me had been discontinued. The patient had developed severe pain once again, and other drugs were given without much confidence or effect. The daughter and husband had hoped that I would come back to treat her. It took three days to organize euthanasia, and the official reason stated for it was "intractable pain." Those of us who had previously been involved with this lady's care, however, knew that the pain was readily treatable and that the drugs we had prescribed should not have been discontinued.

In cases such as this, a palliative care consultant plays a very different role from that of the consultant who is asked to verify that the criteria for euthanasia have been met. The distinction can cause confusion for the family and even for the physician.

Different Types of Patients Requesting Euthanasia

Many patients discuss with us their wish to die more quickly. Most of them are terminally ill and undoubtedly suffering, whether from physical symptoms, psychological distress, or both. My colleagues working outside of the hospice setting would be likely to grant some of their requests without hesitation. Based on our first two hundred patients, we were able to identify specific groups of patients among those who discussed euthanasia with us. Since then, our experience with this model has increased considerably, and many discussions with colleagues in the Netherlands and abroad have made it more mature and complete.

Group A: Afraid

The largest percentage of patients (in our data, approximately 80%) belongs to group A, which stands for "afraid." These people ask for euthanasia because they do not feel safe. They are afraid of something, such as losing their dignity, being abandoned, being in pain, and being in need when their physicians are on holiday. There are thousands of things patients can be afraid of when they are so vulnerable, and things that can seem simple to those who are healthy may appear very complicated to patients who are sick. The reasons for being afraid may be realistic, but equally and not infrequently, they may be very unrealistic. Memories of good and bad things the patients have experienced in the past may play an important role. Here are two examples.

An eighty-six-year-old widow with breast cancer asked to be given a lethal injection. On closer questioning, she revealed that five years previously she had seen an American horror film in which someone had been buried alive. Since then she had been terrified that this would happen to her. When I suggested to her that I would check her for signs of life three times over an eight-hour period after her death, she was reassured. When she died several days later, I kept my promise and her body remained on the ward for eight hours.

An eighty-year-old woman came to see me in the hospice. She was still quite well, but she had recently been diagnosed with colon cancer. She was aware that her condition was expected to deteriorate soon and wanted to arrange everything in advance. She gave me a copy of her will and said, "Please read it first. Maybe you will not want to examine me after reading it." She wanted, in case of extreme suffering, to undergo euthanasia.

She was a very open and sincere lady, and after talking for a while she told me that her father had died of the same disease thirty years earlier. He had suffered terrible pain before he died. She and her sister had begged the physician to give her father morphine to control his pain, but the physician had refused because he felt it might cause premature death. Her father died not because of morphine, but because of the horrible suffering that broke not only him but also his two daughters. She was terrified that when she became terminally ill and developed pain, someone would withhold morphine for similar reasons.

She was admitted to our hospice a week or two later, with total bowel obstruction. We treated her according to our bowel obstruction protocol, and she responded well. She received enough morphine, was not in pain, and was happy with our care. She seemed able to tolerate whatever discomfort she had. She lived another five weeks, but before she died I asked her how she now felt about euthanasia. She said she was not afraid any more. She was with us.

In this group of patients it is important to know how their fear has evolved. This may involve asking about things that have happened in the past and also how they cope with their disease and with pain. Good information, good patient care, knowledge, and continuity will give the patient the feeling of safety and security. The preventability of euthanasia in this group is very high, nearly 100 percent.

Experiences from the past can be a powerful factor in decisions at the end of life. Good experiences with the death of loved ones may decrease anxiety; memories of bad experiences may add to the suffering of those who are dying. And caring for dying patients should always be understood as also caring for the family, who will need to cope with the loss and will carry memories of the experience with them. Providing a good experience may decrease the anxiety they experience when confronting their own death.

Group B: Burnout

This second group of patients is much less numerous, representing only 5 percent of all the patients that we see in the hospice who request euthanasia. This group B ("burnout") consists of patients who suffer a long-standing terminal disease, especially when the disease progression is very slow or absent. Often the term *burnout* applies not only to the patients but also to all those around them.

Janet was a fifty-five-year-old divorced woman with one daughter who was taking care of her. Janet, who had a long history of smoking, developed bronchial cancer. The tumor was diagnosed when she presented with symptoms of cerebral metastases, and she went on to have whole-brain radiotherapy. Following this she was very ill for a period of several weeks, despite having received steroid medication to ease the symptoms of brain edema. The steroids resulted in significant weight gain and muscle weakness. The bronchial tumor did not show any progression, and she had no pain or difficulty breathing. When she came to the hospice, we invested considerable effort into helping her become mobile again, and for three to four weeks Janet remained reasonably well and was able to visit her home and her friends outside the hospice.

The muscular weakness began to increase, so we started to decrease the steroid dose. As this was done her appetite also decreased and she became more and more fatigued. The symptoms of increased intracranial pressure did not return, allowing us to discontinue the steroids completely. This was done with her and her daughter's agreement. She became bed-bound, moving out of bed only to sit at the commode. She became irritable with us and with her daughter and two sisters. She stopped eating and drank only minimal fluids. She experienced recurrent painful mouth and vaginal infections as well as a painful mandibular abscess. On December 31 she asked us to hasten her death. She did not want to go on, and she found little sense in all of our activities and efforts to look after her. Her family supported her fully in her request.

She was imminently dying and in distress with new and progressive abdominal pain. She and her family agreed with our suggestion to provide sedation for symptom control. She slept through the night without pain or nightmares and when she awoke the next morning she asked to remain sedated. She was placed on a continuous infusion of morphine, a pain reliever, and sedating drugs. She died peacefully in her sleep twenty-four hours later.

These patients often have stable disease, with no symptoms to justify aggressive symptomatic treatment. Also, surprisingly, they do not show the typical symptoms of psychological depression, although some psychiatrists consider burnout to be a clinical form of depression. Their suffering is not time limited, and as a result, both the patients and the caregivers are gradually worn down and develop a syndrome of emotional exhaustion that includes a sense of depersonalization toward one's surroundings and a reduced sense of personal accomplishment.[9] Burnout may be seen in survivors of cancer treatment, and it may increase with time.[10] It is to a lesser extent seen as a disease distinct from depression. While in depression the patient feels hopeless, others in the patient's environment may still see realistic possibilities for change and treatment. For the patient with burnout there are no other possibilities or treatment options.

Treatment of burnout may be very difficult, and prevention is by far the preferable option. Many cases of burnout among patients are at least theoretically preventable by timely discontinuation of treatment. However, the same societal force that pushes patients and their doctors in the direction of euthanasia as a solution also does not allow patients or their doctors to discontinue ineffective oncological treatment earlier in the disease course. We are all very familiar with "last resort" treatments in oncology in which patients have to face two stark possible outcomes: to die due to the toxicity of the treatment, or to recover. Even those who do recover may be deeply damaged, physically and mentally unable to carry on with their lives as they were accustomed to before treatment.

Fortunately, the burnout group is numerically relatively small. Continuing psychological care of such patients who request euthanasia is very important. Issues of staff self-support, team building, and communication within the team become paramount. Some of these patients may die peacefully due to progressive disease, yet their existential distress is disproportional to their physical symptoms.[11] Anxiety-relieving medication and sedation may need to be prescribed to manage the anxiety and distress caused by their increasing isolation, but such treatment is intended not to shorten their lives but to control their symptoms.

Group C: Control Oriented

Group C patients are control oriented. This group is small (approximately 1% of our patients) but significant. However, I am convinced that my general practitioner colleagues encounter many more group C patients in their practices than we do. These patients have an intrinsic drive to control all processes, including their death, and are frequently depicted as young, independent managers, with a mobile telephone ringing in their pocket while they lie in the operating room. This stereotyped view is incorrect, as old and frail patients can be equally control oriented.

Tom was seventy-four when he was diagnosed with disseminated thyroid cancer. He had been a well-known artist, and his works were displayed in many museums and galleries. Although I had never heard of him previously, I could imagine how important painting was to him. He came to our hospice in the early stages of his disease, having come for a look around on a previous occasion. He liked the light and the trees and made his decision at that point to come to the hospice. As he had a tracheotomy tube, we were afraid that, in time, he would choke, and our major concern was to protect him from this kind of death.

All of his belongings were moved to the hospice, and Tom enjoyed spending all of his time on his painting. He was very precise in his demands, making clear just when and from whom he needed help. A delay of more than one minute was not tolerated. Despite his demanding nature, we succeeded in caring for him and he felt himself to be safe in the hospice. He could work on his paintings, and his wife, desperate at the time of admission, was able to regain her peace of mind.

Tom created more than fifty paintings while in the hospice, but with time he became very weak. He lost a lot of weight, and his hands would shake while holding a brush. Thanks to good nursing care of his tracheotomy, he did not develop life-threatening complications. One day a good friend, also an artist, visited him. He looked at Tom's works, hanging everywhere in his room. He liked some but found the latest works of inferior quality and made a comment about this. Tom was devastated by it and, after his friend left, he sat at his desk and started to write letters. Knowing our attitude toward euthanasia, he wrote a letter to his internist, who had once promised to "help" him when he needed it. The internist from the local hospital came to the hospice and had a long talk with him culminating in admission to the hospital and euthanasia. His wife came to say goodbye to us, and as a present brought

Karin did not want to see the hospice physician, afraid that the physician would try to talk her out of wanting euthanasia. But she realized that without such a consultation her physician would not cooperate with her. She was seen alone at the hospice, and she told us her full story and all her fears. After interviewing her, we realized that Karin was experiencing a marked depression. Although her physical condition made it likely that she would not live much longer, it seemed possible that she could find satisfaction in the time remaining to her if we could successfully treat her depression. We shared this with her and proposed treatment with antidepressant medication and psychotherapy.

At first Karin refused the diagnosis and refused the treatment. Later, after talking with John and her general practitioner, she changed her mind. We asked our bereavement counselor to start therapy with her and with her husband. Karin tolerated antidepressant medication without problems. Ten days later she started to feel better. Her relationship with John improved dramatically. They would talk with each other for hours. Karin's sleep improved, as well as her tolerance for minor discomforts. On her own initiative, she went to see her general practitioner to tell him that if necessary she would like to be admitted to our hospice rather than to seek euthanasia. She had thought that her husband probably would not be able to cope with her death through euthanasia. She admitted that she wanted to punish him for his treatment of her when she became ill, but felt all this was past now.

She came to the hospice four weeks later with much pain due to her enlarged liver, fluid in her abdomen, and massive swelling of her legs. After the abdominal fluid was drained, she became hypotensive and then comatose and died peacefully three days later. John remained at her bedside the entire time. He was grateful for the process that had given him back his wife before she died.

In the past, the possibilities for treating depression in patients with terminal illness were very limited. The doses of tricyclic antidepressants needed for therapeutic effect often cause significant side effects that are poorly tolerated by this patient population, and the time needed for the antidepressant effect to begin was frequently longer than the patient's prognosis.

Psychotherapy alone was tried but was seldom successful. Therefore, an attitude developed not to bother too much with early diagnosis, because there was nothing to be done. Depression became a part of the problem of dying, a natural part that could be explained by disease progression and the associated losses experienced by these patients. It was seen more as grief than as depression. The use of newer antidepressants with fewer side effects made treatment of depression easier. In my opinion, there is now an urgent need to diagnose and treat depression early, to try to avoid having critical situations occur in the very final stages of disease. Depressed and desperate patients, who may not accept antidepressant treatments, are often encountered on the palliative care ward or in the hospice. However, with early diagnosis of depression, preventability of euthanasia in this group may be high.

Group E: Extreme

The last group of patients requesting euthanasia is group E, for "extreme." Unlike the patients in groups A, B, C, and D, who are classified on the basis of their psychological response to terminal illness, this group's members are distinguished by the severity of their symptoms and their limited responsiveness to palliative treatment. Fortunately, they are a small minority, no more than 3 percent to 4 percent of all patients treated in our hospice. These patients either have not responded to treatment or have refused treatment due to past disappointments and failures. They develop extreme symptoms, such as pain, nausea, itching, and difficulty breathing. One such patient suffered severely due to dry mouth following irradiation of metastases in his jaw.

In these situations, people working in palliative care are very creative in finding solutions, and I believe this is the way to achieve progress. However, each of us is familiar with cases in which such creativity gives only limited results. Sometimes there are further methods of treatment but the patient refuses to participate. In extreme situations, extreme measures should be possible. For patients with excruciating pain who do not respond to large doses of opioids combined with other drugs, the next step of pain treatment may be sedation.

John was forty-eight years old. He had a history of a tumor that had been growing in his right buttock since his thirteenth birthday. Initially it was a benign tumor, and it had been excised many times. However, in the last two years the tumor growth had become malignant and was classified as soft tissue sarcoma. Although there were no metastases and the tumor still was growing slowly, the response to chemotherapy and radiotherapy was very poor, and John eventually refused further therapy.

He told us that as a young man, between the ages of seventeen and twenty-five, he had been addicted to heroin. After successful treatment, he got married and then divorced before moving across the border to Germany to start a flower shop. Now in the face of the malignant disease he had come back to Holland to seek support, first in a hostel for homeless people and later in our hospice.

John experienced excruciating pain in his back, and we started to treat him with opioids, which had only a minimal effect. Local measures were more successful for some time. Despite the escalating doses of many drugs, the pain continued to increase. I looked through all the journals for information about pain treatment in former addicts and could find little to help. John became irritable and unpleasant and could be managed by only one nurse, who had developed a close bond with him. Unfortunately, the nurse left our hospice at the end of the summer and John's pain increased significantly. Sometimes he was without pain and was able to enjoy a glass of wine. Five minutes later he could be in agony, unable to sit in a chair or lie in bed. His pain was bearable only when he was walking but, being weak from his progressive disease, he could not walk for long.

The periods without pain became shorter and shorter, and John was desperate for relief from this misery. Increasing the opioid dose was of little use, as he showed no response to it. Sedating him also seemed impossible, as he did not respond to any of the usual medications. After trying various medications, we felt forced by his extreme pain to agree to put him to sleep with barbiturates. A modest dose of barbiturates was infused intravenously. Before John fell asleep, he told us the pain was gone. He felt himself dying and asked the nurse to polish his shoes so that he would look nice in the coffin. He fell asleep and died two days later.

In this kind of case, the treatment may be criticized. There will always be something that someone could have done better. Using extreme measures like sedation for intractable distress in dying patients in group E can be defended more easily than it can in the case of existential suffering in the burnout group. Existential suffering, which is not physically visible, is always controversial. Sedation at the end of life as an ultimate pain-controlling strategy for members of group E may fully replace the necessity of euthanasia.[13]

What is the benefit of classifying the groups of patients who request euthanasia? I think a better understanding of patients' motives may guide effective prevention and treatment, if you consider a request for euthanasia to be a serious condition that needs to be responded to and treated. If you consider euthanasia a normal occurrence, the result of the patient's autonomous choice, you might not need to do anything.

This classification is flexible. There may be overlap among the groups, and one group may evolve into another. It also seems probable that without treatment patients in groups A, C, D, and E might all evolve into the burnout group, B.

Hospice Rozenheuvel and Euthanasia

Many people in the Netherlands ask why we do not perform euthanasia in our hospice. Do religious beliefs drive us against the stream of Dutch societal developments? Talking about euthanasia with our hospice's patients is a common occurrence. Approximately 25 percent of our patients discuss euthanasia with us, and the majority of these patients do not consider themselves to be religious or to belong to any church. So imposing religious values on these people would be inappropriate.

In addition to the 25 percent of patients who talk with us about euthanasia, we believe that an equally large population are afraid that what we do to them to control their pain will shorten their lives. Many people decrease the dose of their opioids or even discontinue them after being discharged home, and it may be that they do this because they are afraid such treatments will shorten their lives. Because of this, we need to be very clear with our patients about the intentions behind our palliative treatments. The nurse walking through the corridor with a syringe and a needle must never be associated with a patient's instant death or eventual hastened death.

The question that became more important to us was not whether we would or would not participate in euthanasia, but whether we would be able to prevent situations that might lead to euthanasia. This question, in contrast to whether we would participate in euthanasia, can bring people together—those who are in favor of as well those who oppose euthanasia. I believe both groups are united in feeling that euthanasia is an extreme and potentially damaging act. Making it unnecessary should be a common purpose for us all, and if we can make euthanasia unnecessary, that is a pragmatic reason for opposing it. In any case, simply saying "no" to the patient who requests euthanasia is not a good enough response.

An internist from a small Protestant hospital asked me by telephone if I would be able to take over the care of one of his patients. He clarified first that we do not perform euthanasia in the hospice, saying that the patient and her family had been pressing the doctors in the hospital to provide euthanasia, as they did not see the point of her suffering any longer. I agreed to take over caring for the patient and reassured him that we do not perform euthanasia in our hospice.

The next day the patient was brought by ambulance. She was about seventy years old and had cerebral metastases from bronchial cancer. Her brain had been irradiated, and since that time the patient had been confused, anorexic, and dehydrated. She received fluids and nutrition through a tube, which she was vigorously trying to remove, and to prevent this her hands had been tied tightly to the bedsides. On examination, I found fecoliths (fecal stones) in the rectum indicative of chronic and longstanding constipation. Some of them had caused deep ulceration in the rectal mucous membrane, which started to bleed when the stones were removed under sedation. The family said that she had not defecated for as long as four weeks, but because she was dying, nobody considered it necessary to take care of her bowels.

This lack of care forced the family to request euthanasia. Within twenty-four hours, most of the patient's symptoms were being controlled. Her delirium resolved and she was able to say goodbye to her children before she died peacefully without pain.

My initial reaction to this case was astonishment. Had I been that patient, I would have requested euthanasia! Simply denying such a request is not an acceptable response. One has to propose and initiate a way of achieving better care. Saying "no" must not carry a message and implication of abandonment.

The Social Price of Euthanasia

The acceptance of euthanasia has arisen in a modern Dutch society that demands a solution to difficult problems in caring for those who are terminally ill. However, this society needs to be aware that euthanasia seems to have unintended but significant social costs.

What kind of costs are we talking about? Accepting euthanasia or assisted suicide as a normal medical practice for some cases of unacceptable suffering assumes that the process will be controllable. To realistically ensure this, one needs a whole system of rules and laws detailing exactly which cases will be eligible for euthanasia and which will not. Regulation has proved to be difficult if not impossible and is fraught with danger. It also serves to stifle creativity in palliative care and even to make proper care impossible to achieve.

A colleague told me about the following case, which happened in a general hospital several years ago. A fifty-eight-year-old woman was diagnosed with disseminated small cell lung cancer. This is not a curable disease, but treatment can result in a considerable remission. The woman demanded that euthanasia be carried out when she reached a stage where she was suffering and unable to ask for it herself. Her husband fully supported her wish. After a four-month period in which she was free from symptoms, she was admitted to the hospital because she was coughing up blood and had increasing difficulty breathing. She was very distressed and decided with her husband that this was the time to think about euthanasia. The physician in charge suggested trying the second-line chemotherapy treatment, but when the patient refused this he started the euthanasia procedure by asking his colleague to see the patient. At this stage, however, he refused to treat her with subcutaneous morphine because he felt he had not yet fulfilled all the criteria to sanction euthanasia. The woman died before this was done, and in the hours before her death she was in great distress, choked with bloody sputum and terrified.

In this case, acceptance of euthanasia paradoxically blocked what would be considered a basic part of palliative care. In our hospice, we would have no hesitation in starting a subcutaneous morphine infusion at a dose thought appropriate to control the patient's breathlessness. We might also have added a low dose of a drug to relieve anxiety. If necessary, in an acute situation of severe distress, we would also not hesitate to inject higher doses of anxiety-reducing medication intravenously with the aim of sedating the patient to relieve her distress if that was what she wished. In this case, once the decision for euthanasia had been made, the physician's preoccupation with the procedures required to implement it took precedence over his responsibility to care for his patient and to reduce her suffering.

The best way to improve the ability of general practitioners to provide palliative care is to teach them at the bedside of their patients. It is a very effective process, and the teachers are the patients. So besides the time I spend with the patients, talking to and examining them, I need to spend time talking and explaining things to the general practitioner. Afterward I also write a letter to the general practitioner summarizing the consult. The teaching process makes the consultations important. And the teaching process is in danger when euthanasia is considered the ultimate solution to all problems in palliative care.

A general practitioner requested my assistance for a very sick patient with metastasized rectal cancer. The patient refused surgery and had been discharged home. One week later, he developed nausea and began to vomit fecal fluid. The general practitioner attended very quickly and proposed readmission to the hospital, but the patient refused, thinking that he might be pressed to consider an operation. The general practitioner, not knowing what to do next, proposed a good death, meaning euthanasia. The patient, however, was a practicing Roman Catholic and refused this offer. The general practitioner phoned me for advice, saying, "Usually I solve this kind of problem with euthanasia, but this patient seems not to be pleased by this."

I gave the physician our protocol for the relief of bowel obstruction, and he was pleased to be able to ease his patient's distress.

The physician's remark that he usually solves such problems with euthanasia is disturbing. It illustrates how euthanasia becomes a substitute for learning how to relieve the suffering of dying patients. Ordinarily physicians learn more from their patients than from books. By endangering this process, euthanasia has consequences not only for a particular patient, but also for the quality of care in general.

Conclusion

Modern medicine has crossed the invisible border of the command to *do no harm*. We have a chance to cure only by increasing the risk of harm. Patients who respond positively to treatment continue to be treated, while those who do not respond or are damaged by the treatment are often neglected. We have a duty, however, to those who cannot be treated anymore, who do not respond to the treatment, or who are damaged by it—a duty of care like that of a mother who cares, who comforts, who suffers with her child.

Many physicians who choose general practice or nursing home medicine in the Netherlands begin as idealists who believe in the possibilities of care. They believe that there are always ways, if not to cure, then at least to comfort and to care. Modern medicine often makes this impossible for young physicians. They do not have enough opportunity to develop caring attitudes. The caseload in general practice and in nursing home medicine is very high. Instead of the anticipatory, proactive, and preventive medicine that is the key to palliative care, they are forced to react to critical situations that could have been avoided. This means that at the end of the day knowledge that should be available is not and problems that are soluble appear not to be so. If you add to this patients' freedom of choice and the easy option of euthanasia, the choice is often quick and inevitable.

Some people think caring for those who are terminally ill is too heavy and impossible a burden, that it must be horrible to deal with only dying people, never to have the satisfaction of saving someone's life, never to have a grateful patient whom you meet unexpectedly in the shopping mall. However, this is true only when you do not accept death and dying as a normal life event, when you try to deny death in all its aspects. When you accept it, however, you realize that it can be challenging and rewarding to work with dying patients. You discover that it is an extraordinary experience. You grow in this experience while improving your skills. This experience matures you and changes your attitudes toward life. Physicians who perform euthanasia also report being transformed by the experience, but I believe this is a very different sort of transformation.

In the past decade, palliative medicine has developed rapidly in many, mostly English-speaking, countries. Much knowledge has been accumulated worldwide, and the number of scientific journals that deal with pain and symptom management as well as the psychological and spiritual problems of the dying person has increased rapidly. In the Netherlands the benefits of this knowledge are not available. Palliative medicine in the Netherlands is too scattered through all medical and nursing specialties for this improvement to happen. In addition, we need new tools for teaching communication skills, wider dissemination of what we do know about effective treatments, and more research.

Experience gained during consultations done at the request of general practitioners is helpful in understanding the people who request euthanasia as well as the physicians who are willing to perform euthanasia. Instead of judging these physicians and trying to qualify what is "right" or "wrong," we need to depolarize the discussion of euthanasia and move forward. We should concentrate on providing good care and preventing the disappointments and the neglect that terminally ill patients often experience. We will not eliminate euthanasia in the Netherlands, but we can go a long way toward making it not seem necessary by providing better care.

7

The Oregon Experiment

Kathleen Foley, M.D., and Herbert Hendin, M.D.

By a narrow margin in 1994, Oregon voters passed a referendum legalizing physician-assisted suicide. Following a series of legal challenges and a second referendum with a wider margin of approval, the Oregon Death with Dignity Act was eventually implemented.[1] As of November 1997, Oregon became the only state to legalize physician-assisted suicide.* The law permits physicians to prescribe lethal medications to terminally ill patients and differs from that of the Netherlands, where euthanasia and physician-assisted suicide are both sanctioned. Intolerable suffering that cannot be relieved is a basic requirement for assisted suicide and euthanasia in the Netherlands; it is not in Oregon. Simply having a diagnosis of terminal illness with a prognosis of less than six months to live is considered a sufficient criterion. The patient's diagnosis and prognosis of death within six months must be confirmed by a consultant physician.

It was hoped that Oregon would serve as a "laboratory of the states" showing us how assisted suicide would work. This has not occurred, in part because the law was not written with such an aim in mind and stipulates that the information collected by the state will not be open to public scrutiny.[2] Even more troublesome has been the restrictive manner in which the Oregon Health Division (OHD), charged with monitoring the law, has interpreted its mandate. OHD limits its yearly reports to general epidemiological data and collects limited information from physi-

---

*If upheld by the courts, a recent directive by U.S. Attorney General John Ashcroft interpreting federal law to prohibit the use of drugs to assist suicide will override the Oregon law (see Conclusion).

cians who have prescribed lethal medication. Physicians who declined to prescribe the lethal medication, as well as nurses and social workers who cared for the patients, are not interviewed. The second-year report, but not the first or the third, provided some retrospective survey data from a few families. Not all the information collected is made public, and OHD defends its limited data collection and censorship of released information as necessary to protect doctors' and patients' confidentiality. There is no provision for an independent evaluator or researcher to study whatever data are available. This OHD process has prevented a full and open discussion.

Since the passage of the law, various information sources have provided more detailed patient and physician perspectives that suggest a more complex and controversial picture of the Oregon experiment. Compassion in Dying, the major advocacy group for physician-assisted suicide, revealed in 1999 that eleven of the fifteen patients reported as having been assisted in suicide in the first year of the law's operation had come through that organization. Using press releases, a Web site, and public and professional lectures, information on individual patients was made public. Concurrently, Oregon journalists wrote a series of articles based on interviews with the families and physicians of patients who had been assisted in suicide. Three physicians published their personal narratives of experience with patients whom they had assisted in suicide, defending their role in this procedure. Several surveys that captured the experiences of physicians, patients, and families in end-of-life care provided contrasting data to the OHD reports. Physicians who for whatever reason did not comply with patient requests for assisted suicide remained silent, with no forum in which to express their opinions.

Under the Oregon law, when a terminally ill patient makes a request for assisted suicide, physicians are required to point out that palliative care and hospice care are feasible alternatives. They are not required, however, to be knowledgeable about how to relieve either physical or emotional suffering in terminally ill patients. There is no requirement in Oregon for courses in pain management, palliative care, or the evaluation of a suicidal patient for physicians wishing to practice assisted suicide or a certifying exam for physicians who believe they are already qualified. Without such knowledge, the physician cannot present feasible alternatives. It would seem necessary to require a physician lacking such training to refer any patient requesting assisted suicide for consultation with a physician knowledgeable about palliative care. That is not required, however, by the Oregon law.

Under these conditions, offering a patient palliative care becomes a legal regulation to be met, rather than an integral part of an effort to relieve the patient's suffering so that a hastened death does not seem like the only alternative. How this happens is suggested by one of the few Oregon cases about which details have become publicly known. The case was publicized by Compassion in Dying, which featured it as the first case of physician-assisted suicide under the Oregon law.

The First Case

What we initially learned of the case came from newspaper reports of information provided by the staff of Compassion in Dying. Subsequent information came from interviews given anonymously to selected members of the media by the physician who prescribed the medication. On the day after the patient's death, Compassion in Dying held a news conference in which the patient (referred to by her physician as Helen) was described as being in her mid-eighties, having metastatic breast cancer, and being in a hospice program. The conference featured excerpts from an edited audiotape in which Helen said of her impending death, "I'm looking forward to it. . . . I will be relieved of all the stress I have."[3] The tape was said to have been made two days before her assisted suicide.

Helen's own physician had not been willing to assist in her suicide for reasons that were not specified. A second physician also refused on the grounds that Helen was depressed. Helen's husband called Compassion in Dying and was referred to a doctor willing to participate.[4]

Peter Goodwin, medical director of Compassion in Dying, said that he had two lengthy telephone conversations with Helen at the time of the referral and also spoke by phone to her son and daughter. He described Helen as "rational, determined and steadfast" and called "questionable" the opinion of the physician (with whom Goodwin also spoke by phone) who described her as having a depression that was affecting her desire to die.[5] Goodwin felt Helen was "frustrated and crying because she felt powerless." He said she had been doing aerobic exercises up until two weeks before she contacted him but told him she could not do them anymore. She was also unable to continue to garden, which had been one of her favorite activities. He stated she was not bedridden, was not in great pain, and still looked after her own house. Goodwin said the "quality of her life was just disappearing," and he thought it prudent to act quickly before Helen lost the capacity to make decisions for herself. He said she was "going downhill rapidly. . . . She could have had a stroke tomorrow and lost her opportunity to die in the way she wanted."

Goodwin referred Helen to a physician who would help her. That physician referred her to a specialist (we are not told what specialty) and a psychiatrist, both of whom determined she met the qualifications for physician-assisted suicide under the Oregon law. Although the psychiatrist had met Helen only once, Goodwin indicated that the visit was lengthy.

In an interview with Oregon Public Radio, the prescribing physician described his participation as an "extremely moving experience for me."[6] He told a reporter from the *Oregonian* that he was struck by Helen's tenacity and determination. "It was like talking to a locomotive. It was like talking to Superman when he's going after a train."[7]

That physician, who had met Helen two and a half weeks before she died, pictured her as having been in greater physical distress than that described by Goodwin, saying that she had battled breast cancer for more than twenty years and that the cancer had spread to her lungs, causing pain and making breathing difficult. He said that the problem for him was not fulfilling his responsibilities under the law but rather finding a pharmacist to work with him. Eventually he did, and he was with Helen and members of her family when she died.[8] The physician followed a protocol that included an antinausea medication that Helen had taken before he arrived. She then took a mixture of barbiturates (9 grams)[9] and syrup followed by a glass of brandy. She is said to have died within thirty minutes.

The promotional quality of the news conference featuring the taped remarks of the patient offended some, including the patient's family members, who had not anticipated that these remarks and the story would be made public so soon after Helen's death. After the announcement of what was thought to be the first legal assisted suicide in Oregon, the Hemlock Society in Oregon reported that since the Oregon law had gone into effect it had helped arrange an even earlier assisted suicide at some unspecified date for another patient with cancer, but at the family's request no details would be available.[10]

The case of Helen was presented by Compassion in Dying as a model of how well the Oregon law works. Yet even with the limited details supplied by Compassion in Dying and the prescribing physician, there were already disturbing questions raised by the case. The physicians who evaluated Helen offered two contradictory sets of opinions about the appropriateness of her decision. As the decision-making process progressed, it provided no mechanism for resolving the disagreement based on medical expertise, such as that which can be provided by an ethics committee that would hear the facts of the case before going forward. Instead, the opinions of the two doctors who did not support the patient's decision—one who had known her for some time and another who considered that she was depressed—were essentially ignored. Helen and a family member contacted Compassion in Dying to find someone who would agree to assist in her suicide. Goodwin concluded from a phone conversation with Helen that she was not depressed and that her decision was appropriate. He referred her to a physician who would be willing to help her. That doctor did agree, and Helen was then referred to a second physician and a psychiatrist, both of whom supported his opinion. As Barbara Coombs Lee, the director of Compassion in Dying, expressed it, "If I get rebuffed by one doctor, I can go to another."[11]

Patients, of course, have the right to obtain second opinions and to seek out physicians who will provide the therapy that the patients choose. In this case, however, the differing opinions should be allowed to be voiced to understand better the complicated factors that are convincing to some physicians and dismissed by others. We wondered if either Helen's physician or the second physician who diagnosed her as depressed was consulted by the physician who eventually assisted in the suicide.

No information is provided to indicate that the physicians recommended by Compassion in Dying were trying to find any feasible alternatives to suicide. In the taped interview with Helen, her physician tells her that it is important she understand that there are other choices she could make that he will list for her, and in three sentences covering hospice support, chemotherapy, and hormonal therapy he does.

> *Doctor:* There is, of course, all sorts of hospice support that is available to you. There is, of course, chemotherapy that is available that may or may not have any effect, not in curing your cancer, but perhaps in lengthening your life to some extent. And there is also available a hormone which you were offered before by the oncologist—tamoxifen—which is not really chemotherapy but would have some possibility of slowing or stopping the course of the diseases for some period of time.
>
> *Patient:* Yes, I don't want to take that.
>
> *Doctor:* All right, OK, that's pretty much what you need to understand.[12]

During the taped remarks, Helen expressed concern about being artificially fed, a concern that suggests greater vulnerability and uncertainty about her course of action than the physician perceives. He does not assure her that this need not happen in any case. He ignores the remark and instead asks a question designed to elicit a response about her desire to die.[13]

The persistence of the request is one of the requirements for assisted suicide in Oregon, and the physician is impressed by Helen's determination to die. The fact that he describes her as like an unstoppable express train in her unwillingness to wait in hastening death even though she is not in great immediate distress should in itself give him pause. Urgency that brooks no questioning in such a matter is often a sign of irrational motives. Proponents of legalizing assisted suicide maintain that knowledge that patients could control when they die would permit them to postpone death. This Oregonian woman had that option, and the physician is troubled by her haste but unable to resist it. Nor does Helen's family seem to raise any questions as to whether anything could be done to cause her to be less eager to end her life. Certainly the reasons given by Goodwin for haste in effectuating her death are not persuasive.

In reply to a journal article we wrote about the case that asked if the physician assisting in Helen's suicide had consulted her original physician in evaluating the case,[14] we received a response from Dr. Peter Reagan, who had now publicly identified himself as the physician who assisted in Helen's suicide. He wrote, "Before my patient died I didn't personally discuss the case with her regular physician and had only a very cursory contact with her second. I regret this. I don't think either of the previous MDs disagreed with her qualification, but at the time I would have clarified it. Had I felt there was a disagreement among the physicians about my patient's eligibility, I would not have written the prescription."[15] It is noteworthy that Reagan used words like *qualification* and *eligibility* to justify his actions rather than discussing the appropriateness of the decision.

Reagan subsequently wrote an article for the British journal *Lancet* about the case.[16] In it he describes Helen as primarily concerned over anticipated suffering. He informs us that she was influenced by having experienced the lingering death of her husband. This is a frequent factor in the history of those who become suicidal in response to terminal illness. Careful exploration of the circumstances of the earlier death may give a physician the opportunity to relieve anxieties that are motivating the patient's desire to hasten death. There is no evidence that such an exploration was done with Helen.

In his *Lancet* article, Reagan states that he liked Helen immediately, so the thought of her dying so soon was "almost too much to bear, and only slightly less difficult was the knowledge that many very reasonable people would consider aiding her death a crime. On the other hand, I found even worse the thought of disappointing this family. If I backed out, they'd feel about me the way they felt about her previous doctor, that I had strung them along, and in a way, insulted them."[17] Should liking Helen and needing not to disappoint her family be such significant factors in the decision to end her life?

Consulting Physician

Although the Oregon law does require that a second physician evaluate the patient to confirm the diagnosis, prognosis, and voluntariness of the choice, no provision is made for the independent selection of this consulting physician. The Dutch experience suggests that such consultants are likely to be colleagues of the first physician and their evaluations are likely to be *pro forma.* The Royal Dutch Medical Association now recommends that such consultants be independently chosen. Unless the selection is truly independent, the consultant, even if not a colleague of the attending physician, is likely to be a known proponent and practitioner of assisted suicide. In the case of Helen, and in the subsequent cases made public, the fact that we do not know who the consultant is, how the consultant was selected, or what was the basis for the consultant's findings adds to concern about the independence of his or her opinion.

Psychiatric Evaluation

Since Oregon is the first state to legalize suicide as a treatment for medical illness, it would seem to have a special responsibility to protect the significant numbers of patients who become suicidally depressed in response to serious or terminal illness. Medical illness is an important factor in 70 percent of all suicides over the age of sixty. We know also that most suicides and most of those who respond to terminal illness with a desire to hasten death are suffering from depression.[18] Although pain and other factors, such as a lack of family support, contribute to the wish for death, depression is the most important factor, and researchers have found it to be the only factor that significantly predicts the wish for death.[19]

Although a psychiatric evaluation is the standard of care for suicidal patients, the Oregon law does not require it in cases of assisted suicide. Under the law, only if the "physician believes that the patient might be suffering from a psychiatric or psychological disorder or from a depression causing impaired judgment" must the physician refer the patient to a licensed psychiatrist or psychologist for counseling. Depression per se is not considered a sufficient reason for such a referral. The caveat of impaired judgment is strange since depression usually causes patients to see problems in black-and-white terms, overlooking solutions and alternative possibilities.[20] Such impairment of judgment is a basic characteristic of the disorder. In any case, studies have shown that physicians are not reliably able to diagnose depression let alone to determine whether the depression is impairing judgment.[21] A study of cancer patients with moderate to severe depression noted that only 13 percent of clinicians identified depression in the patient population.[22]

That Oregon physicians are experiencing problems in identifying depression in patients requesting assisted suicide is suggested by a 1999 anonymous survey of physicians concerning their experiences since the Oregon Death with Dignity Act went into effect.[23] Oregon physicians reported 221 requests for prescriptions of lethal medications and provided information on 143 of these patients, 67 percent of whom had cancer. The physicians identified depression in only 20 percent of the patients, well under the almost 60 percent found in studies where patients who wish to hasten death are evaluated. National surveys consistently demonstrate the underassessment and undertreatment of depression, particularly in elderly patients.[24] The National Comprehensive Cancer Network has published guidelines for assessing distress in cancer patients and provides a specific protocol for evaluating patients who report suicidal thoughts or ideation.[25] How Oregon physicians assess and treat patients who request physician-assisted suicide is not the subject of the OHD evaluation, preventing a clear assessment of whether quality psychological care is being provided to elderly cancer patients in Oregon.

Not all of the factors justifying a psychiatric consultation center around current depression. Most patients who request assisted suicide are doing so not because of current pain and suffering but out of fear of what will happen to them—such as Helen's fear of artificial feeding. Like Helen's, such fears often derive from the patient's past experiences with the death of those close to him or her, so a history of these experiences should be part of any physician's evaluation of requests for assisted suicide. That evaluation must reflect an awareness of risk factors for suicide, such as alcoholism, a past history of depression, and, of course, any prior suicide attempts.

Most suicide attempts also reflect a person's ambivalence about dying, and patients requesting assisted suicide show an equal ambivalence. Physicians inexperienced in dealing with suicidal patients tend to take requests to die literally and concretely, and may act on them while failing to hear this ambivalence.

The psychiatric consultation as envisioned by the Oregon law is not intended to deal with these considerations but with the more limited issue of a patient's capacity to make the decision for assisted suicide. But there are no criteria and no agreed-on standards for identifying the impairment that may make a patient incapable of such a decision.[26] Nor is there any indication in the law that a determination of impaired judgment in a patient requesting assistance in suicide is an indication of a need for treatment—or any suggestion of an obligation to offer and discuss such treatment. The psychiatrist's role of "gatekeeper" under the Oregon law is narrowly conceived, ignoring his or her ability to explore and relieve the anxiety, ambivalence, and depression that underlie most requests for assisted suicide. Indeed, under the Oregon law such exploration is made to seem irrelevant.

Moreover, when Oregon psychiatrists were surveyed, only 6 percent felt very confident that absent a long-term relationship with a patient they could satisfactorily determine in a single visit whether a patient was competent to commit suicide.[27] In a national survey of forensic psychiatrists, 78 percent recommended a very stringent standard for competency requiring two independent examiners, and 44 percent of those psychiatrists surveyed recommended judicial review of a decision. Of note, 58 percent believed that the presence of a major depression should result in the finding of incompetence.[28] Goodwin indicated that while the psychiatrist saw Helen only once, the visit was "lengthy." But a lengthy visit is no substitute for even a second visit with some time interval in between.

Both the survey of Oregon psychiatrists and the national survey of forensic psychiatrists revealed that the majority of those willing to do an evaluation of a patient's competence for assisted suicide favor the practice. If patients were found not to have a mental condition impairing judgment, the majority of Oregon psychiatrists opposed to assisted suicide were likely to work with the patient to prevent the suicide, while those who supported assisted suicide were likely to support the patient in obtaining a lethal prescription. Because the majority of psychiatrists doing such evaluations will be in favor of assisted suicide, the authors of both studies concluded that "a bias may be introduced into the competency evaluation. On balance the psychiatrists' conclusions may reflect personal values and beliefs more than psychiatric expertise."[29] When advocacy groups, such as Compassion in Dying, are shepherding the cases and the referrals, the likelihood of such bias would seem to be even greater.

Reagan evidently did not consider Helen to be depressed or to have impaired judgment, so the psychiatric referral seems to have been made to counter the opinion of one of the original doctors. Since the Oregon law does not require such consultation, one fears that over time an increasingly smaller percentage of patients will be referred for independent psychiatric evaluation. As we have noted, this is exactly what happened in the Netherlands, where psychiatric evaluation is also not required and only 3 percent of cases are now so referred. In fact, the 2000 report for OHD demonstrates a similar pattern for Oregon, where psychiatric consultations dropped from 31 percent in 1998 to 19 percent.

An Informed Decision

Without a proper psychiatric evaluation, it is not possible even to ascertain if a patient has impaired judgment that would make him or her not "capable" of an "informed decision" as required by Oregon law. Without such a consultation there is less likely to be an attempt made to understand and relieve the desperation, anxiety, and depression that underlie most requests for assisted suicide.

If there has also been no consultation with anyone knowledgeable enough about the patient's symptoms or disease to be able to indicate how the patient's distress might be alleviated, then even if the patient is capable, an informed decision is not possible.

The 1999 anonymous survey of Oregon physicians who received requests for assisted suicide since the Oregon law went into effect gives us some picture of the inadequacy of palliative care consultation in

Oregon.[30] In more than half of the 142 cases for which physicians supplied information, including eighteen of the twenty-nine patients who by that time had been given prescriptions for lethal medications and nine of the seventeen who had died from taking the prescribed medication, there was no palliative care intervention of any kind. In less than half (sixty-eight) of the patients at least one of a variety of measures referred to as "substantive palliative care interventions" is listed as having been suggested: control of pain or other symptoms, referral to a hospice program, consultation (with a chaplain, social worker, palliative care or mental health professional, or a colleague), or giving the patient a trial of antidepressant medication.

In only 13 percent of the 142 cases was there a recommendation for a palliative care consultation, and we do not know how many of these recommendations were actually implemented; we are told that only about half of all palliative care recommendations of whatever kind were implemented. The most frequent consultation (28%) was with a colleague—a referral required under Oregon law to determine patient eligibility for assisted suicide, not necessarily a substantive palliative care intervention.[31]

Without someone knowledgeable enough to assess the pain control measure employed by the physician, we cannot know if care was adequate. Nor can one treat a referral to hospice as a substantive palliative care intervention without knowing what care hospice provided.

Almost half of the patients for whom any interventions were made changed their minds about assisted suicide. How many would have changed their minds had they received adequate assessment and treatment of their requests for suicide is a question that still needs to be explored.

Terminal Illness

The Oregon law specifies that to be eligible for assisted suicide a patient must have six months or less to live. Such predictions regarding terminal illness vary in accuracy depending on the disease involved—high accuracy in cancer, low in cardiovascular disease (a subject discussed in detail in chapter 11).[32] When surveyed, over 50 percent of Oregon physicians indicated that they were not confident they could make such a prediction.[33] Will Oregon patients like Helen be told of the uncertainty of these predictions? The criterion of six months becomes even less clear when the patient exercises his or her right to refuse even treatment that is likely to succeed in prolonging life. Whether the six-month period is to be estimated with or without such treatment is an issue not addressed by the law.

Voluntary Request

The Oregon law strictly stipulates that a patient's request for assisted suicide must be made voluntarily. "A person who coerces or exerts undue influence on a patient to request medication for the purpose of ending the patient's life . . . shall be guilty of a Class A felony."[34] Voluntariness is to be assured by having the patient submit a written request for assisted suicide signed by two witnesses, one of whom must not be a relative, an heir, or the owner or operator of a health care facility where the patient is receiving treatment or is in residence. Neither of the witnesses shall be the patient's attending physician.

The witnesses must attest that the patient is of sound mind and not under duress or undue influence. On what basis is such an assessment made and using what criteria? The Oregon law does not require that the witnesses actually know the patient—proof of the patient's identity is sufficient. The law would permit an heir to be one of the witnesses and a friend of the heir to be another. In proposed statutes in other states, neither of the witnesses can be a beneficiary.[35]

In addition to the written request for assisted suicide, Oregon patients are also required to make two oral requests with an interval of fifteen days in between. Although some proponents of assisted suicide object to the delay,[36] the time interval (if followed) would be a safeguard of some value, since the majority of patients wishing to hasten their death desire less strongly to die when seen two weeks later. How this time requirement is to be monitored has not been addressed, since the only evidence of the oral request that is needed under the law is the physician's own notation in the patient's medical records. In addition, the law does not stipulate that the second request be made in person; an affirmation by phone of the original request and a mailed prescription offer much less protection.

There is nothing in the Oregon law, any more than there is in Dutch law, to prohibit a physician from suggesting assisted suicide to a patient. A task force established by the Oregon Health Sciences University to help physicians understand the law, recognizing that such suggestions compromise voluntariness, recommended that they not be made.[37]

Physicians who believe assisted suicide is a legitimate medical procedure and reasonable option, however, could well feel entitled, if not obliged, to make such a suggestion. Indeed, if physician-assisted suicide is accepted as standard medical practice, as the Oregon law envisions, families could conceivably sue physicians for having caused patients to suffer by not suggesting it.

A Second Case

The lack of safeguards in the Oregon law regarding mental capacity, informed consent, and voluntariness are all evident in the second case in which some detailed information about an assisted suicide case was made available, in this instance by family members who told their story to the *Oregonian* to enlist support for their efforts to obtain assisted suicide for a relative.

Kate Cheney, an eighty-five-year-old widow, was diagnosed as terminally ill with stomach cancer. Kate wanted the option of assisted suicide in case she was in pain or if the indignities of losing control of her body functions became unbearable. Her daughter Erika, a retired nurse who had come from Arizona to care for her mother, went with Kate when she made her request for assisted suicide to her physician at Kaiser Permanente. Erika described the physician as "dismissive" and requested and received a referral to another Kaiser physician. Kate's second doctor arranged for a psychiatric consultation, a standard procedure at Kaiser. Although the psychiatrist who had visited Kate at her home declined to be interviewed, the family released his report to the *Oregonian*'s reporter. The psychiatrist found that the patient did "not seem to be explicitly pushing for assisted suicide" and lacked "the very high level of capacity to weigh options about it." Although the patient seemed to accept the assessment, the psychiatrist noted that the daughter became very angry.

Kaiser then suggested that the family obtain a second assessment from an outside consultant. The psychologist consulted noted that Kate had some memory defects and that her "choices [might have been] influenced by her family's wishes, and that her daughter, Erika, [might have been] somewhat coercive" but felt Kate had the ability to make her own decision. A Kaiser administrator saw Kate and decided that she was competent and was making the decision on her own. Kate received the lethal drugs, which were put under Erika's care.

As time went by and Kate ate poorly and became somewhat weaker, Erika and her husband needed a respite and sent Kate to a nursing home for a week. Kate ate well there, but when Erika visited Kate always asked when she would be going home. On the day she returned from the nursing home she told Erika and her husband that something had to be done, given her declining health. She had considered going permanently into a nursing home but had decided against it. She told them she wanted to use the pills and asked for their help. "When would you like to do this?" her son-in-law asked. "Now," Kate replied. Grandchildren were contacted, those who lived nearby came over, goodbyes were said, and within a short time, with her family beside her, Kate took the pills and died.[38]

Did her daughter's eagerness influence Kate's decision? What would have happened if her family had responded to her request by saying, "We love you and we want you around as long as possible. We want to keep you at home and care for you"? Sending Kate to the nursing home was sending her a message that she was a burden. Were there no other ways for the family to get relief? Sent to a nursing home as a burden to her family, Kate's distress is poignantly expressed in her repeated requests to go home and in her request to end her life on the day she does so. What other option could she choose but to hasten her death? Kate told the Oregon reporter that her family members were not pushing her but felt she should do what she wanted. It would be unlikely for Kate to acknowledge to the reporter anything different about her family, but one can readily see how in the best of circumstances frail elderly patients can feel coerced to die. Caregiver burden leading to depression in the caregiver has now been identified as a serious issue, particularly for women like Erika who are asked to shoulder the work and responsibility of providing twenty-four-hour care to a parent. This particular case raises the question of what real meaning or value is Oregon's prohibition of coercion if it can be circumvented so easily.

The role of a single health maintenance organization (HMO) administrator making the final decision in a matter in which the HMO might have a financial conflict of interest, since continuing care is far more expensive than assisted suicide, was questioned.[39] Would the HMO have asked for a second opinion if the psychiatrist had deemed the patient competent to request assisted suicide? The Kaiser administrator was indignant at a journalist's implication that financial considerations might have influenced both his recommendation to the family to seek an outside consultant and his own final decision. Yet this is a compelling argument for the need for openness and transparency and perhaps even a judicial review because of the competing interests in deciding what was appropriate for this vulnerable elderly patient whose competency was in question and whose family may have been seriously burdened by her care.

Notification of Family

Under the Oregon law, the physician is required to suggest that patients inform their families of their request for assisted suicide, but the patients are not required to do so and are permitted to refuse to inform them. The physician is explicitly instructed in the law not to deny the request on the basis of such a refusal. Even if the patient complies, the physician is not required by law to ask to see the patient's family.

How can any physician be sure there is no coercion unless the physician has met the family and seen the interaction among them and with the patient? The observations by the psychiatrist and the psychologist of Kate's family provided evidence of coercion that should have afforded Kate protection. In Helen's case we eventually learned that Reagan had met her family, but there is no information to the effect that he observed their interaction with Helen or evaluated their motives for favoring assisted suicide.

On the other hand, not informing the family can prevent a caring family from expressing their affection in ways that might alter the patient's decision. It also opens the family up to the devastating grief and guilt that we see in survivors of suicide.[40] Much of that guilt comes from feeling there were things they could or should have done to encourage the person who committed suicide to want to live. Feeling cut off from what a loved one was going through before the act is a major contributor to such anguish. Advocates of assisted suicide argued that legalization, by permitting the family to be part of the process, would ameliorate such suffering.[41] Not informing the family makes this impossible. Does a physician have no responsibility for the consequences?

What if a young husband has made no provisions for his family? One could think of a number of similar situations where a failure to meet the family means that the family will be unprepared for painful consequences. The provision of the Oregon law that states that a patient who declines to inform his or her family "shall not have his or her request declined for that reason" is too sweeping in scope.

Protecting Physicians, Not Patients

A concern with physician rather than patient protection pervades the Oregon law. Under the law, physicians are exempt from the ordinary standards of care, skill, and diligence required of Oregon physicians in other circumstances, such as withdrawing life support. Instead, the physician is immunized from civil or criminal liability for actions taken in "good faith" in assisting a suicide irrespective of community standards in other matters and even if the physician acts negligently.

The choice to apply a good faith standard rather than the higher and customary negligence standard is curious. Good faith is most often used, with varying degrees of success, in the context of a self-defense argument, for example, by individuals who believe they needed to use extreme force to defend themselves. It does not mean they acted reasonably. A person could act negligently or even recklessly, but as long as he or she believed the actions were appropriate, the defense might prevail. It is an entirely subjective standard.

A "negligence" standard, which is customary in professional practices, provides objective guidelines for a particular procedure or the established and objective standards for good practice. If the intent of the assisted suicide law is to protect physicians from accountability for violating the statute's provisions, the good faith standard is ideal. If the intent of the law had been to protect patients, the negligence standard would have been appropriate.

Moreover, there is no enforcement mechanism in the Oregon law should physicians choose not to comply with guidelines set up by OHD for reporting all cases in which medication for the purpose of assisted suicide has been prescribed. The law is "silent on what the Division should do when noncompliance is encountered."[42] Even if the Oregon law were not so permissive concerning reporting, nonreporting would be a serious problem. The Dutch have been able to document that the majority of cases of assisted suicide and euthanasia are not reported. Most nonreporting involves cases in which physicians failed to follow established guidelines for voluntariness or consultation. As we have seen, by continually focusing on this problem, the Dutch have been able to reduce the percentage of unreported cases from 72 percent to 59 percent. Although this means that most cases are still not reported, without such scrutiny the situation would be worse. In Oregon, the question of ascertaining nonreporting has not been addressed.

The purpose of a legal mandate to report all cases would be, of course, to provide a means to sanction physicians who failed to report, as well as to provide the essential statistics on which to do even a minimal research survey. The statute would seem to have been written to preclude both accountability and meaningful data collection.

Secrecy

OHD's focus has been more on doctor-patient confidentiality than on monitoring compliance or abuse. Internal memoranda from OHD to its county vital records offices instructed all employees that they should "neither confirm nor deny if a (physician-assisted) death has occurred in your county." To underscore "how seriously this matter is being taken" by OHD, the memo warned that "any staff within the Center for Health Statistics that reveals any information they are not authorized to release will immediately be terminated."[43] Another internal memorandum from OHD's Center for Health Statistics to funeral homes promises "future plans" to limit all requested copies of death certificates to a new, abbreviated form that eliminates information about the cause and manner of death and underlying disease conditions. These plans, according to the memo, "include a computer generated death certificate and new technology which will allow us to 'mask' our microfilm so we can block out the cause [of death] portion."[44]

OHD has developed measures unique to physician-assisted suicide to protect the privacy of patients and their families. However, the measures appear to be extraordinarily secretive. They also limit the potential for thoroughgoing research into the dimensions and context of this practice as it unfolds.

The Oregon law specifically states that although OHD will issue a report each year based on a selected sample of cases, "The information collected shall not be a public record and may not be made available for inspection by the public."[45] The same provision applies to the death certificates filed in these cases. There is no provision for an independent evaluator or researcher to study whatever data are available.

Since physicians are not asked to report significant medical information about their cases of assisted suicide, and since reporting is not mandatory, OHD itself does not know very much. OHD's restriction of access to whatever information is available means that other Oregonians will know mainly what advocacy groups involved in the cases or participating physicians choose to reveal.

The anonymity and secrecy about physician practice of assisted suicide goes counter to all standards of medicine, which depend on openness about facts, research data, and records to assess the appropriateness of treatment. If physician-assisted suicide is to be part of the medical treatment for terminal illness, why are existing patient-doctor confidentiality rules not sufficient to protect physicians in this setting? Restricting access to information about the indications for assisted suicide, patient data, radiologic documentation, and specific drug therapy limits the opportunity to establish a standard of care, providing excessive protection to the physician while, in the name of confidentiality, leaving the patient vulnerable. The vulnerability of the patient becomes a real concern when we begin to focus on any potential conflict of interest or bias of the treating physician.

Patient privacy is and should be protected by law, but nothing in law, ethics, or medicine requires or suggests that the identity of doctors participating in any particular medical procedure should be concealed. We do not know how physicians are diagnosing and managing patients who are requesting assisted suicide. The information we have about specific cases or from the anonymous survey of physicians is disturbing. Care appears to be provided arbitrarily and is being protected in secrecy by the law, preventing a clear assessment of the true quality of care of patients with serious medical illness in Oregon. The secrecy encouraged by the lack of a detailed evaluation of the quality of care patients who request physician-assisted suicide receive at the end of life prevents a full assessment of whether the overall process is working well or poorly. Perhaps most important, the process prevents us from knowing whether all patients who request such assistance are receiving quality care at the level of national guidelines for the evaluation and treatment of psychological distress, symptom control, and social support.

Don't Ask, Don't Tell

In keeping with its mandate under Oregon's physician-assisted suicide law, OHD issued its first yearly report in March 1999. In a public document,[46] an article in the *New England Journal of Medicine*,[47] a National Press Club Briefing, and visits to various congressional offices, OHD argued that physician-assisted suicide was being carried out safely under the state's Death with Dignity Act. The report was marked by its failure to address the limits of the information it had available, overreaching its data to draw unwarranted conclusions.[48] The second report, issued in February 2000 and published in the *New England Journal of Medicine*, continued to provide limited data but attempted to offer some insight into the perspectives of families of patients who were aided in death.[49] This additional information further exemplifies the poor methodological design of OHD's monitoring process: questions to families were restricted on the grounds that the families were unable to distinguish between various symptoms in patients. The palliative care literature, however, is replete with studies to show the reliability of families in reporting and distinguishing patient symptoms. No family perspective is provided in the 2001 report from OHD, which lists only the minimal data set obtained through physician completion of the forms and physician interviews. The report appears on the OHD Web site, and a short summary was published in the New England Journal of Medicine.[50]

Perhaps what is most striking and least justified has been OHD's contention, without substantiating data, that patients who requested assisted suicide were receiving adequate end-of-life care. OHD's own data from family interviews, newer surveys of families of patients receiving end-of-life care in Oregon, and new surveys of physicians' experience are all in stark contrast to the narrow focus of the state's official report. These conflicting studies emphasize that we know little about the physical, psychological, and existential needs of patients requesting assisted suicide, the capabilities of the physicians responding to such requests, and the context in which these patients live and are cared for. We do know, however, that based on physician interviews in the 2000 report, patients in higher numbers—63 percent compared to 26 percent in 1999 and 12 percent in 1998—express concern about being a burden.

Limited Data

The data OHD has collected are largely epidemiological: the assisted suicide cases were divided between men and women; the median age of the patients was seventy in 1998, seventy-one in 1999, and sixty-nine in 2000.

All of the patients were white, and most of them had cancer. Although in 1998 and 1999 patients who chose assisted suicide were more likely to be divorced or to have never been married, the proportion of married patients increased significantly in the 2000 report. The demographic characteristics of those who were assisted in suicide in 2000 "resembled those of Oregon residents who died of similar underlying diseases in 1999, with a single exception: as their level of education increased their likelihood of choosing physician-assisted suicide increased."[51] The statement, made without elaboration, seems intended to leave the reader with the implication that those who choose assisted suicide are smarter than those who do not. Of course, the overwhelming percentage of college graduates dying of these diseases did not choose assisted suicide. And more to the point would have been the education in palliative care of the physicians involved, since patients with physicians who are so educated are less likely to feel they need or want assisted suicide.

Physicians participating in assisted suicide are not asked to provide OHD with significant medical information about their patients. They are merely asked to check off a list on an OHD form indicating that such statutory requirements as a written request for the lethal dose of medication, a fifteen-day waiting period, and consultation with another physician have been met.

Only one line on the form is provided for both diagnosis and prognosis, although a terminal illness and a prognosis of death within six months are the essential requirements for assisted suicide in the state. The form does not inquire on what basis the physician made the medical diagnosis—for example, review of x-rays, written material, pathology reports, or other information. Nor are physicians asked to report on what basis they made the prognosis—what tables they have used, what experts they have consulted. The form does not even inquire as to the patient's reasons for requesting assisted suicide. The data provided do not make it possible to know what transpired in any particular case.[52]

To supplement the meager information required by formal reporting, OHD asked physicians who participated in assisted suicide to respond in person or by phone to a questionnaire that was also given to physicians of a comparison (control) group of patients who died in 1998 of similar illnesses without assisted suicide. (No control group was used in the second or third report.) OHD does not tell us who asked the questions, what training they had, or whether any follow-up questions were asked. But the questionnaire (published on the Internet) and the reports show that these efforts were also flawed. Significant medical information was not asked for or provided.

In the absence of medical data, how does OHD reach its conclusion that patients who requested assisted suicide were receiving adequate end-of-life care? It used the facts—derived from the physician questionnaire—that the proportion of patients who had advance directives, had health insurance, and were enrolled in hospice programs was comparably high for both the case and comparison groups, and that neither worry about pain control or nor financial concerns drove patients' request for assisted suicide. But advance directives, health insurance, or enrollment in a hospice program does not provide proof of competent assessment and treatment—the essential components of adequate care—any more than patients' apparent silence about palliative care or financial concerns. Such figures cannot substitute for direct knowledge of patients and their illnesses. Although the physicians questioned reported that more patients requesting assisted suicide were concerned with loss of autonomy or loss of control of body functions than were the control group, physicians were not asked how these concerns were expressed or addressed. Without such information it is not possible to judge whether the care these patients received was adequate.

The reports indicate that in six of the fifteen cases in 1998, and in eighteen of the twenty-seven patients for whom the information is available in 1999, the first physician seen by the patient did not agree to assist in the suicide; none of these physicians was contacted by OHD. In 1999, ten patients received prescriptions from a second physician. Eight went to a third or fourth physician. OHD justifies not collecting information from physicians who did not agree to prescribe the medication on the ground that many physicians are opposed to assisted suicide. But surveys indicate that a significant majority of Oregon physicians support the practice. In any case, one would want to know the reasons of those who declined to write a prescription. Were they opposed to assisted suicide in all cases? Did they consider that viable options were available? Did they consider the patient not competent to make the decision? Did they think the patient was being coerced?

To fairly evaluate the adequacy of the end-of-life care provided these patients, OHD investigators would have needed to interview these physicians as well as those who participated in the assisted suicide. Instead, the OHD report treats physicians who declined to assist patients' suicides as though their opinions reflected a personal bias rather than perhaps a considered but different medical opinion.

Any evaluation by OHD of the end-of-life care that such patients received would have to be conducted by physicians trained in palliative care, able and willing to inquire about the nature of the patient's illness and concerns and what was done to address them. Those administering the questionnaire are not more likely than the physicians assisting in suicide to have had such training. As it now stands, untrained physicians are being assessed by untrained evaluators.

The 1999 report stressed the fact that only one of the fifteen patients expressed concern about inadequate pain control at the end of life. The report's authors believe this may reflect advances in palliative care in Oregon and the fact that the state ranks high in the use of morphine for medical purposes. Yet fifteen of the forty-three control patients were worried about end-of-life pain control, suggesting the concern is frequent among those who are terminally ill. In 1999, seven of twenty-six patients expressed concern about inadequate pain control as their disease progressed, a figure that the authors regard as low. Yet in 2000, 30 percent report concern about inadequate pain control. The OHD investigators state that this concern was not correlated with patients' actual experience of pain.

But the figures are themselves suspect. They are based on physicians' responses long after the fact to the question whether patients volunteered such concerns about pain. The physicians did not directly ask the patients about their pain. The inadequacy of relying on physicians' perceptions of patients' experiences has long been documented, particularly with regard to pain: in numerous published studies physicians underestimated what patients were experiencing.[53] In surveys of barriers to effective pain relief, patients reported that they did not want to use their time with their doctors to discuss pain relief but rather to discuss their treatments.[54] This is particularly apt to be true of patients requesting assisted suicide, who, if successful in persuading physicians to give them a lethal prescription, would have no need to be concerned about future pain. A study surveying cancer patients with pain or depression showed how differences in their attitudes toward physician-assisted suicide would affect their choice of physicians. Patients with pain reported they would change physicians if they knew their physician participated in physician-assisted suicide.[55] Those with depression were more likely to seek out such physicians.

The anonymous survey of Oregon physicians contrasts with the findings of OHD that pain was not a significant problem for patients requesting physician-assisted suicide. Oregon physicians reported that 43 percent of the 143 patients requesting assistance in death had pain as one of the important reasons for such a request.

Surveys of family members of dying patients can also provide insight into the adequacy of palliative care services. OHD's 1999 report failed to cite the Oregon Board of Medical Examiners (BME) survey of 475 surviving family members listed as informants from a stratified sample of Oregon death certificates for 1997 that showed a statewide trend of higher rates of moderate to severe pain reported by family members of patients in acute care hospitals throughout Oregon.[56] The BME viewed the trend as a "worrisome" statistic that suggested inadequate palliative care. Responding perhaps to criticism of their failure to interview family members, a single family member of nineteen of the assisted suicide patients was interviewed in the second report. Unfortunately, that member was chosen by the physician who assisted in the suicide, which compromised the integrity of the process. The absence of family data on the 2000 report does not make it possible to correlate the physicians' perceptions with patient and family realities.

The Lethal Prescription

The reports, however, do help settle one debate that went on between advocates and opponents before implementation of the law. Opponents of legalizing assisted suicide in Oregon pointed out that because there was no reliable information about the lethal dose for medically ill patients, physicians assisting suicide would essentially be experimenting on patients. In Dutch studies, 20 percent of patients given 9 grams of barbiturates, considered to be a lethal dose, lived for more than three hours.[57] A recent Dutch report provided evidence that in 18 percent of cases such delays caused Dutch doctors to intervene with lethal injections,[58] a practice that would be illegal in Oregon. In a number of reported cases in this country, after swallowing presumed lethal doses of barbiturates, patients did not die and families intervened with pillows or plastic bags.[59] In a telephone survey of American oncologists, Emanuel and his colleagues found that 15 percent of attempts at physician-assisted suicide were unsuccessful.[60]

Advocacy groups denied the validity of such accounts and of the Dutch findings, although recommending the 9-gram barbiturate dose, which was given by physicians to fourteen of the first fifteen Oregon cases. OHD notes without comment that four of the fifteen patients in 1998 lived longer than three hours and one lived as long as eleven, figures that are consistent with the Dutch experience. In 1999 three patients lived longer than eleven hours and one lived as long as twenty-six.

In discussing the 1999 Oregon report in an editorial in the *New England Journal of Medicine,* Sherwin Nuland noted that the Oregon investigators did not inquire on the frequency of other complications of assisted suicide (such as nausea and vomiting) and expressed the opinion that they were therefore ignoring the complications that inevitably arise when debilitated patients take lethal prescriptions.[61] Perhaps in response to such criticism, in 2000 some minimal data are provided. The report refers to a patient who regurgitated 10 milliliters of the suspension before dying seven minutes later. The report goes on to say that among patients on whom information was received all were unconscious within thirty minutes of ingesting the medication. The incompleteness of the data makes the report difficult to interpret. For example, in only fourteen of the twenty-seven cases in 2000 were physicians present at the time the patient ingested the lethal medication. For the other thirteen patients, the incomplete data provided were indirect and culled from a variety of family and attendant sources to the prescribing physician.

In all three years, more patients received prescriptions for lethal medication than used them. It would have been valuable to compare interviews with physicians of six patients the first year, five the second, and eight the third who requested assisted suicide but who died of their underlying illnesses without using the lethal prescriptions given them. Yet these nineteen are essentially dropouts in the study, a group that investigators normally wish to compare with their cases. Such patients might provide further information about the complicated aspects of patient requests.

Economic Factors

The pitfalls that result from OHD's inadequate methodology are nowhere more apparent than in the report's conclusion that economic factors did not influence the choice of assisted suicide. OHD informs us that apprehensions that assisted suicide would be chosen by those "fearful of the financial consequences of their illness" were unjustified. This may or may not be true, but OHD is not in a position to know. The Oregon law does not ask physicians to inquire about patients' economic or social circumstances, nor does OHD require physicians to report such information.

On the basis of the physician questionnaire, the first OHD report concluded, "None of the case patients or control patients expressed concern to their physicians about the financial impact of their illness. We found no significant difference between the case patients and the control patients with regard to insurance at the time of their death."[62] A recently published study to understand patient and caregiver economic and other burdens of terminal illness noted that there were significant disparities in care according to sex, ethnicity, age, and income, but not according to insurance status.[63] Economic hardships arise from the high care needs of terminally ill patients and are independent of insurance status. OHD does not assess the high care needs of patients who requested assisted suicide, nor does it assess the caregiver burden. Thus its strong conclusion that economics did not appear to influence patients' decisions is based on inadequate and irrelevant data.

In the 2000 report, 36 percent of patients were receiving either Medicare or Medicaid, yet 88 percent were in hospice programs. Given the median age of seventy-one in this cohort, it would suggest that a higher percentage of patients might well be receiving Medicare and a better display of the data would be to indicate the type of insurance associated with the patients' age. Of note: physicians, when interviewed, knew that patients had insurance but not the type, and in two patients they had no knowledge of the patients' insurance status.

The apparent lack of difference between the case and control groups is more likely to reflect the lack of sensitivity of the model and the superficiality of the data collected. It is very unusual for physicians to have a clear understanding of the financial issues facing their patients. More commonly they are unaware of patients' out-of-pocket expenses or of other family and personal considerations. Physicians have little time to discuss these issues, and patients have strong needs (out of pride) not to provide this information to clinicians. Although a patient requesting assisted suicide may also feel that the request is less likely to be granted if the physician feels that the patient is making the request because he or she cannot afford proper care, in point of fact a survey revealed that Oregon physicians were more likely than Dutch physicians to be responsive to a request for assisted suicide based on financial hardship.[64] The authors reasonably conclude that this difference in attitude may reflect the reality that economic hardship is a more critical factor in end-of-life care decisions in this country than it is in the Netherlands. In any case, when a patient requests assisted suicide one would expect physicians to inquire about the patient's ability to afford adequate care, whether or not the patient raises the question and even though the Oregon law does not suggest that physicians should ask.

Even among the insured there is compelling evidence to suggest that the cost of end-of-life care can contribute to financial hardship. In a comprehensive study of end-of-life care, more than half of the families involved reported at least one financial burden, ranging from loss of family savings, to loss of income, to changes in educational plans or employment status.[65] High deductibles, copayments or coinsurance, and limits of coverage can all contribute to high out-of-pocket expenditures. Medicare covers only 83 percent of typical charges for lung cancer and 65 percent of typical charges for breast cancer; it does not reimburse for out-of-pocket drug expenses, which can be particularly burdensome. And hospice provides only limited nursing care (four hours per day) unless the patient is imminently dying. Although OHD reported that none of the cases in either the 1998 case group or the control group expressed financial concerns, an *Oregonian* reporter who reinterviewed the family of Helen was told that the patient was concerned that her financial resources not be dissipated by her care.[66]

In the 2000 report, the observation that patients increasingly expressed concern about becoming a burden to family or caregivers does not exclude the possibility that they may have viewed this as a financial burden. No attempt was made to tease this out in interviews with physicians.

Psychiatric Concerns

How does OHD monitor the process to see that depressed patients are adequately protected? Buried in tables but not discussed in the report is the fact that only five of the fifteen cases in 1998, ten of the twenty-seven cases in 1999, and five of the twenty-seven cases in 2000 were referred for psychiatric or psychological evaluation. Since all of the cases went forward, we are to conclude that there was no case in any group in which depression or any other mental illness was considered to be compromising the patient's judgment.

OHD does not appear to have wished to know about the psychiatric status of the patients requesting assisted suicide. Psychiatrists who may have examined patients and found them to be incompetent are not even asked to file a report with OHD. If OHD wished to monitor the psychiatric evaluation, a trained psychiatrist or psychologist should have interviewed both the prescribing physicians and the psychiatrists who saw the referred patients. Questions need to be asked. Were the reasons for requesting assisted suicide explored? How did the physician evaluate them? What was the physician's response? Was the patient depressed? What were the symptoms? Was treatment offered? What was the patient's response? What other risk factors for suicide were present, such as a family history of depression and/or suicide, alcoholism, and any past suicide attempts? What was the patient's past experience with the death of those close to him or her? Did the patient—like most of those who commit suicide and assisted suicide—express any ambivalence about suicide? If so how was this expressed and how was it dealt with?

OHD might well consider that the psychiatric consultation as envisioned by the Oregon law is not intended to deal with these considerations but the more limited issue of a patient's capacity to make the decision regarding assisted suicide. But then at a minimum OHD would need to monitor on what basis clinicians were making the decision to refer patients for psychiatric evaluation and whether these decisions were appropriate. The psychiatrists approving the assisted suicide would have to be interviewed to learn how well they knew the patient, whether the patient was seen more than once, and on what basis they decided the patient was competent.

A Third Case

The story of Joan Lucas, whose suicide was facilitated and publicized by Compassion in Dying, strikingly points out how the way the Oregon law was written and is being monitored undermines the potential value of a psychiatric consultation. Not only are such consultations requested infrequently but, as the Lucas case illustrates, psychological and psychiatric consultation often seem to be requested to protect doctors rather than patients. The case also raises a question as to what is Oregon's standard of care for paramedics called to evaluate someone who has attempted suicide.

Joan Lucas, a patient with amyotrophic lateral sclerosis, attempted suicide. Paramedics were called to Joan's house but her children sent them away, explaining "We couldn't let her go to the ambulance. They would have resuscitated her."[67] Joan survived her attempt and was assisted in suicide eighteen days later by a physician who gave interviews about the case to an Oregon newspaper on condition of anonymity. He stated that after talking with attorneys from the Oregon Medical Association and agreeing to help aid Joan in death, he asked Joan to undergo a psychological examination. "It was an option for us to get a psychological or psychiatric evaluation," he said. "I elected to get a psychological evaluation because I wished to cover my ass. I didn't want there to be any problems."[68]

The doctor and the family found a cooperative psychologist who asked Joan to take the Minnesota Multiphasic Personality Inventory, a standard psychological test. Because it was difficult for Joan to travel to the psychologist's office, her children read the true-false questions to her at home. The family found the questions funny, and Joan's daughter described the family as "cracking up over them." Her son added: "Those were some of the best last moments we had with Mom."[69] Based on these test results, the psychologist concluded that whatever depression Joan had was directly related to her terminal illness—a completely normal response.[70] His opinion is suspect, the more so because while he was willing to give an opinion that would facilitate ending Joan's life, he did not feel it was necessary to see her first. OHD neither interviewed Joan Lucas's primary care physician who refused to assist in her suicide, nor assessed the quality of her psychological evaluation, nor evaluated the paramedics' role in addressing Joan's suicide attempt.

Conclusion

OHD monitoring reflects the law's predilections, so that OHD seems determined not to ask the tough questions and not to ask them of the right people. Patients are not asked to provide any information to the state. Over 70 percent of the patients were in hospice care, but since OHD did not interview hospice staff, hospice nurses and social workers who might have the most knowledge of the patients were given no voice in the monitoring process. And the information physicians provide is far too limited to be relevant to those wanting to understand the end-of-life care these patients receive. Although the questionnaire given to physicians provides three lines for them to reply to a question as to why their patients chose to request assisted suicide, if the physicians had not previously explored the matter with their patients—something they are not required or asked to do under the law—those replies would be of questionable value.

The physicians who did not agree to assist in suicide and were not interviewed by OHD cannot, on the basis of doctor-patient confidentiality, speak publicly about the reasons for their refusal. This is in contrast to physician advocates, some of whom talk and write publicly about the treatment. One wonders if they have their patients' permission to do so. We are told by Compassion in Dying that Helen's family gave permission for the release of the tape recordings. Did Helen also consent? If there was adequate consent, why release only excerpts of an edited version of the tapes? Did the doctors discussing the case with the media have the patient's or the family's consent for them to do so? If so, why should doctors assisting in suicide give interviews to media representatives and not be questioned by their peers? Particularly when a procedure is new and untried, physicians customarily present what they are doing to colleagues so they can learn from the feedback.

Fifteen cases in the first year and twenty-seven in each of the next two years was seen as a small number and as such interpreted by proponents of assisted suicide, including the governor of the state, as indicating that the law was not likely to be abused. In such a controversial procedure, however, one might expect patients and physicians to be hesitant about participating. Although we do not have figures for the early years in the Netherlands when assisted suicide and euthanasia were first given legal sanction, they appear to have been practiced at first relatively infrequently. It was only after the practice became generally accepted for some years that the numbers seem to have risen significantly.

Some of the early Dutch patients were advocates of assisted suicide who used their deaths partly to make a statement on behalf of a cause in which they believed. There has been some question as to whether the Oregon patients were advocates or disproportionately shepherded by advocacy groups to chosen physicians. The physician questionnaire partly addressed this latter concern in asking, "Was the patient specifically referred to you regarding PAS by an organization such as Compassion in Dying or the Hemlock Society?" Inexplicably, OHD did not publish the answer and seemed reluctant to reveal it. Only after Compassion in Dying revealed that eleven of the fifteen patients assisted in suicide in the first year of the law had been referred by its organization did OHD confirm that fact. One other referral was acknowledged by the Hemlock Society. The question was asked again in subsequent years, but neither OHD nor Compassion in Dying chose to release the information.

After information about Helen's case had been made public, the chair of the Subcommittee on Guidelines for the Death with Dignity Act of the Oregon Health Sciences University told the *Oregonian* that too much information had been revealed about the first case. "They (the public) wanted to know (the law) worked in general and other than that they were almost embarrassed to read about details."[71] She went on to say that would seldom happen in the future. Her attitude, which seems to reflect the desire of so many Oregon officials to keep from public scrutiny the facts about assisted suicide in Oregon, is particularly troublesome. From what we have learned so far, despite the efforts at concealment, details about how the law operates would probably be more embarrassing to OHD and to advocates of assisted suicide than to the public.

Particularly disturbing in Oregon—and most similar to the Netherlands—is that those administering the law and those sanctioned by government to analyze its operation have become its advocates and its defenders. The over-reaching conclusions in the OHD reports and the public relations campaign that accompanied the release of the first report—from the National Press Club briefing to the visits to various congressional offices—seem to belie its authors' claims that they are simply a "neutral party" collecting data.

OHD has a higher responsibility, to present what it knows and admit what it does not. The ideal solution would be for OHD to appoint a task force made up of physicians from outside the state who are experts in palliative care, psychiatry, and medicine to review the assisted suicide cases—perhaps even to embark on a prospective study. Unless physicians are going to be asked to report more than they are now required to under the law, and unless properly trained independent physicians can question the physicians and examine the data, we will not learn much from the Oregon experiment. Nor will we be assured that patients who choose assisted suicide are receiving appropriate care at the end of life.

Under the Oregon law, physicians have been given authority without being in a position to exercise it responsibly. They are expected to inform patients that alternatives are possible, without being required to be knowledgeable enough to present those alternatives in a meaningful way or to consult with someone who can. They are expected to evaluate patient decision-making capacity and judgment without a requirement for psychiatric expertise or consultation. They are expected to make decisions about voluntariness without having to see those close to the patient who may be exerting a variety of pressures, from subtle to coercive. They are expected to do all of this without necessarily knowing the patient for longer than fifteen days. Since physicians cannot be held responsible for wrongful deaths if they have acted in good faith, substandard medical practice is encouraged, physicians are protected from the consequences, and patients are left unprotected while believing they have acquired a new right.

Oregon's Culture of Silence

N. Gregory Hamilton, M.D.

On Tuesday, November 8, 1994, medical practice in Oregon faced an unexpected ethical challenge. That day in a referendum physician-assisted suicide was voted into law by a slim margin. Yet the Oregon Health Sciences University Department of Psychiatry, of which I had been a member for over ten years, had never discussed, much less debated, this important issue.

As the director of the psychiatry outpatient clinic, I had long advocated training residents and medical students to treat aggressively depression, pain, and other problems in those who are seriously ill and without ever condoning suicide in these medically ill individuals, any more than we would in anyone else. I championed open discussion of medical issues and looked forward to our next faculty meeting less than a month after assisted suicide became legal in Oregon. Then, I believed, we would finally have an opportunity to discuss this life-and-death issue within the department. This opportunity, rather than materializing, however, was lost—a fact that illustrates the official approach to institutionalized assisted suicide. Instead of promoting clinical discussion, legalization of physician-assisted suicide inaugurated a new culture of silence.

Before the election, the only statement made by department administrators was that faculty members were not to use their titles or mention their employer if they commented on the assisted suicide referendum before the voters. The reason given for silencing the academic community was that we were state employees. Surprisingly, there was no outcry from this faculty defending academic freedom, but acceptance of a generic role as state employee. Meanwhile, the Center for Ethics in

Health Care at Oregon Health Sciences University remained officially "neutral," without acknowledging that ethical "neutrality" could be interpreted as actually favoring the legalization of assisted suicide.

But now a law had passed and we were no longer dealing with a ballot measure. Surely department members would speak as medical experts. After all, that was the reason the public paid our salaries, not merely to gain knowledge and to form opinions, but also to make our expertise available, to openly and freely debate important issues.

In the many years I had spent teaching outpatient psychiatry, we discussed such things as why a doctor's attitude toward a patient has a profound effect on the likelihood of the patient's suicide. We discussed topics ranging from how people find hope and meaning in life to how, once a patient becomes discouraged and suicidal, a combination of talking, empathy, social support, and antidepressant medication, sometimes even hospitalization, can help restore the patient's sense of life being worth living.[1] I established an outpatient psychiatric morbidity and mortality conference to discuss every suicide attempt, as well as other adverse outcomes, to determine what, if anything, could have been done better to restore the patient's will to live.[2] We felt proud of how infrequent suicide attempts were among our patients.

On Friday, December 2, 1994, the faculty meeting began with the usual collegial chatting. The chair then broke with ordinary procedure by turning the meeting over to a faculty member, who instructed us that we would be discussing how to implement the new assisted suicide law. We would not, it was emphasized, discuss whether the new law could or should be implemented in our clinics. The only question allowed would be what committees and referral systems would be set up to process requests for suicide. The room fell silent.

The meeting was carefully guided. Going around the room, each psychiatrist had on average less than a minute to give advice about implementation. Most said nothing. A few mentioned forming a referral system composed of individuals with varying views to do consultations. A tense silence gripped the room.

At the same time, in Eugene, Oregon, a legal challenge hung on the horizon.[3] This legal action was being brought by a patient with a progressive neuromuscular disorder, along with other plaintiffs. She had previously become depressed and vulnerable to suicidal ideation and with treatment had recovered from those feelings, as most patients do. She pointed out that the assisted suicide law discriminated against her and threatened her life, because once her disorder progressed to the point of meeting the definition of a "terminal illness," she would no longer be afforded the same protection against her suicidal impulses that others are granted.[4] If her depression recurred, as it was likely to do, this time she could be given an overdose instead of help. Her challenge raised serious questions about how difficult it is to tell when depression is affecting decisions about assisted suicide and the impossibility of protecting those who are depressed and other mentally ill individuals. A similar concern would soon be raised by 94 percent of Oregon psychiatrists surveyed, who said they were uncertain they could determine in a single visit when depression or other mental disorder was affecting decisions about assisted suicide.[5] None of these obvious psychiatric concerns were addressed in the state's only medical school department of psychiatry. Such issues were off the agenda.

After years of teaching students and residents to advocate on behalf of vulnerable patients, I was being told I could not talk about whether to implement a fatal procedure. Yet the cries for help from those who were vulnerable and depressed, even suicidal, regardless of their state of physical health, needed to be heard. They needed a voice.

The turn to comment circled the room. Now it was time to speak—or say nothing. With as much diplomacy as I could muster, I pointed out that we had not yet studied this suggested new procedure, a procedure that some now claimed might be somehow within the scope of physician practice, although virtually every national medical and nursing group disavowed it as unethical. We had not even given this lethal procedure the consideration we had recently given to whether we should require new patients to fill out a screening paper-and-pencil questionnaire. I reminded my longtime colleagues that it might seem cavalier, perhaps even arrogant, to implement a lethal procedure without the kind of study and consideration we would afford any other clinical change. If some of the colleagues believed giving a patient a lethal overdose could be called treatment, then they were obliged to study the indications for such a procedure, to study issues of safety and efficacy to protect vulnerable individuals, as they would with any other new procedure. But none of this had been done.

Other experts who had studied the issue had raised important concerns. In 1994, a New York State Task Force on Life and the Law study group of experts with widely divergent views and backgrounds concluded that regardless of one's philosophical, political, or religious views, assisted suicide, once introduced into institutionalized medicine, cannot be regulated and controlled—and therefore poses a threat to public health and safety.[6]

Since I was one of the senior faculty members and one of my functions at that time was to oversee all the clinical services, not just my own clinic, I was given more than the accustomed one minute. One option in dealing with an administrative request to implement a new procedure, I suggested, would be to study the proposed procedure more carefully. If there was a request from outside the department for implementation, we could legitimately decide that the first step in introducing any procedure would be to study its safety and efficacy. I acknowledged that I suspected that if we looked at the issues and problems carefully we could better understand the complex reasons patients were requesting physician-assisted suicide.

The silence broke suddenly and briefly. A single pro–assisted suicide faculty member declared, "The voters have spoken!" He asserted that I, as the clinic director, had a moral obligation to carry out the will of the people, regardless of my personal and professional opinions. One other faculty member countered that regardless of the vote, assisted suicide was unethical, according to the American Psychiatric Association's own ethics committee, and that we have an obligation to follow those ethics, regardless of a law allowing us to do otherwise.

The squall of controversy passed as quickly as it struck. The chairperson closed the discussion. A dark cloud of silence again closed over the room. In subsequent years the topic has not appeared on the agenda of the Oregon Health Sciences University Department of Psychiatry.

The result? A parallel consultation system outside normal channels was created bypassing the clinic director. Only those in favor of allowing assisted suicide were included in clinical discussions. This arrangement was made even though department researchers were soon to reach an obvious conclusion: "Our data raise the concern that psychiatrists who are proponents of assisted suicide and would support the patient in obtaining a lethal prescription may fail to recognize the patient's ambivalence. . . . Psychiatrists who too quickly or easily support the patient in obtaining a lethal prescription may also be responding to an agenda, not the patient's needs."[7] Yet the possibility of allowing for open clinical deliberation including those opposed to assisted suicide in the discussion of cases as a safety check to compensate for any possible "agenda" and failure to "recognize the patient's ambivalence" was disallowed. Thereby, meaningful discussion was effectively stifled.

There was no further deliberation. The implementation system had been created. It seems likely that this approach was taken primarily as an administrative expedient, an avoidance of open conflict and institutional embarrassment during a difficult period in the department, rather than as an orchestrated attempt to promote assisted suicide and euthanasia. That is one of the dangers of medicalized assisted suicide. Institutions, by their very nature, are self-sustaining systems, sometimes to the peril of those whom they were designed to serve.

An "Experiment" with Secret Results

Assisted suicide and euthanasia advocates promised Oregon voters that legalization of assisted suicide would bring this previously rare and clandestine practice out into the open. Some assisted suicide advocates, such as Dr. Marcia Angell, emphasize that physician-assisted suicide should be an experiment conducted in the "laboratory" of the states.[8] Yet the culture of silence that has developed around assisted suicide in Oregon has led to the results of this practice largely being kept secret. Closely guarding knowledge of the outcome of a new intervention is in contrast to the openness to outside, independent review of valid medical research. The extent of secrecy about the outcome is nowhere clearer than in the Oregon Health Division (OHD) report of the first year's experience.[9]

As discussed in the previous chapter, those individuals in OHD assigned to monitor the safety of the law have become its apologists, if not its advocates.[10] Implementation of assisted suicide is being treated as a potential political embarrassment to be justified, rather than as a health concern to be frankly reported. Under such political pressure, the authors of the health division report made exaggerated claims of safety and withheld vital information.

For example, the first report failed to mention that depression played a part in any of that year's fifteen cases, while the medical literature documents that at least one case was diagnosed as depressed.[11] The patient was nevertheless given assisted suicide by her Compassion in Dying doctor in less than three weeks.

The report also claimed economic factors did not influence patients, contrary to an *Oregonian* verification that economic factors did motivate

at least one of those cases.[12] OHD cited evidence that the majority of patients had some kind of medical insurance as proof that they were not
under economic pressure. The report entirely ignored the fact that Oregon's rationed health plan denies payment for 171 needed services, while
it fully funds assisted suicide for the poor. Neither did it reveal that over
38 percent of Oregon Health Plan members find barriers to obtaining
mental health services[13] or that within weeks of the assisted suicide law
being implemented, whether inadvertently or not, the state placed barriers in the way of funding some of the most widely used and needed
psychiatric medicines for the poor.[14] The report indicated there were no
economic pressures but failed to note that private Oregon insurance
companies had responded to federal laws forbidding discriminatory
dollar limits on mental health benefits by translating those dollar limits
directly into number of visits; and Oregon, unlike many states, has failed
to provide parity for mental health care.[15] This lack of information, this
silence about the kind of insurance provided, allowed Oregon officials
misleadingly to reassure the public. Following OHD's lead, a year later,
a survey that did list general types of insurance failed to divulge crucial specifics about capitated care arrangements, profit-sharing incentives restricting care, and known severe limits on palliative care benefits
that favor assisted suicide over good care.[16]

OHD also remained entirely silent about the results of one vital question it asked. Assisted suicide activists had reassured the public that once
the law was passed, patients would make this life-and-death decision in
collaboration with a doctor with whom they had a long-term and trusting relationship. They claimed such a relationship might provide some
kind of safeguard. On the other hand, opponents of assisted suicide
pointed out that it would often be given by doctors who barely knew the
patient or who had a strong interest in advocating assisted suicide.

Because of this controversy, it made sense that OHD would ask how
many patients got assisted suicide from their own doctor versus how
many obtained the fatal overdose after referral from an assisted suicide
group, such as Compassion in Dying or the Hemlock Society. Yet OHD
left the answer to this question, and this question alone, out of the report.[17] It was later determined that the first fifteen assisted suicide cases
reported involved fourteen different doctors. Compassion in Dying, an
out-of-state assisted suicide group that moved to Oregon just weeks after
the law was implemented, claimed eleven of the fourteen doctors were
theirs.[18] The *Oregonian* also documented that at least one additional case

came through the Hemlock Society.[19] So at least twelve of fourteen, or 86 percent, of the assisted suicide cases were handled by groups politically active in promoting legalization of assisted suicide. This unsettling fact was the one held back, suggesting to many that OHD had become selective in its silence, failing to report disturbing facts and emphasizing the reassuring.

Secrecy in the Classroom

Reticence to talk openly about the results of Oregon's venture into assisted suicide has not been confined to departments of psychiatry or highly publicized official reports. It has even permeated small classrooms in community colleges.

On December 3, 1999, Cathy Hamilton, a licensed mental health counselor, took a continuing education class on how to counsel patients about assisted suicide at Portland Community College.[20] She was surprised to find that all the teachers in the day-long seminar were widely known, politically active assisted suicide proponents, only one of whom was actually a practicing clinician. No faculty member was there to discuss how to help patients overcome suicidal despair. When, despite careful editing of cases, several disquieting facts about actual assisted suicide attempts were revealed, one of the instructors went so far as to demand that students not talk to anyone about anything that was said during the class.[21] The counselor was dismayed when George Eighmey, the executive director of Compassion in Dying in Oregon, followed her down the hall insisting that she not reveal important clinical problems raised in the class. Despite the fact that no patients had been named or identified in the discussions, as soon as some clinical problems became apparent, this assisted suicide activist suddenly switched from touting his cases to demanding silence.

Such selective insistence on silence has also been demonstrated in national continuing education classes taking place in Oregon. For example, a Compassion in Dying speaker openly criticized a co-panelist at a national meeting of medical board regulators for discussing a previously published case. This conference included central agency administrators, professional board members, even some legislators, as well as investigators. The moderator said he had organized the panel because Oregon, by its statute legalizing assisted suicide, had provided a "laboratory" for the concept of assisted suicide. To further the discussion, the panel had been titled "Oregon's Death with Dignity Act: Health Care Professionals Speak Out on Its Impact." Yet when the only health care provider on the panel did speak out about problems with the adequacy of treatment and with complications in one case, Eighmey chastised, "And it is unfortunate that Dr. Hamilton refers to that case."[22] It is highly unusual in medical and scientific circles to attempt to silence discussion about complications in any procedure, yet the political environment created by legalizing assisted suicide has created a taboo against candid discussion.

The Patrick Matheny case, which Eighmey did not wish to have openly discussed, was originally brought to light by assisted suicide activists themselves. These political advocates obviously hoped to promote it to the media as an "ideal" case—before things went amiss.

Newspaper reports revealed that Matheny, a man with amyotrophic lateral sclerosis (ALS), was highly ambivalent about assisted suicide and changed his mind at least once.[23] There were indications that he might be suffering from the effects of untreated alcohol addiction or abuse (a leading contributing cause of suicide of all kinds), since it was stated that he had always expected to die not from ALS but from liver failure caused by excessive alcohol consumption. Issues of diagnosis and treatment of potential causes of his suicidal feelings receded into the background. The major question in his life now increasingly seemed to be framed by those closest to him and by the press as one of when he was going to take the lethal overdose of drugs he had received in the mail—not how he was going to live as well as possible, whatever life remained for him.

It is not known if appropriate referrals for a life-sustaining palliative care consultation or antidepressant medication, psychotherapy, alcohol treatment, or family support were made or not. Such knowledge would be important, considering the finding that even in Oregon 46 percent of those who receive such interventions change their minds about assisted suicide.[24] The fact that a large percentage of Oregon patients receive no such intervention[25] is an indication that end-of-life care in Oregon is inadequate for patients who finally become so desperate as to ask for assisted suicide.

When Matheny did eventually undertake suicide, with no doctor in attendance, because of his medical condition he had difficulty swallowing the large number of pills. He could not complete his suicide attempt and tried again the next morning. After he could not complete the second attempt, his brother-in-law said he "helped" him die and complained that Oregon's suicide law discriminates against those who cannot swallow.[26]

Immediately, doctors and other citizens demanded that the prosecutor investigate the death, because suffocation of the patient or lethal injection, both of which are illegal, even in Oregon, have been the most frequent methods of "helping" someone whose assisted suicide attempt fails. The body, however, had been cremated within a day; consequently, no autopsy could ascertain the actual cause of death. And the Coos County prosecutor refused to pursue the case, apparently without ever questioning the only witness. Instead, he made public comments that individuals who are disabled by being unable to swallow should have the "right" to assisted suicide, as long as they are otherwise qualified.[27] It is clear that the assistance the prosecutor had in mind was lethal injection. But the Oregon public had been promised assisted suicide would not include lethal injection, because that clearly gives power and control to doctors and nurses and the organizations for which they work.

This case raised the important issue those opposing legalized assisted suicide had been mentioning throughout Oregon: once assisted suicide is allowed, the practice cannot be limited to oral assisted suicide alone. Through judicial revision, as assisted suicide and euthanasia activist Stephen Jamison strategized,[28] legalized oral assisted suicide will inevitably bring in lethal injection for those whose attempts fail, and, consequently, for others.

In response to further inquiry about this case from Senator Neil Bryant of the Oregon state legislature, Oregon's deputy attorney general issued an official opinion[29] indicating that lethal injection may need to be accepted once assisted suicide is accepted, because Oregon's assisted suicide law does not provide equal access to its provisions for disabled people who cannot swallow and thus may violate the Americans with Disabilities Act.[30] He issued this opinion much to the dismay of advocates for the disabled in Oregon.

No wonder assisted suicide activists did not want this case discussed once it went awry. The case prematurely made obvious to many what opponents of assisted suicide had observed from the beginning, and even some assisted suicide activists admitted:[31] that assisted suicide is a strategy to introduce lethal injection or infusion and other more efficient forms of medicalized killing once the failure of oral overdoses is recognized. The use of lethal injections when assisted suicide attempts have failed has been documented by Dutch investigators,[32] and the rationale for accepting euthanasia as a consequence has been put forth in the *Oregon Health Law Manual*,[33] a publication of the Oregon Bar Association.

Forty-Eight Hours to Death

While members of the assisted suicide movement considered it "unfortunate" that anyone should continue to discuss the Matheny case, Compassion in Dying had another case on which it wished to focus. The case was described as follows by Eighmey in a talk given to state regulators about Oregon's experience with physician-assisted suicide:

> I conclude with just one example of one patient who used Oregon's Death with Dignity under our guidance and direction and assistance. I received a call from a woman who was desperate, while driving back from Coos Bay, after visiting another patient, Pat Matheny, in fact. She said, "I can't take it any more. My husband is begging me to kill him. I cannot stand his continued suffering any more. I love him too much." I begged her to wait and she said, "Unless you're at the door with the pills, don't come." I said, "I cannot be there with the pills, I don't do that." But wait—I arrived at her door, she opened the door, and as with a lot of people who are in emotional states, she saw me and started laughing and crying simultaneously and I hugged her and I walked in and we sat for three hours, talking to her husband and to her at length about the process. Fortunately, her . . . ah . . . his physician had already noted in the file that he had asked for Oregon's Death With Dignity fifteen days prior, so the time had elapsed. So we said, you have to ask for it a second time and you have to put it in writing. And then forty-eight hours after the writing you may obtain the prescription. The day that he obtained the prescription we three Compassion in Dying members were present, the wife, the two friends across the street, and we were preparing everything. He came up and asked, "What do I wear, and where do I go?" We said, "You might do it in bed, or do it wherever you wish, but we recommend that you do it in bed." And he said, "You know what I'm going to wear?" And I said, "No." "Well, my wife gave me a pair of silk pajamas twenty-five years ago and I have never worn them." So he slipped on his silk pajamas, crawled into bed, and we left [him] and his wife together for a while. We came in with the medication and we said, "Now you have the choice to change your mind at any time. Please, please do not feel compelled to do this." And he said, "I want to do it. I have had a beautiful life, I have had a loving wife, and it is my time. I said goodbye to this earth." We handed it to him; he took it and he turned to his wife and said to his wife, "I love you very much. We had a good life." In five minutes he was in a deep coma,

and died in seventeen minutes. And that is what being open and honest and above-board and regulated by a state statute means in the state of Oregon. We have compassion for people who wish to die with dignity.[34]

Eighmey made no apparent attempt to disguise this case using available medical guidelines to protect patient confidentiality; nor did he mention whether he had obtained written permission from the patient, his family, or the doctors involved to discuss the case. This case raises some important questions about the psychological state of the patient's wife, the assessment of the patient's competency in making decisions, and the role of advocacy groups and a lay advocate acting as a support to the patient and family. What were the medical issues involved? What were the psychological issues? Was the patient appropriately evaluated?

Perhaps the fact that Eighmey mistakenly identified the physician as the wife's doctor and then had to correct himself to say that it was the patient's doctor was a small and insignificant error. On the other hand, it may illustrate what is so clear in most Compassion in Dying cases: that the primary alliance seems to be with the healthy family member, not with the vulnerable patient.

What is certain, however, is that this assisted suicide proponent considered it fortunate that the normal fifteen-day waiting period, could, in his view, be circumvented. This case suggests that assisted suicide proponents have little respect for the fifteen-day waiting period, which had been written into the law as a safeguard against impulsive suicides. And this speaker had found a loophole to circumvent it. The clock had been set in motion and was ticking. It was only forty-eight hours to death.

Perhaps the speaker felt confident using this loophole because he trusted his own impressions so implicitly. As is common with some individuals new to a medical setting, he had become unduly impressed with his own ability to understand and interpret the facts. As he put it, patients "tell me more in [a] half-an-hour phone call than they sometimes will tell their physician or their spouse. I know more about their life history in that half an hour than a lot of other people close to them." Evidently, such confidence led him to feel quite sure of his understanding of the life-and-death issues very quickly.

It is not known why the attending physician did not think assisted suicide was appropriate for this case. Neither is it clear why he noted the request for assisted suicide in the chart. Perhaps he was documenting suicidal ideation as a symptom of depression. Perhaps he did not agree to the assisted suicide because he considered the patient ineligible. There is no way to tell.

We know only what this assisted suicide activist said about the case. He made no mention of whether the patient's doctor was even consulted, much less his reasons for not agreeing to the assisted suicide, only that assisted suicide was somehow noted in the chart more than fifteen days previously.

This case is also typical in that once an assisted suicide group was contacted, there was little mention of making arrangements for additional consultation from a palliative care or pain care clinic, much less a social worker to help the wife deal with her distress or a psychiatrist competent in treating depression or anxiety in those who are seriously ill. It is not known whether this was one of those many Oregon cases that do not receive a "substantive palliative intervention" and consequently do not change their minds about assisted suicide.[35] Undoubtedly, mention of palliative care was made on the written form, but a concerted effort to improve palliative care was unlikely to have been made, as has been documented on previous tape-recorded interviews.[36] Instead of a considered and life-sustaining approach, it was simply gratitude at the fact that the fifteen-day requirement could be circumvented.

At the end of this discussion, the moderator reminded the audience that Oregon has provided a "laboratory" for assisted suicide. Yet at this discussion of the assisted suicide "laboratory experiment"—a term many consider dangerously cold and sterile—the results of the "experiment" were a closely guarded secret, with only assisted suicide proponents claiming freedom to discuss the cases.

Kaiser Permanente Speaks Out for Silence

Health maintenance organizations (HMOs) have joined the chorus demanding that the shroud of secrecy draped over assisted suicide in Oregon not be lifted, except when it serves their purposes to do so. As an example, Kaiser doctors and administrators freely discussed a case involving a woman named Kate Cheney with the press, even releasing copies of confidential psychiatric consultation reports to the area's largest newspaper.[37] They made no attempt to disguise the case. Neither did they mention written consent to discuss the details, although, as will be seen, it is far from clear that the patient would have been competent to provide such consent. Kaiser officials moved forward in revealing selective details of the case until an outcry about possible mishandling of this case arose from doctors. Then, Kaiser suddenly claimed public discussion of the case was no longer appropriate.

Cheney (whose case is presented in more detail in the previous chapter) was an eighty-five-year-old woman with growing dementia who had cancer. The psychiatrist who evaluated her found her ineligible for assisted suicide because of her obvious cognitive impairments and because her family appeared to be pressuring her. She could not remember recent events and people, including the names of her hospice nurses and her new doctor. When the psychiatrist said she was not eligible for assisted suicide, Cheney appeared to accept the decision without protest. The daughter and the new doctor (who had been obtained at the daughter's, not the patient's, request) did not accept the opinion as the safeguard it was intended to be. Instead, they sought another opinion from a second mental health professional. This psychologist also determined that the patient could not remember when she was diagnosed with terminal cancer, although it had only been a few months ago. She wrote that the patient's "choices may be influenced by her family's wishes and that her daughter, Erika, may be somewhat coercive." Nevertheless, she approved the suicide. The final decision about which mental health consultation to accept was made by a single Kaiser physician-administrator, Dr. Robert Richardson. He approved giving a lethal overdose to this elderly woman under pressure from her family.

Kaiser Permanente is a fully capitated HMO with cost-saving incentives for its doctors. Whether Richardson's loyalty to his organization during this era of cost containment, not to mention a personal profit motive, might have played even the smallest role in contributing to his motivations and biases concerning this case cannot, of course, be determined. Nevertheless, several people pointed out that this case illustrates how once assisted suicide is legalized, there is no way to protect those who are vulnerable and mentally ill from social or even financial pressures.[38]

Once public discussion of this case turned less than flattering to the HMO's handling of the case, suddenly Kaiser officials claimed there should be no more discussion. Richardson quickly sent a nationally broadcast e-mail claiming that medical comments unfavorable to his handling of the case were "hurtful," "deeply offensive," and "mean-spirited."[39] The regional medical director of Kaiser Permanente, Allan Weiland, even jumped into the fray by writing an opinion piece in the *Oregonian* in an apparent attempt to quell public discussion.[40] In it, he called for silence, chastising *Oregonian* journalist Dave Reinhard, claiming that he should not raise questions about or worry about Kaiser's conduct, but that, instead, "he should worry about the impact of his opinions on Kate Cheney's family . . . and on the health professionals." While all of us would like to protect the family of a deceased patient and health care professionals, Weiland failed to recognize that it was Cheney herself, the vulnerable patient, who most needed protection.

After this case was revealed, Kaiser no longer mentioned that Richardson and others at a Kaiser conference titled "When the Diagnosis Is Terminal"[41] had proclaimed that four of the cases in the first Oregon report were Kaiser HMO cases. The clarion call was for silence.

Silence about Cases Referred for but Not Given Assisted Suicide

Even the few available surveys veil secrets behind their statistics. Little is known, for example, about the adequacy of treatment of the large number of patients whom studies show may request assisted suicide yet are not given the lethal overdose by their doctors.

There is no mention of the woman in her mid-fifties with severe heart disease who requested assisted suicide from her cardiologist, despite having little discomfort and good mobility. She was referred to another doctor, who in turn referred her to a physician willing to provide assisted suicide. That doctor determined that the woman had more than six months to live, according to his best estimate. Therefore, she was eventually dismissed as ineligible. Rather than inquire further into possible causes of or treatments for suicidal despair in this patient, the physician apparently considered his job finished, his responsibility ended. With no more ado, he told her to go back and make yet another appointment with her original physician and dismissed her. She killed herself the next day.

In this case, even the doctors involved retrospectively recognized that the adequacy of diagnosis and treatment of suicidal despair in this ill woman was interfered with by framing the case solely in terms of the question, Is this woman or is she not eligible for assisted suicide? There was little thought given to the psychological effect of her doctors' being preoccupied with the legalities of assisted suicide instead of remaining clinically focused on how to help this woman overcome her suicidal feelings. Instead of receiving the careful diagnostic inquiry and treatment she needed, she was passed from one doctor to another and eventually dismissed as "ineligible," only to then kill herself the next day. I know of this case because one of the physicians involved told me about it and gave me permission to publish it provided the patient's identity was disguised. How many more such tragic deaths hide behind the few available statistics?

Subsequent Oregon Reports Hide More Than They Reveal

With the shortcomings of the first OHD report, one could have hoped that subsequent reports would have been more forthcoming. Instead, OHD has again confined its data collection to information provided by those needing to justify their recent participation in a patient suicide, although in 1999, but not 2000, OHD included the physicians who wrote lethal prescriptions and a few family members selected by these physicians.[42]

No independent review of the adequacy of palliative care or treatment of depression was done. The report merely listed the number of cases and provided reassurances that overlooked known failures to protect the mentally ill, involvement of HMOs in assisted suicide, and family pressure to commit assisted suicide.[43]

Nor did OHD report a known case of an assisted suicide attempt that failed. In this case, after a man took the prescribed overdose of barbiturates, with no doctor present, he lingered, suffering to the point where his wife called 911. Medical technicians helped save him and brought him to a hospital When he recovered he was released to a care facility where he was said to have later died, presumably of natural causes.[44]

This failure to report problem cases calls into question the credibility of all the OHD reports. In the same issue of the *New England Journal of Medicine* in which the second report appeared, Dutch researchers revealed that at least 18 percent of physician-assisted suicides in the Netherlands result in serious complications or fail to work at all.[45] These findings caused American euthanasia proponent Sherwin Nuland to write an editorial in the same issue, stating, "This is information that will come as a shock to the many members of the public—including legislators and even some physicians—who have never considered that the procedures involved in physician-assisted suicide and euthanasia might sometimes add to the suffering they are meant to alleviate and might also preclude the tranquil death being sought."[46]

With a sampling of sixty-nine reported cases over three years purporting to represent 100 percent of the cases, it would be exceedingly unlikely to find no cases of complications, with a base rate of serious complications estimated between 15 and 25 percent in the Dutch experience.[47]

Conclusion

A culture of silence has surrounded legalized assisted suicide in Oregon. It has permeated medical university departments, governmental agencies, continuing education classes, national discussions, and large HMOs. Attempts have even been made to silence open political debate in the press—except when the examples flatter those promoting or participating in assisted suicide.

Imposed silence about assisted suicide and euthanasia is not merely a technical implementation problem. The requirement of silence is at the very heart of the assisted suicide and euthanasia movement. Silence is required when assisted suicide is legalized, because medicine is regulated by the consciences and conventions of physicians more than by statute.

The Oregon Medical Practice Act, like laws regulating the practice of medicine in every state, mandates that physicians shall not engage in unprofessional conduct. The law goes on to define unprofessional conduct as being determined by the medical profession itself. It is medicine's ethics that are upheld by statute. The medical ethics outlined by the American Medical Association Code of Ethics have been widely accepted "as the primary compendium of medical value statements in the United States"[48] and as such have legal bearing on all physician behavior, regardless of whether a particular doctor belongs to that organization. Also, the standards and ethics of other professional organizations are taken into account in defining ethical professional conduct and legitimate medical practice.

With Oregon assisted suicide, however, not only is the giving of lethal overdoses to patients taken out from under the purview of the medical organizations, which clearly define it as unethical, the law actually forbids medical organizations to censure physicians for unethical conduct in this area. To censure does not mean to punish. It only means to criticize, to speak out, to protest verbally. So medical organizations can no longer even criticize physicians in Oregon who break the medical standards endorsed by virtually every medical organization in the country. This restriction not only applies to medical organizations, it applies to individual doctors and nurses, who are called "providers" under the law. No medical "provider" may criticize another for unethical conduct in this area.

This abridgment of free speech is at the very heart of Oregon's assisted suicide law.[49] If it were not for this prohibition against speaking out critically, the profession of medicine itself would limit, control, and make practically nonexistent assisted suicide, as it has numerous other unethical practices, without recourse to state criminal laws. For example, only a few states have statutes forbidding doctors from having sexual relations with their patients, yet public censure by colleagues, and medical societies and boards, sometimes followed by malpractice lawsuits, has drastically limited this abuse of power in the doctor-patient relationship. Consequently, those who wrote the Oregon assisted suicide law forbade medical organizations, and even individual physicians or nurses, from upholding their ethics and from declaring their opinion.

Some observers contend that a culture of silence about assisted suicide has developed in Oregon because of political pressure for and against it. Others assert that physician-assisted suicides are taking place under the cloak of secrecy in Oregon because even apologists for assisted suicide somehow sense that it is actually wrong or shameful and therefore almost instinctively hide it. Still others assert that the pall of silence merely arises from governmental and organizational expedience, another concession to what is sometimes termed "political correctness." Regardless of what other causes may also exist, it seems clear that the very nature of the Oregon assisted suicide law itself has contributed to, even laid the groundwork for and insisted on, a culture of silence.

The Oregon assisted suicide law states, "No professional organization or association, or health care provider, may subject a person to censure, discipline, suspension, loss of license, loss of privileges, loss of membership or other penalty for participating or refusing to participate in good faith compliance with ORS 127.800 to 127.897."[50] It is not an oversight that among all the other words of this long sentence are included the words "health care provider" and "censure." These words have been included because silence is the only basis on which legalized assisted suicide and euthanasia can continue. Once assisted suicide is allowed on this basis, the practice, in itself, demands more and more secrecy. Contrary to its promoters' promises, legalized assisted suicide has become a major contributor to Oregon's new culture of silence.

9

Deadly Days in Darwin

David W. Kissane, M.B., B.S., M.P.M., M.D.,
F.R.A.C.G.P., F.A.Ch.P.M., F.R.A.N.Z.C.P.

Seven patients entered Australian medical folklore during 1996–97, when for a period of nine months euthanasia was a legal medical treatment within the Northern Territory, a large, sparsely populated and mostly desert region of the north-central part of the country. Two men and two women died making use of this legislation, while three others attempted to but died from other causes. All seven people were patients of the euthanasia advocate Philip Nitschke, who subsequently permitted the author to go over each of their stories with him to prepare them for publication so that these historic medical facts could be placed on the public record.[1] This chapter reviews this unique Australian social experiment, looking especially at the clinical histories and decision-making processes involved for these seven patients, the role and effect of the relevant legislation, and the sociopolitical climate in which this remarkable tale evolved.

The Northern Territory, Australia

Representing one-sixth of the country's landmass, the Northern Territory has a population of nearly 180,000 people, one-quarter of whom are indigenous people. Like the Australian Capital Territory centered on Canberra, the Northern Territory does not have the full legislative powers of Australian states, and its laws are subject to review by the Commonwealth when it can be shown that its acts are in conflict with the views of the nation. However, it does have a parliament of twenty-five elected members, which sits in its capital, the modern city of Darwin—a city rebuilt after its 1974 destruction by tropical cyclone Tracey.

Many of the residents of the territory are transient and young, moving to the tropics to gain work for a few years before returning south again. Almost half of the deaths in the Northern Territory are of indigenous people, whose health status is often very poor. Thus the infant mortality rate is nearly twice that of the rest of the country, and the median age at death for men (53.9 years) and women (64.0 years) is almost twenty and sixteen years below the national Australian figure, respectively.[2] Aboriginal Australians die more commonly than other Australians from diabetes, circulatory, respiratory, infectious, and parasitic diseases as well as external trauma. Their languages do not have words for suicide or euthanasia, and there is a lack of interpreters to have their health needs addressed.[3]

The Anti-Cancer Foundation gave evidence to the territory's Select Committee Inquiry on Euthanasia about the lack of palliative care in the Northern Territory.[4] There was no dedicated oncology unit, no radiotherapy, and no dedicated palliative care unit or hospice before the legislation was introduced. A palliative care home nursing service was subsequently initiated in October 1995. There was the perspective that elderly, poor, and socially disadvantaged persons lacked access to good medical care, yet the barriers preventing such access were not investigated by this Select Committee on Euthanasia.[5] Key politicians moved headstrongly to create an act they termed the Rights of the Terminally Ill (ROTI) Act 1995, Northern Territory of Australia.[6] It was passed by thirteen votes to twelve on May 25, 1995, and enacted through passage of its regulations on July 1, 1996.[7] Australia became the first country in modern times to practice legalized rather than just sanctioned euthanasia.

The ROTI Act

Under this legislation, terminally ill patients who were experiencing pain, suffering, or distress to an extent deemed unacceptable could ask their medical practitioner to help them to end their lives. The provision of an opinion on the existence and terminal status of the illness was required by a second medical practitioner, a resident of the territory, who needed special expertise in the illness and qualifications in a medical specialty recognized by fellowship in a specialist college in Australia.

If the first medical practitioner did not have special qualifications in palliative care, defined by the regulations as either two years' full-time practice in palliative medicine or not less than five years in general practice, then a third doctor with such qualifications was required to give information to the patient on the availability of palliative care.

Finally, a psychiatrist was required to examine the patient and certify that he or she did not have a treatable clinical depression. The act required that a period of seven days pass between the initial request to end life made to the first doctor and the patient's signing of an informed consent form, witnessed by two medical practitioners. A further forty-eight hours later, assistance to end life could be provided.

A death as the result of assistance under the act was not taken to be unnatural, but a copy of the death certificate and relevant section of the medical record relating to the illness and death in each case had to be forwarded to the coroner. The coroner was subsequently required to report to the parliament the number of patients using the act.

The Euthanasia Activist, Nitschke

The intention of the law was that the person's usual doctor would occupy the role of the first medical practitioner, but instead it became filled by one doctor only, Philip Nitschke, a public advocate for euthanasia who volunteered to assist these patients. I first met Nitschke at educational meetings, where as a psychiatrist and professor of palliative medicine I was asked to debate issues involved in physician-assisted suicide and euthanasia. I expressed interest in learning more about the clinical details of his patients so that these could be written up as a historical record. He eventually agreed to my visiting him at his home in the outer suburbs of Darwin. A fellow academic with experience in ethnographic research, Annette Street, a medical sociologist, accompanied me, and, having obtained formal consent from Nitschke as prescribed by the university's ethics committee, we audiotaped eighteen hours of interview with him. As he reviewed his medical records, we explored the medical decision-making processes and reviewed the specialist opinions he had obtained. Analysis was also undertaken of documents from the coroner's court, public texts created by patients in the form of letters and televised documentaries, and other comments made by the media, rights groups, and politicians. Nitschke reviewed transcripts of the taped interviews for validation and carefully reviewed the clinical material that was jointly published in the first instance.[8]

Nitschke had not previously been involved with the care of terminally ill patients, having been a mature medical graduate from the University of Sydney in 1989. In earlier life, he had completed a doctorate of philosophy in physics from Flinders University in South Australia and then worked as a political activist for the Aborigines in the Wave Hill uprising against the pastoral company Vestey's. He spent a period as a ranger in the Northern Territory, living off the land whenever he "went bush." Once he had graduated as a medical practitioner, he did his internship at the Royal Darwin Hospital. There he led a protest by the junior medical staff of the hospital opposing nuclear disaster drills during the visit of a U.S. nuclear-powered ship into the Darwin harbor. In the following year, he was not reappointed to the junior medical staff and initiated Discrimination Tribunal action against the Darwin Hospital; eighteen months later, he won. In the interim, he had worked as a locum general practitioner and became a member of the Northern Territory's Voluntary Euthanasia Society.

When the Australian Medical Association, Northern Territory branch, declared its opposition to the ROTI Act, he publicly declared his willingness to assist patients with euthanasia. From that day, he became a constant media personality campaigning for the introduction of the regulations and availability of the act. Patients began to seek him out for assistance in accessing the ROTI Act, and he developed what he called his "deliverance machine," a computer that asked patients to confirm their intention to die and wish to proceed by further pressing the computer's spacebar. His publicized technique involved the insertion of an intravenous line and preparation of a barbiturate to induce sleep, which was then followed by a muscle relaxant medication to induce paralysis and respiratory arrest, leading to death. Via simple machinery, the computer regulated the introduction of these agents into the intravenous fluid, once the patient had again confirmed his or her desire to die.

Nitschke was constantly traveling because of his political activities, and he was not generally able to provide continuity of care as the regular care attendant to patients who sought him out. Rather, he solicited opinions from specialists to meet the regulations of the act and thus coordinated the preparation of the patients for euthanasia. Before the act officially became law on July 1, 1996, two patients made dramatic public appeals to hasten the passage of the regulations, each supported by Nitschke as an advocate for their right to access euthanasia. The first of these, a woman named Marta Bowes, appeared on the *60 Minutes* television show,[9] while the second, Max Bell, made a dramatic 3,000-kilometer journey from Broken Hill to Darwin, documented by the Australian Broadcasting Commission as *The Road to Nowhere*.[10]

Cries for Euthanasia

The stories of these two patients are indicative of people who seek euthanasia.

Marta was a divorced sixty-eight-year-old teacher and member of the Hemlock Society who flew to Australia from New Mexico declaring that she had terminal cancer. Her postmortem revealed that this was not true. Early-stage bowel cancer had been newly diagnosed in the United States, but Marta declined surgery, fearing altered body image should a colostomy prove necessary. She made a serious suicide attempt in Albuquerque following her diagnosis of cancer, taking an overdose of insulin that necessitated admission to intensive care. There appeared to be deep-seated reasons for her unhappiness, including the death of her daughter in earlier years and estrangement from her son in recent years. Alienated and with few friends, her campaign on national Australian television and through letters to the press argued passionately for access to managed death. Her eventual suicide from barbiturate overdose concluded a life latterly marred by an untreated depressive disorder, masked by her dramatic campaign for euthanasia.

Wanting to comply with the requirements of the ROTI legislation, Nitschke arranged for Marta to be examined by a psychiatrist-in-training, who returned the observation that she denied feeling depressed. His records showed no elaboration of details about her rift with her son, but Marta later broke down with a television reporter when pressed for details about this relationship. That very evening she became further distressed and called Nitschke, threatening immediate suicide. He dissuaded her from impetuous action, but she maintained her desire to die and did commit suicide three weeks later.

The autopsy confirmed an early-stage bowel cancer and death from barbiturate overdose, supplemented by asphyxia. The coroner determined that Marta had committed suicide on September 24, 1995, in a hotel room in Darwin. In the coroner's file was a copy of a letter, dated August 25, 1995, to a member of the Voluntary Euthanasia Society of New South Wales, describing that Marta now had a kit with enough barbiturate to kill, and adding, "Now I have advice that I have the correct amount and I will have a relative and a doctor with me until I am gone. I plan my final exit at the end of September." The coroner's file included an English translation of a book of her Spanish poetry written in earlier years, which was found on a coffee table beside her in the hotel room in which she died. Among these poems were some describing her nostalgic and loving feelings for her son.

The second person involved in the public campaign in the lead up to the ROTI Act was Max Bell, who drove his taxi 3,000 kilometers from his outback home to Darwin, also seeking euthanasia. Single, isolated, and somewhat cantankerous, this sixty-four-year-old man described on national television the meaninglessness of his life.[11] He said, "I'm just existing. I can't see the point anymore. I've seen my time. I'm ready for the sweet long sleep." A gastric cancer had been diagnosed one year earlier. Bell believed he could access the ROTI legislation if he traveled to Darwin, but as appeals were proceeding through the Supreme Court and doubt existed at that time that the legislation would become law, this man returned to Broken Hill. He subsequently died a natural death.

The sad plight of these individuals as they told their stories showed the force of tragic human narrative in influencing public opinion. The euthanasia societies used every opportunity to capitalize on the sensational press over this period. Such reporting promoted adversarial and entrenched positions, which may have actively prevented such individuals from accessing the medical care that might have appropriately assisted them. For example, the medical reports provided by Nitschke to the coroner in his investigation into the death of Marta Bowes cited twelve consultations with her between July 4 and September 23. His prescriptions included analgesics for pain relief and a tranquilizer and a barbiturate for sleep. His record on September 16 noted, "Increasingly talking of ending her life, tried repeatedly to dissuade her to no avail, became angry when I persisted." On September 23, his record concluded, "No sign of depression. Repeated her intention to carry out her wish, unable to convince her otherwise." She died twenty-four hours later. Nitschke did not invoke the Mental Health Act to protect Marta from being a danger to herself in wanting to commit suicide, which one could argue was his duty of care. Rather, he believed in her right to commit suicide and lamented the unavailability of legislation that would assist her to achieve her wish. For others that followed, however, that legislation became law.

The ROTI Act Becomes Law: Bob Dent's Death

The first patient to make use of the ROTI Act was Robert Dent, who suffered from metastatic prostate cancer and died in his Darwin home from euthanasia on September 22, 1996. A prominent Sydney psychiatrist, John Ellard, subsequently told the media of his willingness to fly to Darwin to examine Dent and certify, as required by the ROTI Act, that he was not suffering from a treatable depressive disorder. Dent himself published a posthumous letter to the nation in which he said:

> For months I have been on a roller coaster of pain made worse by the unwanted side effects of the drugs. Morphine causes constipation—laxatives work erratically, often resulting in loss of bowel control in the middle of the night. I have to have a rubber sheet on my bed, like a child who is not yet toilet-trained. Other drugs given to enhance the pain-relieving effects of the morphine have caused me to feel suicidal to the point that I would have blown my head off if I had had a gun.
>
> I can do little for myself. My red cells are decreased in number and deformed because of the cancer in the bone marrow. This anaemia causes shortness of breath and fainting.
>
> My own pain is made worse by watching my wife suffering as she cares for me; cleaning up after my "accidents" in the middle of the night, and watching my body fade away. If I were to keep a pet animal in the same condition I am in, I would be prosecuted. I have always been an active, outgoing person, and being unable to live a normal life causes much mental and psychological pain, which can never be relieved by medication.[12]

During his middle years as a carpenter, a building venture in Adelaide led to financial difficulties and a period of depression, treated with medication and counseling for some time. During his latter years in Darwin, Dent watched colleagues die "bloody horribly" and feared a similar fate.[13] Visiting nurses noted that he wept frequently; Nitschke observed angry exchanges in Dent's household. The full complexity of his circumstances was not, in my opinion, well understood through a single assessment by a visiting psychiatrist supportive of the euthanasia legislation.

Dent's prostate cancer was metastatic on diagnosis in 1991 and managed with antiandrogen approaches. In 1995 he first needed transurethral resection of the prostate for blockage of urinary flow. While he traveled to Perth for unproven therapies utilizing microwaves, he did not travel to Adelaide for radiotherapy for bone pain. However, Nitschke did not consider his pain to be excessively troublesome, but rather recalled him weeping, saying he felt it pointless to continue suffering. Dent's regular care providers were not told that he was being assessed for euthanasia, and they were shocked to learn of his death. Although Dent's wife was present, his sons who resided in another state were unaware. Cremation was excluded under the ROTI Act but was sought in the Buddhist tradition. The coroner was therefore required to hold an inquiry to determine cause of death before permission was granted for cremation.

Janet Mills, The Second Euthanasia Death

The second person to receive euthanasia had also become a public figure. Janet Mills was a small fifty-two-year-old married woman who wore a beanie on her head during national media presentations. Although she had been ill for twelve years with mycosis fungoides, it had become systemic since 1994 and was treated with chemotherapy without resolution of her skin itch. Her general practitioner had treated her depression with an average dose of an antidepressant. Records of her psychiatric examination revealed loss of interest and pleasure, lowered mood, poor concentration, insomnia, reduced reactivity to her surroundings, hopelessness, helplessness, a sense of worthlessness, and a strong desire to die. Clearly, she suffered from a severe major depression with poor response to initial antidepressant treatment. Unfortunately, a forensic psychiatrist who lacked experience in working with those who are medically ill reviewed her case. He judged her depression to be "consistent with her medical condition" and added that side effects might limit further increases in the dose of her antidepressant medication. This judgment blocked her access to a range of potentially effective treatments that might have altered her subsequent choices.

When Mills first traveled from another state to Darwin, Nitschke looked for a specialist who would provide the second medical opinion. Two surgeons agreed to see her and then withdrew; one physician assessed her and declined to certify that she was terminally ill. There was no attention to her depression over this time, as the focus was on bureaucratic processes. After Mills made a public appeal on national television for a specialist to come forward and confirm that she was terminally ill, an orthopedic surgeon was driven to compassion and agreed to see her, subsequently certifying that the ROTI Act had been complied with.

Having obtained the necessary signatures, she returned home to bid farewell to her family before returning to Darwin to receive euthanasia on January 2, 1997. The coroner of the day ignored the breaches of the regulations.

The Next Two Deaths

The identities of the next two people to make use of the ROTI Act have remained confidential. The third, a man, appeared totally isolated, while Nitschke obtained permission from the son of the fourth patient, a woman, to tell her story in an anonymous manner.

The first was an isolated English migrant who lacked family in Australia. He had suffered from gastric cancer and developed jaundice from compression of his common bile duct by tumor. Usual management options involving stenting of his common bile duct did not appear to be pursued. This man was indecisive over a two-month period, commenting on the pointlessness of his life but not able to make the final decision. His exploration of access to the ROTI Act appeared based on a sense of hopelessness and meaninglessness and a demoralized mental state, but not a formal depressive disorder. A superficial examination by a psychiatrist, which did not occur until the day of his death and which lasted only twenty minutes, provided indirect confirmation of his sense of his life's pointlessness. From the psychiatrist's office, he was taken home to a musty house that had been shut up for several weeks. Nitschke had to hunt for sheets to cover the bare mattress. It rained heavily in Darwin that summer afternoon, and in administering euthanasia Nitschke felt sadness over the man's loneliness and isolation.

The fourth euthanasia patient was flown in from another state. Suffering from breast cancer, this seventy-year-old divorced mother of five had recently watched her sister's death from the same cancer and been horrified by what she perceived to be the indignity of double incontinence. She feared she would die in a similar manner. She was also concerned about being a burden to her children, although all three daughters were trained nurses. She had stayed with one daughter over six months of chemotherapy treatment for retroperitoneal lymphatic spread of her tumor that caused lymphedema of her legs. There appeared to be little response to her chemotherapy, and so her son arranged her transport to Darwin. All five children traveled with her and were present to say farewell in the hotel apartment before she died.

Esther Wild: Final Case at the Closure of the Act

The seventh case in this series was a woman, Esther Wild, who met the requirements of the act but deferred her death until she was ready; in the interim, the act was repealed. She was a fifty-six-year-old woman with advanced cancer. Following initial diagnosis in 1977 and a prolonged period of remission until 1991, she then needed extensive abdominal surgery to resect the tumor but was left with bilateral leg swelling. She retired from her nursing job at that stage. Further recurrence in 1996 necessitated bowel bypass surgery to overcome an obstruction, but she was left with a colostomy. She developed an antibiotic-resistant infection of her wound drain tube, leaving her with a smelly persisting discharge through a permanent fistula. She was troubled with its odor, but fortunately medication lessened the discharge.

Over subsequent months, she gradually became more and more unhappy. She stopped reading, ceased letter writing, and withdrew from friends. Having thought increasingly about euthanasia, she completed the necessary documentation, but she did not yet want to die. A team of nursing friends supported her in her home with the help of her general practitioner. In the interim, on March 25, 1997, the Commonwealth government repealed the ROTI Act. One month later, her general practitioner's medical record described her as mentally and physically exhausted, more distressed than ever before, and now actively suicidal. As she sat with a fixed gaze, she displayed psychomotor retardation indicative of a serious depression. No one seemed to consider treatment of her depression.

Instead, as a protest at the repeal of the legislation, a television documentary was made about her death from prolonged sedation. Film clips were shot every few hours, interspersed with a commentary by Nitschke about progress in getting her to die. Nitschke administered massive doses of narcotics and sedatives. The autopsy showed death from bronchopneumonia with mixed drug overdose, but the coroner decided in the difficult political climate to take no further action. Such management of a patient clearly involved a poor standard of medical care and the classic mistake of failing to obtain a second opinion when the management appeared hard going. Esther Wild died prematurely, and although she consented to the treatment she received, she was not in my opinion fully informed of other potential options of care. Her depression, the cause of much of her suffering, went untreated.

Although not a large series, these seven deaths are important for their completeness as a sample of patients who actively sought euthanasia during this period of controversial legislation in Australia. Moreover, because their clinical histories have been able to be examined, the effectiveness of the legislation can now be assessed from a much more informed position.

Safety and Effectiveness of the ROTI Legislation

The legislation did not precisely define what was meant by "the terminal status" of a patient, leaving this up to the judgment of the two key medical practitioners involved. This cast them in a gatekeeping role. The second medical practitioner was to be a specialist with expertise in the patient's disease. One might have expected this to be a medical or radiation oncologist for patients with cancer, but instead we found that surgeons filled this role. Clearly they are involved in the diagnosis and initial management of cancer, but in Australia, ongoing care is usually then transferred to a cancer specialist. There was one oncologist working in Darwin by the time the act became law, but Nitschke found that within this community only surgeons were willing to certify that the patient was terminally ill, a curious state of affairs!

The purpose of the regulations was to protect the broader community and in particular vulnerable patients while permitting a mentally healthy and rational individual to choose euthanasia for him- or herself. A key intent of the legislation was, however, to ensure that the patient did suffer from a terminal illness. The above cases illustrated how problems developed with this assessment of prognosis, best exemplified when different specialists gave varied estimates of Janet Mills's potential length of life. There was no capacity within the regulations to deal with such a difference of opinion. Moreover, when an orthopedic surgeon came forward following Mills's public appeal for a certifying specialist and he did not have expert knowledge of mycosis fungoides, a rare tumor involving both the skin and lymphatic systems but not the bones, this was ignored by relevant authorities. Such breaches of the regulations were permitted by a legal system wanting to facilitate the legislation, thus removing the very safety features that had been designed to protect vulnerable patients.

The other gatekeeping role was that of the psychiatrist, required to protect a patient whose rational choice might be marred by a depressive disorder. This was the part of the certification schedule most feared by patients, and Nitschke reported that all seven patients saw this step as a hurdle to be overcome.[14] Fear of the power of the psychiatrist militated against the development of a therapeutic alliance, a trusting relationship through which one's story can be openly and honestly discussed, as is necessary for a thorough assessment. The protective intent of the legislation was not accomplished because of this barrier. Indeed, four of the seven deaths in Darwin revealed prominent features of depression, highlighting its strong role in decision making by those seeking euthanasia. Alarmingly, these patients went untreated by a system preoccupied with meeting the requirements of the act rather than delivering competent medical care to depressed patients.

Demoralization: An Unrecognized Yet Highly Pertinent Factor

Review of these patients' stories highlighted for me the importance of demoralization as a significant mental state influencing the choices these patients made.[15] They described the pointlessness of their lives, a loss of any worthwhile hope and meaning. Their thoughts followed a typical pattern that appeared to be based on pessimism, some exaggeration of their circumstances, all-or-nothing thinking, and negative self-labeling, and they perceived themselves to be trapped in their predicament. Often socially isolated, they were hopeless, leading to a desire to die, sometimes as a harbinger of depression, but not always with development of a clinical depressive disorder. It is likely that the mental state of demoralization influenced their judgment, narrowing their perspective about available options and choices. Furthermore, demoralized patients may not make a truly informed decision in giving medical consent. The third person to receive euthanasia in Darwin (name withheld) was an example of a demoralized patient, as was Max Bell.

Demoralization syndrome has been considered, albeit briefly, in the consultation-liaison psychiatry literature and is an important diagnosis to be made and actively treated during advanced cancer.[16] It is recognized by the core phenomenology of hopelessness and an inability to find meaning in life. The prognostic language within oncology that designates "there is no cure" is one potential cause of demoralization in these patients, a cause that can be avoided by more sensitive medical communication with those who are seriously ill. While truth telling is needed, hope must also be sustained so that life may be lived out as fully as possible. Patients with advanced cancer can be guided to focus on "being" rather than "doing," savoring the present, so that purpose and meaning in life are preserved through inherent regard for the dignity of the person. Active treatment of a demoralized state by hospice services would involve counseling and a range of complementary therapies, and use of community volunteers and family supports, all designed to counter isolation and restore meaning.

Fear of Loss of Dignity, Burden, and Dependence

Just as the Dutch mention fear of unworthy dying as a prime reason for euthanasia,[17] this Australian cohort considered concern about loss of dignity, becoming dependent on others, and potentially being a burden as prominent reasons for the request for euthanasia.[18] A considerable challenge exists in cancer care to protect patients from perceptions, based on earlier experience as onlookers, that their own journey and death will be similar to others'. Research has repeatedly shown how quality of life is appraised differently by patient, caregiver, and clinician.[19] A patient with cancer can adjust to the experience of gradual frailty over time, so long as adequate reassurance is given about the thoroughness of care along the way. Family onlookers can have a more difficult task, especially when the onlookers work or worked in medicine and have a variety of memories of decay, bodily disintegration, and disability, sometimes associated with revulsion and disgust.

One of the silent discourses within the medical community is the story of disgust at what is witnessed during everyday care. Bedsores, gangrenous limbs, smelly fistulas, and stomas—medicine is replete with horror tales of rotting bodily decay. Little research has evaluated how staff members cope with and adjust to these experiences by repressing the ugly in favor of the value of the whole person whom they have come to know. Undoubtedly for some, this experience is not easy. Families also need help to adapt to such predicaments, helping them remember the complete person rather than focusing on the failing bodily part. Open communication about such reactions is a vital means of debriefing, normalizing human response and affirming the courage involved. Family meetings occur all too infrequently, thus denying the opportunity for members to share feelings and transcend their initial human responses to adversity.

Acceptance of euthanasia by a family, as exemplified by case four, where five children traveled to Darwin with their mother, might subtly confirm to the patient that he or she would indeed be a burden, interfering with busy lives, and that any remaining length of life was unimportant. These unspoken messages have further profound effects on morale. Many elderly patients fear being a burden but seek reassurance and expression of gratitude for efforts in years gone by. Families are challenged to take care that they do not misunderstand a tentative suggestion by a family member that he or she might be a burden. As a clinician, I believe that patients who are convinced they are a burden have lost perception of their own worth, sacrificing their lives heroically to advantage their families. Exploration of such stories invariably reveals a demoralized perspective.

Repeal of the ROTI Act

Rather than a bill prepared by a political party, it was a private member's bill, the Euthanasia Laws Bill 1996, introduced into the Commonwealth Parliament of Australia on September 9, 1996, that sought to repeal the ROTI Act. It was introduced by Kevin Andrews, a member from Victoria, and parliamentarians were permitted a conscience vote rather than having to follow party line. While territorians attempted to argue that it was an issue of states' rights, most commentators focused on the appropriateness of the legislation itself. In Australia, the federal parliament can overrule the laws of its territories, although it cannot overrule state laws. Before this bill of repeal came into effect on March 25, 1997, the issue was thoroughly explored by a Senate Legal and Constitutional Legislation Committee.[20]

This body received 12,577 submissions, a record for our country, 93.3 percent of which were opposed to euthanasia.[21] Noteworthy were those from the indigenous community, which comprises nearly one-quarter of the Northern Territory's population. Concepts of euthanasia were unfamiliar to Aborigines, many dialects having no words for it. Providing assistance to make a person die was considered likely to be an instrument of sorcery or payback within their culture and traditionally regarded as morally wrong. Evidence was received that hospitals had become feared as places in which Aborigines could be killed without their consent. A submission from Reverend Djiniyini Gondarra stated, "Our ancient

Law/*Madayin* <u>does not empower</u> our Traditional *Närra*/Parliaments, to create Law/*Wäyak,* that gives an individual the right to take the life of another."[22] The Senate committee concluded that the ROTI Act had an unacceptable impact on the attitudes of the Aboriginal community toward health services.

Many other submissions testified to the importance of improving palliative care services and aiming at the delivery of quality medical care rather than empowering doctors to kill. Concern was expressed at the change that euthanasia would bring to this delivery of medical care, alluding to the complex decision making that goes on within a doctor's mind when he or she determines that a patient's life is no longer worthwhile. It was pointed out that the boundary transgression involved when a doctor has sex with a patient is similar to that involved when a doctor kills a patient.[23] The Commonwealth Parliament strongly upheld the bill that rescinded the ROTI Act.

The Euthanasia Debate in Australia

As in other countries, euthanasia societies were more active in Australia during the second half of the twentieth century, sponsoring a range of medical treatment bills similar to ROTI in state parliaments across the country.[24] Public opinion polls emphasized fear of pain and suffering in generating a rising tide of support for euthanasia.[25] Bioethicists Helga Kuhse and Peter Singer, amid others, surveyed doctors' and nurses' attitudes regarding voluntary euthanasia, using questions that blurred the boundary between respect for a natural dying process and killing the patient.[26] Community support for voluntary euthanasia was rising, while palliative care remained in its infancy in many sectors of the country.[27] Since ROTI, some of this has changed, with greater funding being made available for palliative care. The Northern Territory has developed a dedicated palliative care service in Darwin and other aspects of the region, but nationally there is still much to be done.

Our society's unspoken attitude toward dying merits some understanding. There is a reduced role for religion in promoting acceptance of dying for many in the community, and the belief that death is a transition to a heaven or another life has been replaced with the simple notion that life for that person ends. For such individuals, however, there is a wish, and indeed, a community expectation that they will die a heroic death.[28] With awareness of death approaching, such a patient, accompanied by family or caregivers, is encouraged to display acceptance calmly and courageously. However, for others whose death is feared to lie outside this script of insightful courage—those facing a death with too much suffering, loss of dignity, or feelings that their lives are meaningless—medically managed deliverance is perceived to bring welcome relief from a feared predicament. Euthanasia or physician-assisted suicide thus returns this person to an experience of heroism in the choice of a managed death, holding considerable public appeal to those otherwise contemplating some undignified manner of dying. Such attitudes continue to prevail in our Australian culture, in which medicine is perceived to omnipotently provide the technological solution to all suffering.[29]

Within this climate, Kuhse and Singer sought to further expose end-of-life decision making in Australia through a comparison of our medical practice with that reported by the Remmelink Commission appointed by the Dutch government in 1990 and restudied in 1995. The Netherlands and Australia have fairly similar populations and annual death rates. In conducting their study, Kuhse and her colleagues administered an English version of the retrospective questionnaire used by the Dutch, but without interviews to verify understanding.[30] Furthermore, they varied the wording of key questions to combine both actions or omissions that did not seek to prolong life with those aimed at hastening death. In the process they combined normal care that is respectful of natural dying with actions that hasten death. This conflation of the arguments about allowing to die and killing led to their grossly flawed conclusion that in 36.5 percent of all Australian deaths, a medical end-of-life decision was made with the explicit intention of ending the patient's life. The incorporation of actions or omissions aimed at not prolonging life would include a doctor who appropriately decided not to initiate futile intensive care or ventilatory support for a patient dying from terminal cancer. The wide range of ordinary treatment decisions that have nothing to do with intention to kill but were included in their questions, rendered any comparison with the Dutch meaningless.

Moreover, their utilitarian thinking equated the decision not to treat and the cessation of futile treatment with killing. Such thinking is flawed. For an action involving the omission of a treatment to carry culpability for causing death, the treatment must be proven to be clinically effective in the circumstances and the underlying condition potentially reversible.

As the dying process unfolds in a terminal patient, the condition becomes irreversible, and interventions could cause harm through prolonging the dying if they were inappropriately applied. "Moral equivalence" arguments based on outcome cannot ignore the assessment of clinical proportionality and appropriateness.

A sad consequence of their survey was the evidence it provided for widespread misunderstanding among Australian doctors about the contribution of morphine to death. Kuhse and colleagues claimed that 30.9 percent of deaths resulted from a probable life-shortening effect of opioids.[31] There is no determinative fatal dose of morphine; rather, it is the increment in dose relative to a prior dose that is relevant.[32] In pain management, gradual dose escalation by 50 percent to 100 percent of the previous dose is usual practice, although patients who are not new to the drug can usually tolerate substantially higher increases. Despite a sustained international campaign by the World Health Organization, appropriate opioid usage is surrounded by myths and fears among the general public and health care professionals, appearing to be largely attributable to the nonmedical use of this class of drug.[33] The survey work and public comment by Kuhse and Singer has sustained this mythology about opioids in a misinformed and damaging manner.

Palliative care is inevitably drawn into debates about euthanasia and physician-assisted suicide, creating an unfortunate comparison that proffers hospice as *the* solution, perpetuating the myth of an available answer to all suffering. Palliative care as an emerging new specialty has much to offer in providing excellence of care at the end of life, for indeed, there is much that can still be done. Major tasks remain to ensure broad coverage of palliative care in medical and nursing school curricula and to advance the distribution of hospice services so that they become equitably available to all. While we remain unable to guarantee the quality of medical care within our societies, there can be no place for euthanasia, but a vital need does exist for good palliative care.

Conclusion

The brief period of legalized euthanasia in Australia provided a useful window of opportunity to view the experience of such a social experiment. Despite considerable legislative effort to draft safe regulations that would protect vulnerable patients, review of the clinical accounts of patients who sought access to this legislation, made possible by the interviews with Nitschke, revealed blatant failure of the ROTI Act to achieve its purpose. Given the level of error that does occur in medical practice, this experience suggests it would be impossible to safely legislate for doctors to kill. Certainly, the gatekeeping roles designed by this act failed to protect depressed, isolated, and demoralized patients. Cast in a legislative and bureaucratic stance, these gatekeepers ceased to practice the craft of medicine, to the detriment of the patients they sought to serve.

Important lessons can be learned from this social experiment. They point to the need to develop palliative care, something that was a major failure of the government in the Northern Territory. They also highlight the distress that exists in society, the challenge that this brings to medicine, and the comprehensive responses—fiscal, social, political, and medical—that are needed to respond to suffering in our world.

We are challenged to better understand the dignity of the person, and fear of dependence, loss of control, and bodily decay, together with systemic responses that include family-centered care and adequate means of staff support. Disorders of hope and meaning warrant greater study alongside depression in those who are medically ill. But if there was a key lesson from the act permitting euthanasia in the Northern Territory of Australia, it was that it does not appear possible to safely legislate to grant autonomy for the few without creating danger to many other vulnerable individuals in society. We should continue to work to prevent suicide, including physician-assisted suicide by those who are medically ill.

Reason to Be Concerned

10

Not Dead Yet

Diane Coleman, J.D.

I n recent years, the disability community's opposition to legalization of assisted suicide and euthanasia has become increasingly visible. On June 22, 1996, members of the national press covered a protest by about forty disabled activists and nondisabled allies at the Michigan cottage where Jack Kevorkian lived.[1] This action was the first publicized announcement of the formation of the national grassroots disability rights group Not Dead Yet, created to give voice to this opposition. From the U.S. Supreme Court[2] to the U.S. Congress,[3] from medical, legal, and bioethics conferences to state legislatures and local news desks, more and more people have acknowledged that the disability community should have a seat at the debate table. While the struggle for a place at the table is far from over, the greater challenge may be to communicate the basis of our opposition to legalization of physician-assisted suicide in a manner that can be understood by nondisabled society as not only relevant but central to the debate.

In 1983 the case of Elizabeth Bouvia first dramatized the issue of physician-assisted suicide for the disability community. Bouvia, a woman in her mid-twenties with cerebral palsy, used a motorized wheelchair for mobility and had a slight speech impairment. Having already built a successful life, in spite of the damage done by being put in an institution at age ten, Bouvia went through a series of devastating ordeals. In the two years preceding her request for help in ending her life, her graduate program in social work at San Diego State University violated her federally protected civil rights.[4] Reportedly, one of her professors told her she was unemployable and that if they had known just how disabled she was, they would never have admitted her to the program. So Bouvia dropped out of school, and the state department of rehabilitation repossessed her wheelchair lift–equipped van.

Meanwhile, she married and kept her marriage secret from social welfare authorities in order not to run afoul of the "marriage disincentives" that would have cost her essential financial aid. She got pregnant, had a miscarriage, separated from her husband, decided to divorce him, and learned that her brother had drowned and that her mother had cancer.

At this point, Bouvia checked herself into the psychiatric unit of Riverside County Hospital and said she wanted help to starve herself to death while receiving morphine and comfort care. Bouvia's lawyers, led by Richard Scott, distorted the nature of her disability, likening her to a terminally ill patient. Instead of urging her to fight the university's discrimination, Scott, a Hemlock Society cofounder, wrote the following in his brief: "Were Plaintiff Bouvia an 84-year-old woman whose life was prolonged solely by various tubes and numerous machines, and she sought to end such an existence, it is doubtful that this Court would even be involved. . . . Plaintiff should not be denied that same right merely because she is 26 years of age and does not yet require a machine or machines (other than her wheelchair) to prolong her pitiful existence."[5]

A psychologist named Faye Girsh was one of a few mental health professionals who provided testimony that Bouvia was "competent" and her desire to die was rational, that her desire was based on her suffering from her permanent disability rather than any temporary despair caused by her recent traumas. A nondisabled woman facing similar traumas would have been found suicidal and therefore "incompetent," but Girsh, who later became the executive director of the national Hemlock Society, argued that Bouvia was "competent" and should not be treated as suicidal.

The disability community in the Los Angeles area wrote articles published in the local press[6] and even held a disability rights rally to protest the fact that the way Bouvia was being treated was different from the way a nondisabled woman would be treated. A disabled psychologist experienced in disability and suicide, Carol Gill, provided expert court testimony to refute that of Girsh and the other professionals. Ultimately, however, the appellate court found that Bouvia was like a terminally ill person, was not suicidal, and should have a so-called right to die. The court distorted Bouvia's medical problems in stating the following: "Petitioner would have to be fed, cleaned, turned, bedded, toileted by others for 15 to 20 years! Although alert, bright, sensitive, perhaps even brave and feisty, she must lie immobile, unable to exist except through the physical acts of others. Her mind and spirit may be free . . . but she herself is imprisoned and must lie physically helpless, subject to ignominy, embarrassment, humiliation and dehumanizing aspects created by her helplessness."[7]

In addition to inaccurately characterizing her medical condition, the *Bouvia* opinion expressed archaic views of disability, essentially ruling that disability was a sufficient basis to deny an individual the equal protection of laws and public policies related to suicide prevention. Fortunately, the court case took several years and, with time for her suicidal feelings to dissipate, Bouvia did not exercise her newly won right. The obviously erroneous court opinion, however, has been cited as precedent up to the present time.

Legal Aftermath

After *Bouvia*, a series of court challenges were brought involving people with nonterminal disabilities. These cases redefined terminal illness, heroic measures, suicide, and competence in a manner that gave legal sanction to the deaths of disabled individuals. A series of these cases in different parts of the country was increasingly referred to in the disability community as the "give me liberty or give me death" cases. In the last half of the 1980s, several disabled people presented that demand to society. Many people with high-level quadriplegia, who depend on ventilators to breathe, live independently in their own homes and apartments with "attendant services" or "personal assistance services" (the disability community's terms for "home care"). However, then and now, many ventilator users have been forced into nursing homes for lack of adequate insurance coverage of these services.[8] Since the 1960s, each state has legally been required to fund nursing home services but has had the flexibility to limit, or even exclude, Medicaid coverage for long-term in-home services. Both Medicare and private insurance have limited home health and long-term care services as well.

A number of individuals on ventilators who were involuntarily trapped in nursing homes were ignored when they demanded liberty, the freedom to live in the community. Others were ignored when they asked for the assurance that a family caregiver's illness or death would not rob them of their freedom and force them into nursing homes. But when David Rivlin, Larry McAfee, Kenneth Bergstedt, and others gave up the demand for freedom and asked to die,[9] there was no shortage of euthanasia advocates and lawyers to take their "right to die" cases to court: In each of these cases, the courts followed the *Bouvia* precedent. Courts compared these men, who clearly asked for freedom from nursing homes, to people who were imminently dying and asking for a natural death free of unwanted medical interventions (the ventilators these men had lived with for years). Courts ruled that their wish for death was not suicidal by definition (a legal fiction) and that the state did not have the usual interest in preserving their lives that would apply to a healthy person. It is clear that if Bergstedt had enjoyed sound physical health but had viewed life as unbearably miserable because of his mental state, his liberty interest would provide no basis for asserting a right to terminate his own life with or without the assistance of others.[10]

Rivlin and Bergstedt died when their ventilators were disconnected as a result of the court rulings. Only McAfee lived, not because the Georgia court ruled differently from courts in the other cases but because the disability community was able to mobilize the resources he needed to move from the nursing home into the community and return to computer-aided engineering before it was too late[11]—when McAfee got the freedom he demanded, he did not want death. He later testified before the Georgia legislature: "You're looked upon as a second-rate citizen. People say, 'You're using my taxes. You don't deserve to be here. You should hurry up and leave.'"[12]

These highly publicized cases were a "wake-up call" for the disability community. They demonstrated in no uncertain terms that the "right to die" movement did not confine its political agenda to people who were imminently dying from a terminal illness.

Although these cases involve the right to refuse treatment rather than assisted suicide—particularly since the U.S. Supreme Court ruled in *Cruzan* that all competent adults have a constitutional right to refuse treatment[13]—they highlight how prejudice regarding disability and failure to provide humane care for those who are disabled deprives patients who might otherwise want to live of the feeling that they have a choice. If an individual depends on a ventilator to live, the law concerning refusal of treatment recognizes no difference between someone who is imminently dying from a terminal illness who has not routinely used a ventilator, on the one hand, and someone who has used a ventilator successfully for years or decades, on the other. The decision-making or basic "competency" standard is the same and bears no resemblance to the standard applied to nondisabled suicidal people. Precipitating factors for suicide are not at issue. No questions need be asked about why the individual wants to die, simply whether he or she understands the medical diagnosis and prognosis. Disabled people have been criticized for challenging this simplistic application of the right to refuse treatment in the context of disability prejudice and discrimination, a cost-cutting health care system, and a medical profession abysmally ignorant about disability.

Not Dead Yet recognizes the need for laws permitting competent people to refuse treatment based on meaningful informed consent and meaningful availability of health care and related alternatives. Disabled people are intimately familiar, however, with the "gloom and doom" scenarios common in health care providers' descriptions of disability. Disabled people are intimately familiar with how frequently our legal rights are violated in the health care system. A superficial application of treatment refusal law virtually guarantees a lack of informed consent in the disability context. With 7,800 new spinal cord injuries each year[14] and an estimated 80,000 people acquiring long-term disability via head injuries yearly,[15] the risks to newly disabled people are staggering. Of equal concern, little or no data are being gathered to assess how these laws are in fact being implemented.

Although publicity in these cases has become rare, in 1999 two attracted public attention. The case of Georgette Smith involved a woman in Florida whose mother shot her after the mother overheard her daughter and her boyfriend planning to put her in a nursing home.[16] The mother was charged with attempted murder, but when Smith, who was now quadriplegic and on a ventilator, stated that she wanted her ventilator to be turned off less than three months after the injury, the implications for the criminal prosecution brought press attention. A local reporter contacted people at Shepherd Spinal Center, people involved in saving McAfee years before, questioning whether Smith could make a truly informed choice this soon after the injury. Quadriplegics using ventilators stated that in time she would change her mind but that at least six months was needed just to get through the medical trauma and initial phase of realization and adjustment. Under now-settled legal precedent, the potential, even the likelihood, that Smith would change her mind about wanting to die after a reasonable adjustment period to her disability had no bearing on when Smith's request to turn off the ventilator would be granted. More disabled than her mother at this point, she may have believed that she too had no meaningful alternative to a nursing home. Truly informed consent became irrelevant. The issue of Smith's death was settled quickly in the courts. Smith was able to have her ventilator shut off before disability advocates had a chance to see if explorations of her options would have changed her mind in favor of living.[17]

Another case arose in Rochester, New York, involving Bill White, a man who had been confined in a hospital for thirty-two years. No explanation was provided for this long-term confinement, although ventilator users who live in and around New York City pointed out that there appear to be no such individuals living freely in Rochester. White's mother, his primary visitor, had died two years before. When he had tried to commit suicide by spitting out his ventilator mouthpiece (he was not connected to the ventilator through a tube in his throat), he had asked for the mouthpiece back. This time he asked for medication to sedate him to preclude this reaction. This would have occurred without coming to the attention of the courts or the public, but for the fact that a friend of White's complained to the district attorney. This led the hospital to await a ruling from the authorities.[18]

During the days that ensued, the Disability Rights Center in Rochester rallied and held vigil, objecting to White's thirty-two-year confinement. The center alleged that this violated his civil rights under Titles II and III of the Americans with Disabilities Act of 1990,[19] which requires that people with disabilities receive long-term care services in the most integrated setting appropriate to their needs. The Disability Rights Center was denied legal standing to raise these civil rights violations in federal court as grounds for finding a lack of informed consent, which might have delayed White's death until he could first experience adult life outside a hospital. The hospital provided White the sedation he asked for to enable him to commit suicide by spitting out his ventilator on August 13, 1999.

Active Measures to Cause Death

Beginning in 1990, Jack Kevorkian provided a further wake-up call to people with disabilities—disabilities like multiple sclerosis, quadriplegia, and chronic fatigue syndrome. According to a study conducted at Wayne State University, 70 percent of Kevorkian's victims were people with nonterminal disabilities, applying the predicted-to-die-within-six-months definition.[20]

Kevorkian's last acquittal, in 1996, involved a forty-four-year-old woman with multiple sclerosis, a nonterminal disability that includes treatable depression among its common symptoms. Sherry Miller had been abandoned by her husband and lost custody of her children. She needed assistance in daily living activities and was forced to move in with her parents to get it. Kevorkian's defense was that he was only relieving suffering.

Without a doubt, Miller was suffering, but what were the causes of that suffering? Many people who acquire disabilities, especially women, lose their predisability spouse. In time, however, many establish new, more secure and enduring marriages and other relationships.[21]

Many disabled parents face child custody battles, and courts are notorious for custody-related discrimination.[22] In the Miller case, an ignorant press and public assumed, without question, that Miller could not participate meaningfully in the rearing of her children when she herself needed help in physical activities. But with appropriate consumer-directed in-home supports (less costly than nursing home care), the most severely disabled people have proven themselves successful parents. Because of social rejection and discrimination, Miller lost the relationships most important to her.

And then Kevorkian entered the scene, exploited her despair, and made her losses permanent. The press, public, judge, and jury agreed that he was motivated by compassion, in spite of ample evidence from his own writings about his actual policy agenda. In *Prescription Medicide*, Kevorkian explained his primary goals of live human experimentation and organ harvesting.[23] In a medical journal article, he discussed these goals in connection with death row prisoners, as well as adults with Alzheimer disease and babies with spina bifida.[24] His written testimony from his first prosecution also mentioned his motive to *"enhance* public welfare" through the "voluntary self-elimination of individual and mortally diseased or crippled lives taken collectively."[25] Nevertheless, increasingly popular with celebrities and the press, Kevorkian was released again.

Within a month of the Miller acquittal, Not Dead Yet was formed. During the next three years, Kevorkian assisted in the deaths of scores of people with nonterminal disabilities. It was as though "open season" had been declared on disabled people. Legal authorities refused to act. There were occasional questions raised, for example, when he assisted in the death of a woman who had previously called 911 regarding alleged spousal abuse,[26] or when he assisted the twenty-one-year-old paralyzed African American whose mother was a struggling single parent,[27] or when he did an amateurish job at removing a man's kidneys.[28] None of these individuals was terminally ill, but that was almost never mentioned or discussed in the public debate.

For charges to be brought that eventually put Kevorkian behind bars, he had to admit to committing active euthanasia and arrange for a videotape of the act to be broadcast on *60 Minutes,* along with an interview in which he dared the prosecutor to try to stop him. Charges were brought. For the first time, Not Dead Yet activists were able to attend a Kevorkian trial from start to finish. Outside the courthouse, the group distributed leaflets that included the following quote: "I will argue with them if they will allow themselves to be strapped to a wheelchair for 72 hours so that they can't move, and they are catheterized and they are placed on the toilet and fed and bathed" (Jack Kevorkian, *Time* magazine, May 1993).

Underneath the quote, the leaflet said, "This time, we're here, and we demand the equal protection of the law. Jail Jack." The group also spread over the ground outside the courthouse a giant "quilt" of posters depicting each Kevorkian victim; blue squares for those identified as terminally ill in the Wayne State University study, yellow for those identified as not terminally ill. The "quilt" was over two-thirds yellow.

"Death with dignity" is part of the title given to most legislative efforts to legalize assisted suicide. In the summer of 1996, Janet Good, the founder of the Michigan Hemlock Society and a collaborator in Jack Kevorkian's activities, told the *Washington Post:*

> Pain is not the main reason we want to die. It's the indignity. It's the inability to get out of bed or get onto the toilet, let alone drive a car or go shopping without another's help. I can speak for literally hundreds of people whose bedside I've sat at over the years. Every client I've talked to—I call them "clients" because I'm not a medical professional—they've had enough when they can't go to the bathroom by themselves. Most of them say, "I can't stand my mother—my husband—wiping my butt." That's why everybody in the movement talks about dignity. People have their pride. They want to be in charge.[29]

In other words, when asked to describe the "indignities" that assisted suicide would help people to avoid, proponents describe disability—that is, "substantial impairment of a major life function," specifically the life function known as "self-care." The need for assistance in the basic activities of daily living, especially in the bathroom, is the most fearsome "indignity." Allegedly, it assaults one's pride and deprives a competent person of the ability to be in charge, in control, of his or her life. This is the dreaded image of the "indignity" of disability, a form of "imprisonment" from which the only "escape" is death. Disability is feared far more than death.

This widespread public image of severe disability as a fate worse than death is not exactly a surprise to the disability community. Disability rights advocates have fought against these negative stereotypes of disability for decades in the effort to achieve basic civil rights protections. What has been a surprise for many advocates is the boldness with which these stereotypes are asserted as fact by proponents of assisted suicide, and the willingness of the press and the public to accept them, without even checking them against the views of people who themselves live with severe disabilities. Numerous studies have documented that people with disabilities almost universally attribute their "suffering" to societal attitudes about disability rather than to disability itself.[30]

These stereotypes then become grounds for carving out a deadly exception to longstanding laws and public policies about suicide prevention. This is not a comment on the quality or quantity of suicide intervention services, which leave much to be desired, but on the issue of discrimination in public policy. Legalizing assisted suicide means that some people who say they want to die will receive suicide intervention, while others will receive suicide assistance. The difference between these two groups of people will be their health or disability status, leading to a two-tiered system that results in death to the socially devalued group. For every completed suicide, there are sixteen failed attempted suicides,[31] but people eligible for assisted suicide will be guaranteed a successful demise, without the mess of a violent suicide to clean up afterward, and with the social sanction that avoids questions or recriminations among those who continue living.

Proponents of assisted suicide assert that this two-tiered system, which can be (and, in Oregon, is) applied to kill individuals whether or not they depend on life-sustaining medical treatment, can be implemented with safeguards to ensure that death is voluntary and uncoerced. In support, they assert that there is no evidence of abuses in connection with withholding and withdrawing of treatment. In fact, little systematic evidence about withholding of treatment exists at all. We know that the overwhelming majority of surrogate decision makers base their decisions on the doctor's recommendations.[32] Other factors correlated with death by withdrawal of treatment have not been studied to a meaningful extent, not even to determine whether economic or insurance status, or any other socially mediated factors, are influencing decisions.

Initially, proponents claimed that assisted suicide should be limited to people with terminal illnesses, that is, illnesses predicted by at least two physicians to cause death within six months. For example, the Hemlock Society, the leading U.S. lobby group for assisted suicide, responded to the concerns of the disability community by posting the following on its Web site in 1997:

Hemlock Society Challenges Disabled on Opposition to Assisted Dying

The Hemlock Society USA, a 17 year old grass roots, right to die organization with more than 25,000 members in 80 chapters, takes issue with organizations representing the disabled in their opposition to the right of dying patients to seek help from their doctor in hastening their death. While recognizing the needs of the disabled community to achieve recognition and medical assistance, we support legislation which insures that a request for assistance in dying is voluntary, enduring, monitored, and from a person who is already in the dying process.

The Hemlock Society has many members who are disabled. Indeed, having a chronic, terminal illness generally renders a person disabled. People join Hemlock to support the idea that when death is inevitable they can retain their dignity in the face of irreversible suffering and degradation by making a choice not to prolong the dying process. . . .

NDY and ADAPT [American Disabled for Attendant Programs Today] argue that people with severe disabilities are denied equal protection of the law since assisted suicide would only apply to people with illnesses and disabilities. If the courts were to recognize a right to assisted suicide, they argue, the provisions should apply universally regardless of health or disability status. This is an absurd logic. We are talking about the ability of people who are already dying to ask for help in hastening death—not everyone who is suicidal. If it were the case that assistance in dying were universally available the disabled and the able-bodied would indeed be in jeopardy.

Disabled persons have every right to protect their interests—but *not* at the expense of the rest of us. The majority of Americans agree with the legalization of physician aid in dying for mentally competent, terminally ill people who request it. This has been Hemlock's mission for 17 years. No proposed legislation has included people with mental or physical disabilities *except* if he or she were terminally ill and because of their suffering chose to *ask* for help to die. The right to die movement will never have the intention to eliminate vulnerable populations, including the disabled. Hemlock has made it clear that this must be a *voluntary, personal* choice in the context of *safeguards* against abuse.[33]

While acknowledging that most terminally ill people are disabled, Hemlock claimed to limit assisted suicide to people already in the dying process. In contrast and at the same time, the Hemlock Web site also included the Harvard Model Statute to legalize assisted suicide, which proposes two eligible groups: (1) people with terminal illnesses (using the "six months to die" definition), and (2) people with incurable conditions who claim that their suffering is unbearable.[34] The nature and cause of such suffering is not defined, reducing the eligible class to people with incurable conditions. In a number of legislative sessions, the Hemlock Society supported an "aid-in-dying" bill (SB 44-FN) in New Hampshire that defines "terminal condition" as any incurable condition that shortens one's overall life span.

At the time of this writing, most major pro–assisted suicide groups in the United States do not include a requirement of "terminal" status in their eligibility criteria for assisted suicide. For example, the Death with Dignity National Center, a member of the Death with Dignity Alliance, explicitly requires only that "The patient's condition is incurable."[35] Most, however, continue to assert that safeguards to ensure voluntariness can prevent abuses.

The Oregon Law

The Oregon assisted suicide law has been hailed as a model statute, legalizing a purportedly narrow right to assisted suicide, with safeguards carefully crafted to prevent abuses and coercion. The law has been discussed in detail by Foley and Hendin in chapter 7, but I would like to make some additional comments on it from a disability perspective.

The Oregon law provides that physicians must inform patients who request assisted suicide about feasible alternatives, including, but not limited to, comfort care, hospice care, palliative treatment, and pain control. However, this safeguard presumes that physicians are knowledgeable about these alternatives and that they are motivated to disclose them to patients (regardless of managed care contracts and other financial disincentives to disclosure). The life experiences of people with disabilities are filled with evidence of the unreliability of medical and professional opinions about either physical or psychological issues. Many of us were expected to die but lived—and lived to enjoy life with our disabilities. Moreover, there is no proposed requirement that desired treatment alternatives actually be paid for, not even as a "last resort" in the absence of adequate insurance or payment options.

Medicare already does not pay for prescription medications, except for those in hospice. The nation's top health maintenance organizations have been pulling out of publicly funded health care programs that serve poor, elderly, and disabled people. Federal courts have also been upholding the rights of private health insurance companies to cap HIV/AIDS benefits at severely reduced levels, for instance, $25,000 (one other court case says $100,000, and there are others), in policies that cap other benefits at $1 million.[36] This threatens to force individuals with AIDS into the weakening publicly funded system. According to the U.S. Court of Appeals for the Seventh Circuit, there is no legal reason that such caps could not be contractually placed on cancer and other expensive conditions as well.[37]

Nor is there any requirement that sufficient home and community-based long-term care services be provided to relieve demands on family members and ease the individual's feelings of being a "burden." The Medicare hospice benefit is often insufficient to meet individual and family needs regarding personal care. Nor does Medicare cover personal care needs for people with nonterminal chronic conditions. The inadequacy of the in-home long-term care system is central to the assisted suicide and euthanasia debate.[38]

Most proposals to legalize assisted suicide do not require a psychological consultation, but physicians may be asked to document that the patient's request for assisted suicide is not the product of "impaired judgment" caused by a mental illness. While purporting to ensure a "voluntary" request, this criterion involving mental illness utterly fails to address the more prevalent but subtle forms of social coercion. A conscious, "competent" person knows that society considers the need for assistance in activities of daily living to be degrading and undignified. A conscious, "competent" person might overhear the "kitchen talk" and feel like an economic and physical burden on family members.

Disabled people note that psychological consultations were sought in the withholding of treatment cases in the 1980s as well, but these consultants failed to distinguish the effects of environmental pressures (involuntary confinement in nursing homes) from the disability itself. Even though Rivlin, McAfee, and Bergstedt all said enough about the nursing home issue that the courts and press all referred to the problem, the "expert" consultants never saw it as an external and correctable precipitating factor in suicide. Common social stereotypes appear to have overcome professional objectivity and insight.

Studies also show that medical professionals assess the quality of life of disabled people to be dramatically lower than disabled people themselves do.[39] Yet in the face of documented inadequacies in medical knowledge, as well as documented economic pressures in the health care system, these medical professionals are the gatekeepers of the safeguards. These medical professionals determine who is voluntarily choosing assisted suicide. And the law does not preclude "doctor shopping" until a gatekeeper is found who will open the door.

A purported "safeguard" of the Oregon law provides that no physician will be subject to any form of legal liability for assisted suicide if he or she acted in "good faith." A claimed "good faith" belief that the requirements of the law are satisfied is virtually impossible to disprove, rendering all other safeguards effectively unenforceable.

The Oregon statute calls for no enforcement provisions, reports, or procedures that would enable monitoring of compliance with the safeguards. Patient confidentiality ensures that legalizing assisted suicide will not bring the practice out into the "light of day," as advocates have often claimed. Instead, it simply creates a new form of legal immunity and shifts the legal and medical defaults in connection with the deaths of old, ill, and disabled people. A few forms in the medical chart, no questions asked.

Proponents of assisted suicide now offer studies of the first few years under the act as proof that all is well. Based on brief interviews with physicians who reported assisted suicides, perhaps the most striking information from the first fifteen study cases is that pain was not a significant issue for this group. The primary issue was fear of future increased loss of bodily function and the assumption that such loss would mean loss of dignity and autonomy. In other words, the issue was fear and prejudice about disability.

Take, for example, the assisted suicide involving a woman in the beginning stages of dementia reported in the *Oregonian* in October 1999 (see chapter 7 for more details). Kate Cheney's physician had requested a psychiatric consultation because of her dementia, and the psychiatrist declined to support the assisted suicide because of concern that the woman's daughter seemed to be a strong advocate for her mother's assisted suicide, raising questions about how voluntary the request was. A second opinion was sought and a psychologist, after making a similar observation about the daughter, concluded that Cheney was acting voluntarily. A prescription was issued. Sometime later, Cheney's family wanted respite from caregiving responsibilities and placed her in a nursing home for a week. Shortly after her return, she took the lethal dose.

The case produced a flurry of editorial comment, including from a physician involved in Cheney's care, Dr. Robert Richardson. Through the Internet, I wrote to Richardson:

> In my role as a long term care advocate, I have heard for years of Oregon's claim to operate the most progressive long-term care programs in the country, model programs that emphasize in-home and community based services, even for the most frail elderly. What in-home services was Ms. Cheney receiving? How is it that Ms. Cheney had to spend a week in a nursing home to give her family respite from caregiving? Did Ms. Cheney and her family know of other respite options? If not, who failed to tell them? How can their actions have been based on the informed consent promised in the Oregon law? Or did the family choose the nursing home respite option with knowledge of other alternatives (an even more disturbing possibility)? What ongoing support options were explored to reduce the daily need for family caregiving? There are many ways to resolve the feeling of being a burden on family, and the family's feelings of being burdened. In what depth were these issues explored? In this context, family relationships are complex, and the emotional dynamics could not realistically be uncovered in a brief consultation.
>
> It appears from the newspaper account, as well as your response to Dr. Hamilton, that these issues were not meaningfully addressed. Ms. Cheney appears to have been given the message that she had three choices—to be a burden on family, to go to a nursing home, or to die. After a week in a nursing home, an experience I wouldn't wish on my opponents except perhaps to educate them, it appears that Ms. Cheney felt she had only one option. How is this a voluntary and uncoerced decision based on informed consent?

I did not receive a response.

At Risk

The prevalence of elder abuse presents another challenge for those who allege that safeguards can ensure that assisted suicide is voluntary. According to a study by the National Elder Abuse Center, in 1996 there were 450,000 cases of abuse or neglect perpetrated on elderly people.[40] In cases involving known perpetrators, 90 percent were family members. Among these, the majority were a spouse or an adult child.

In the face of the harsh realities of our society, even the staunchest advocates of assisted suicide must admit that abuses will occur in the implementation of the right they seek. Apparently, fear of poverty and abuse is too remote a concern for these advocates, who are more likely to be white and affluent than the majority of the population.[41] How much abuse is difficult to assess. Nor does the Oregon law provide a means through which abuses may be identified. How many individuals who request assisted suicide would change their mind if given better health care, more individually tailored social supports, more respect? How many had families who needed help and did not get it? Were these lives expendable? In *Freedom to Die: People, Politics, and the Right-to-Die Movement*, Derek Humphry and Mary Clement conclude that economics, not liberty interests, will move their agenda into accepted practice: "Similar to other social issues, the right-to-die movement has not arisen separate and distinct from other concurrent developments of our time. In attempting to answer the question Why Now?, one must look at the realities of the increasing cost of health care in an aging society, because in the final analysis, economics, not the quest for broadened individual liberties or increased autonomy, will drive assisted suicide to the plateau of acceptable practice."[42]

But is society really ready to ignore the risks, tolerate the abuses, marginalize or cover up the mistakes, and implicitly agree that some lives—many lives—are expendable, in order to enact a law that immunizes health providers and other participants in assisted suicide?

A Duty to Die

Evidence is mounting that the euthanasia movement may not limit its message to subtle forms of coercion. In the spring of 1997, for example, the *Hastings Center Report*, a leading bioethics journal, featured a cover article by John Hardwig entitled, "Is There a Duty to Die?" which began like this: "Many people were outraged when Richard Lamm claimed that old people had a duty to die. Modern medicine and an individualistic culture have seduced many to feel that they have a right to health care and a right to live, despite the burdens and costs to our families and society. But in fact there are circumstances when we have a duty to die. As modern medicine continues to save more of us from acute illnesses, it also delivers more of us over to chronic illnesses, allowing us to survive far longer than we can take care of ourselves."[43]

For individuals who internalize the social oppression that declares severe disability to be undignified, the legalization of assisted suicide may convey the message that suicide is the best way to reclaim their dignity. It may even convey the message that suicide is the most honorable way to make one last contribution to a society that increasingly operates from a "lifeboat" mentality, a mentality that tells the disenfranchised and despised to get out of the way, without ever seriously questioning the decisions and motives of the policy makers who shape the culture we live in.

Nor is a "duty to die" understood to fall only on competent, hitherto nondisabled adults. During the first decades of the last century, the eugenics movement enjoyed significant popularity in the United States. This movement passed forced sterilization laws that affected both disabled and nondisabled people, especially those who were poor and uneducated. Over thirty states passed laws that later served as the template for similar laws in Germany.[44]

Euthanasia of disabled people also became a legitimate topic of professional discourse at that time. Foster Kennedy wrote the following in 1942 in the *American Journal of Psychiatry*:

> I believe when the defective child shall have reached the age of five years—and on the application of his guardians—that the case should be considered under law by a competent medical board; then it should be reviewed twice more at four-month intervals; then, if the board, acting, I repeat, on the applications of the guardians of the child, and after three examinations of a defective who has reached the age of five or more, should decide that that defective has no future or hope of one; then I believe it is a merciful and kindly thing to relieve that defective—often tortured and convulsed, grotesque and absurd, useless and foolish, and entirely undesirable—of the agony of living.[45]

Reaction to the Holocaust limited further development of this line of thought, which favored active euthanasia of disabled children, at that time. Nevertheless, as time passed, nonvoluntary euthanasia through the withholding of medical treatment from disabled infants and children became increasingly common. This passive euthanasia raised serious questions about misguided quality of life judgments and became a topic in a 1989 report of the U.S. Civil Rights Commission entitled *Medical Discrimination against Children with Disabilities.*

Among the information considered by the commission was an experiment conducted from 1977 to 1982 at the Children's Hospital of Oklahoma. Doctors there developed a "quality of life" formula for babies with spina bifida that took into account the socioeconomic status of the baby's family to determine what to advise them about a simple but life-and-death procedure. Better-off families were provided a realistic and optimistic picture of their child's potential, while poor families were provided a pessimistic picture. Four out of five poor families accepted the doctors' advice, and twenty-four babies lost their lives. The U.S. Civil Rights Commission stated the following: "To accept a projected negative quality of life . . . based on the difficulties society will cause . . . rather than tackling the difficulties themselves, is unacceptable. The Commission rejects the view that an acceptable answer to discrimination and prejudice is to assure the 'right to die' to those against whom the discrimination and prejudice exists."[46]

Again, while Not Dead Yet does not oppose all forms of surrogate medical decision making, we recognize the inherent risk, in fact the certainty, that wrongful decisions will be made by nondisabled family members, based on biased professional advice, cultural stereotypes, and social and economic pressures. We urge society to retain the *relatively* "bright line" distinction between passive measures that cause death and active measures that cause death, and then work to minimize the damage resulting from professional, cultural, and economic factors in the context of refusal of treatment.

In the *Vacco v. Quill* Supreme Court case, Quill argued that the distinction between passive euthanasia (withdrawal of treatment) and active euthanasia (administration of a lethal medication) wrongfully deprives competent adults who do not depend on life-sustaining treatment of a simple and legal method of suicide. But this argument ignores "end-of-life sedation," whereby a competent individual may execute a living will opposing food and water by tube and then receive only palliative care, including sedation, until death occurs. Given the clear legality of this option (reaffirmed by the Supreme Court in *Vacco*), "competent" individuals already have a "right to die." An additional right to kill, an immunity statute for those who provide an affirmative means to die, is not necessary.

Taking the argument a few steps further, on December 3, 1997, the Hemlock Society issued a press release advocating the expansion of surrogate decision-making law to include the possibility that people who do not depend on life-sustaining treatment can be actively euthanized. The press release quoted Girsh: "In the case of a minor or an incompetent adult, the law now allows life or death decisions to be made by a designated health care agent and/or a family member in most jurisdictions. . . . Some provision should be made for a situation in which life is not being sustained by artificial means but, in the belief of the patient or his agent, is too burdensome to continue. . . . A judicial determination should be made when it is necessary to hasten the death of an individual whether it be a demented parent, a suffering, severely disable [sic] spouse or a child."[47]

In a subsequent newsletter, Girsh referred to the case of Robert and Tracy Latimer to exemplify the need for these and other changes in public policy.[48] Tracy Latimer was twelve years old. She had severe cerebral palsy and was unable to speak. She was known to enjoy activities and friends in spite of the pain she experienced in her hip. In 1993 Robert Latimer, a farmer in Saskatchewan, stayed home with his daughter Tracy while the rest of the family went to church.

While they were gone, Robert Latimer carried Tracy to the barn, put her in the front seat of his truck, ran a pipe from the exhaust into the cab of the truck, turned on the ignition, closed the barn doors, and left her there. Once she was dead, he carried her body back to the house and put the body in bed. He informed the family and authorities that she had apparently died in bed.

The coroner was somewhat suspicious and performed an autopsy. The autopsy made it clear that Tracy died due to carbon monoxide poisoning rather than any natural cause. Once confronted with the evidence, Robert Latimer confessed to the murder. He claimed to have killed Tracy for her own good. She experienced chronic pain in her hip and was due for another bout of surgery to help with the pain. Latimer claimed that he did not believe the surgery would help her. Almost immediately, the press and the public seemed to embrace Latimer's sincerity and even to support his assertion that the killing was a loving act.[49] Latimer was embraced by the Canadian Right to Die Society, whose leader, Marilyn Seguin, was quoted in the *New York Times* challenging a prison sentence for Latimer as unconscionable, since he had already served a twelve-year sentence, the length of Tracy's life.[50] Although Latimer has been convicted twice of second-degree murder, as of this writing, he remains free pending an appeal of the mandatory prison sentence.

Children are not the only potential victims. George Delury's wife, Myrna Lebov, had multiple sclerosis. She needed help in the activities of daily living, and a personal assistant provided sixty hours per week of in-home services to address this need. Ms. Lebov experienced depression, for which she was prescribed antidepressants.

Her husband kept a diary documenting her mood swings, as well as his own reflections, as the couple agreed that they would plan her assisted suicide.[51] Delury stockpiled the antidepressants and tested them in various mixtures. He discouraged Lebov from writing another book, something she had previously done successfully. He told people at a wedding that she was a burden to him, in front of her. He wrote in his diary that she was a "vampire sucking his life" and showed the passage to her.

In the month before she died, she told her physical therapist that she had changed her mind about suicide and wanted to live. When she appeared to die of assisted suicide, Delury claimed responsibility, was charged with manslaughter, and entered a plea bargain for a six-month sentence, of which he served four months. The Hemlock Society provided him a legal defense fund, and Delury contributed the proceeds from the publication of his diary to the Hemlock Society.

The couple's story was the subject of two hour-long *Dateline* episodes. In the second of these, Delury had served his sentence when he revealed that Lebov had eaten only about half the deadly mixture he prepared the night before her death. In the morning when the assistant was scheduled to arrive, she was still alive, though asleep or unconscious, so he used a plastic bag to kill her and hid it from the police.

The Hemlock Society press release that advocated expanded surrogate decision making to enable nonvoluntary euthanasia, also called for the creation of a lesser class of homicide to address these cases in which ill and disabled people are killed by relatives who claim to be acting out of love: "Even with such a[n assisted suicide] law, there are many people suffering from chronic and terminal illnesses who beg either to have their lives ended or who are not competent to make this decision and are in those instances assisted by a loved one. . . . We suggest that, if these cases are to be prosecuted, they should be treated as special crimes of compassion and evaluated separately. The criteria might include the person's wishes to die, the person's medical condition, the family's concurrence, the alternatives available, and the motives of the person being tried."[52]

There are already tremendous disparities in the sentences meted out to parents who kill their children, depending on whether the children are disabled or nondisabled. Sentences for murder of children in general average thirty years, and fifteen years for negligent manslaughter.[53] In a review of sentencing patterns in thirty-five cases of homicide involving a child with a disability, fifteen of the thirty-five received no jail time at all. An additional eight received up to five years. Twelve received sentences of over five years. To what extent might assisted suicide laws be viewed by the public as social permission to hasten the deaths of burdensome family members even without the involvement of health care providers? In evaluating Girsh's call for a lesser class of homicide, it is important to note statistics on homicide by family members. According to the Federal Bureau of Investigation, 55.9 percent of all homicides of children eleven or younger are committed by family members, and 21.2 percent of homicides of individuals age fifty and over are committed by family members.[54] Overall, approximately one in seven of all homicides are perpetrated by members of the victim's family.

Assuming that the Hemlock Society does not wish to encourage outright involuntary euthanasia (as distinguished from nonvoluntary euthnasia, which it clearly supports for people who are not deemed "competent"), how does this assumption reconcile with the proposed lesser class of homicide? In fact, as the Delury and Latimer cases demonstrate, as well as recent multiple murder cases in hospital and nursing home settings,[55] society has already communicated tremendous tolerance for these killings.

Despite the far-reaching nature of its policy recommendations, the Hemlock Society press release received little or no media attention at the time it was issued. The disability community has subsequently provided copies to national and local media outlets, in the context of a disability protest at a national Hemlock Society conference and at the Kevorkian trial (attended by Girsh, who opposed conviction). But the media has failed to raise any questions concerning the implications of the policies recommended, or to question the scope and breadth of the political agenda—the allegedly "progressive" agenda—of the assisted suicide movement.

Support for such an agenda comes from respected academics as well, for example, Peter Singer, the Australian philosopher best known, perhaps, for his groundbreaking work in animal rights. A credible academic working from a utilitarian perspective and now holder of the Ira W. DeCamp chair in bioethics at Princeton University, Singer has also achieved recognition for writing books that are appreciated by many people, both inside and outside of academia. He is known for being clear and direct.

Singer offers a philosophical framework, a "moral" justification for euthanasia.

> We often use "person" as if it meant the same as "human being." In recent discussions in bioethics, however, "person" is now often used to mean a being with certain characteristics such as rationality and self-awareness.[56]
>
> The term "person" is no mere descriptive label. It carries with it a certain moral standing. Just as, in law, the fact that a corporation can be a person means that a corporation can sue and be sued, so too, once we recognize a nonhuman animal as a person, we will soon begin to attribute basic rights to that animal.[57]
>
> The right to life is not a right of members of the species Homo sapiens; it is . . . a right that properly belongs to persons. Not all members of the species Homo sapiens are persons, and not all persons are members of the species Homo sapiens.[58]

Human "nonpersons" include infants as well as children and adults who cannot demonstrate that they view themselves as a consistent being over time. The latter group would include some people with significant cognitive disabilities, mental illnesses, brain injuries, and dementia. In Singer's view, and that of many bioethicists, individuals who cannot demonstrate that they meet the criteria for personhood can be treated without moral consideration and may be killed based on the preferences of their families or society.

Like other proponents of legalizing assisted suicide and euthanasia, Singer rejects the legal distinction between passive and active measures to cause death. He asserts that if society accepts death by withholding treatment as moral, then society should also allow death by active killing. Unless the benefit to the people who love these "nonpersons" outweighs the emotional and financial burden to individuals and society of keeping the "nonpersons" alive, they can safely and deliberately be killed. He compares the ethical revolution he advocates to the Copernican revolution of scientific thought. Both, he notes, were or are resisted by religious tradition. Both, he claims, were or are advanced by the inevitable progress of science.

But Singer focuses on a very narrow range of scientific evidence in reaching his conclusions. Missing are sociological and psychological evidence on suicide, homicide, abuse, disability, geriatrics, health care, long-term care, economics, and law enforcement, to name a few. Singer claims that he is saying only what most people think, that it should be considered moral and right to kill some ill and disabled people because those around them feel socially or economically burdened by their existence. He is as direct in saying this as the underpublicized Hemlock Society press release.

Still at the Margins of the Debate

The disability rights movement has lagged behind the other antidiscrimination movements. Our legal protections against federal discrimination were passed more than eighty years after laws prohibiting such discrimination against African Americans. Our education rights were established a few decades later than *Brown v. Board of Education*. And a full generation passed after the Civil Rights Act of 1964 before the Americans with Disabilities Act (ADA) declared that state and private discrimination based on disability is wrong.

Most people do not know very much about the history of the disability rights movement. Our struggles have been fought on the margins of society's awareness. Few are aware of the hundreds who were arrested and jailed in the fight for passage of the ADA. We have rarely been on the media's radar screen, except as human interest stories of tragedy and courage. The public knows little of the public policy war we are now waging to free disabled people, old and young, from forced placement in nursing homes and institutions. As far as the network news is concerned, our political movement does not exist.

When disability news stories arise, comments are rarely sought from leaders in the disability movement. More often, physicians and other nondisabled professionals are viewed as the experts to consult on disability issues. Perhaps similarly, before the gay and lesbian rights movements achieved a certain degree of public and media acceptance, homosexuality was primarily treated as a psychiatric illness, not as a social or political identity affected by significant discrimination, even from within a gay or lesbian individual's family. However, disability is still almost universally seen as a medical issue. Disability discrimination is rarely viewed as wrongful. In fact, it is often viewed as justified, and there is a fairly widespread "backlash" against the ADA.[59] Negative family reactions to disability, including abandonment and even killing, are seen as understandable.[60] The societal role assigned to disabled people—of tragic victims who would be better off dead, or courageous overcomers who never complain of discrimination—leaves little room for serious discourse. Many ask, How could disabled people be competent to contribute in a significant way to the public debate on assisted suicide? And Hemlock says, how dare *they* try to stop the legalization of assisted suicide for the rest of *us?* From the standpoint of euthanasia advocates we seem to be expendable.

The Disability Opposition Grows

Since the formation of Not Dead Yet, as of this writing, ten other national disability rights organizations have taken formal positions on the issue of legalization of assisted suicide, all opposed:

1. American Disabled for Attendant Programs Today (ADAPT), which advocates for the civil rights of people with disabilities, old and young, to receive consumer-controlled long-term care services in the community instead of being warehoused in nursing homes and institutions

2. Association of Programs for Rural Independent Living (APRIL), an association of nonprofit service and advocacy organizations working with people with disabilities who live in rural areas

3. Disability Rights Education and Defense Fund, Inc. (DREDF), a national law and policy center dedicated to protecting and advancing the civil rights of people with disabilities through legislation, litigation, advocacy, technical assistance, and education and training of attorneys, advocates, persons with disabilities, and parents of children with disabilities

4. Justice for All, which, with an extensive e-mail network, was formed by Justin Dart, Jr., to defend and advance disability rights and programs in the U.S. Congress

5. National Council on Disability (NCD), an independent presidentially appointed body making recommendations to the president and Congress on issues affecting fifty-four million Americans with disabilities

6. National Council on Independent Living, the national association of hundreds of consumer-controlled centers for independent living,

nonresidential grassroots advocacy and service organizations operated by and for people with disabilities

7. National Spinal Cord Injury Association, an international nonprofit organization for people living with spinal cord injury, whose mission is to enable people with spinal cord injuries to make choices and take actions so that they might achieve their highest level of independence and personal fulfillment

8. TASH (formerly the Association for Persons with Severe Handicaps), a civil rights organization for, and of, people with diagnostic labels of "mental retardation," autism, cerebral palsy, physical disabilities, and other conditions that "make full integration a challenge"

9. World Association of Persons with Disabilities, a membership organization that advances the interests of persons with disabilities at national, state, and local levels and in the home

10. World Institute on Disability, an international public policy center founded by Ed Roberts, the "father" of the independent living movement, and dedicated to carrying out cutting-edge research on disability issues and overcoming obstacles to independent living

Each of these organizations has worked, in some cases for decades, to fight the social stigma attached to disability, to push society to accept disability as a natural part of the human experience, to welcome people with disabilities as part of the diverse human community. Each has worked to advance laws and public policies that guarantee our civil rights. Long defined by medical professionals as tragic failures of science, objects of pity and charity, disabled people have worked to demonstrate that we are like other minority groups and that the difficulties we face are more a product of oppressive social attitudes than biological destiny. Although we have made significant progress in achieving these goals in some arenas, the media, the courts, and public opinion have not shifted much in their conviction that disability is at least a dreaded permanent tragedy, often a fate worse than death. Public and media responses to Kevorkian, Delury, Latimer, Singer, and others have demonstrated unequivocally to these organizations that the lives of people with disabilities are at stake.

Conclusion

Fear of disability, and the social and economic consequences that currently accompany disability, are at the heart of the public debate over assisted suicide and euthanasia. Individuals fear future disability, be it their own or that of someone close to them. Most have little or no knowledge of the reality of disability and know even less of the social policies that affect the experience of disability or how these policies can be changed.

Leaders in the movement for assisted suicide and euthanasia have capitalized effectively on these fears, while at the same time obscuring their source. They talk about "end of life," but they have won most of their legal advances by advocating killing people who were not dying but disabled. The assisted suicide and euthanasia debate is not simply about the role of medicine at the end of life but, at a fundamental level, about the role of disability in society.

Euthanasia advocates talk about loss of dignity, but they are the ones who claim that it is undignified to need assistance in self-care. They work hard to exclude the disability voice from the debate, portraying the issues as a simple dispute between compassionate progressives on the one hand, and the religious right and medical establishment on the other. Under this formulation, the issue is simply one of personal "choice."

The broader social effects of legalizing assisted suicide or euthanasia for a class of people based on health or disability status are obscured and ignored. The economic and social pressures, and human character flaws, that already lead to abuse and killing are dismissed as correctable by safeguards.

There are, perhaps, two essential reasons for which society should reject the arguments being made by assisted suicide and euthanasia proponents: First, as human beings, by now we should know ourselves and each other well enough to recognize that people, whether individuals or corporations, cannot be trusted with the right to kill other people, especially people who are socially devalued. The problem is big enough already without making it legal and easier than it already is.

Second, we have no idea what it would be like to live in a society that welcomed and accommodated each individual, regardless of his or her abilities and disabilities. We should try that first—respecting and valuing everyone by according them real dignity and real human rights. People will feel much better if they do not have to fear being devalued and disrespected, or abandoned by families, friends, and health care resources, with nowhere to turn and no one to turn to for support. We can do better than that. In the meantime, the right to a natural death is sufficient. The right to be killed, or to kill another, is premature at best.

Vulnerable People:
Practical Rejoinders to Claims in Favor of Assisted Suicide

Felicia Cohn, Ph.D., and Joanne Lynn, M.D., M.A., M.S.

Though everyone recognizes that death is a certainty, few know how to live with fatal illness. The realities of dying are difficult, for serious illness usually lasts many months, with substantial burdens and expenses. Death itself is not a choice, but its timing sometimes is, or could be. For those persons who conclude that they do not wish to endure the suffering and the costs associated with prolonged dying, physician-assisted suicide seems to offer an answer. It appears to provide individuals the chance to prevent suffering and maintain control over what once seemed uncontrollable.

For others, however, physician-assisted suicide conjures fear that someone else will determine what is to be considered excessive suffering or costs, and that others might seek to eliminate the suffering or the costs by eliminating those persons who are perceived to be suffering or costly. The elderly and the poor are particularly vulnerable to the effects of inadequate health care resources and the attendant constraints on medical decision making. The issue of physician-assisted suicide, however, is not merely a matter for "other" groups. "The poor" is a lifelong or end-of-life reality for many Americans; "the elderly" is a group that most of us would eventually like to join; and "the dying" is a category we cannot reasonably avoid.

Care of those who are elderly, particularly those approaching the end of life, has proven to be expensive. Indeed, more than $2 in every $8 spent on Medicare are spent in the last year of life, and $1 in every $8 is spent in the last month. Those with cancer have approximately 20 percent higher than average costs. As of 1993, end-of-life care consumed 10 percent to 12 percent of all health care expenditures. Over a quarter of Medicare expenditures are spent on about 5 percent of the Medicare beneficiaries who die during a given year.[1]

Health care providers and institutions face increasing pressure to reduce the costs of care. Medicare benefits, for example, remain a regular political issue, sparking controversy over the costs of preserving the program and the introduction of additional benefits deemed desirable or necessary. In an era when resources are increasingly being squeezed while the population ages and health care needs increase, the elderly and the dying compete against other portions of the population for health care services.[2] Given the high and seemingly disproportionate costs of health care for the elderly and those in the final phase of life, these "users of excessive medical resources" may be the targets of cost-saving efforts.[3]

Those with adequate personal finances may be able to purchase supplemental insurance or pay for services. Those without such resources, however, may have to choose among recommended services, face bankrupting their families, or go without much-needed health care altogether. The "haves" in our society may be immune to the potential for coercion that the choice of assisted suicide creates for the "have nots." However, the majority of the population, the "have nots" or the "have not enoughs" and their families, living with the reality of unaffordable health care needs, remain vulnerable to the possibility of avoidable suffering and premature death. In fact, the argument that a duty to die exists when a seriously ill individual faces the likelihood of financial hardship has made its appearance in the bioethics and policy debate.[4]

While costs alone do not drive health care decision making and policy, costs cannot be ignored. As the population ages, both the proportion of elderly persons in society and their health care needs increase. Ideally, health care would change to reflect the real needs of these changing demographics; but such change, when it occurs, occurs very slowly. Our current health care system, focused as it is on acute care needs and high-tech procedures, is largely neglectful of the growing and expensive need for chronic and palliative care. Explicitly or implicitly, arguments from cost savings are emerging, despite the lack of evidence that such savings will become a reality and studies that indicate that physician-assisted suicide will have a negligible effect on health care expenses nationally.[5] Major public policy innovations to improve end-of-life care have relied heavily on methods that were promoted in part to reduce costs—advance directives and hospice, for example. The vaunted savings have not been realized, at least not to the extent anticipated, but these innovations persist for other good reasons.[6] The unproven assumption that physician-assisted suicide would lower costs, and continued public sentiment in favor of self-determination, are powerful forces behind the movement to legalize physician-assisted suicide. While no one would admit to a willingness to see his or her own aging and frail mother die in order to save money, the elderly as a group may not have such stalwart defenders.

A number of voices have emerged that speak to the potential for abuse of physician-assisted suicide against members of various groups (e.g., people with disabilities, AIDS patients, members of minorities). Though these people do not speak with one voice, either within or across communities, their insights help us to demonstrate why nine of the most common and most compelling arguments for legalizing physician-assisted suicide are unpersuasive or misleading.

1. The Public Wants Physician-Assisted Suicide

One opinion poll after another has indicated that a majority of the American public favors legalizing physician-assisted suicide.[7] However, a survey by the American Medical Association demonstrated that support for physician-assisted suicide reverses when respondents are given information about abuses in the Netherlands and about other options for care at the end of life.[8] Applying the rate of physician-assisted suicide in the Netherlands to the American population indicates that physician-assisted suicide could account for over 61,000 deaths in the United States annually. The Dutch experience also reveals that there are a significant number of unreported cases and instances in which physician-assisted suicide was provided without patient request or consent, contrary to stated guidelines.[9] When presented with Dutch data, one-half of those who supported legalizing physician-assisted suicide reversed their positions. Once provided with descriptions of hospice and palliative care options, only 14 percent said they would still opt for legal access to physician-assisted suicide.[10]

Furthermore, reports of the polls hide the distribution of preferences among various subpopulations of our society. Those favoring legalization of physician-assisted suicide tend to be young, male, and white.[11]

Those opposing legalization of physician-assisted suicide are often elderly, female, or from minority groups—some of the very people who face progressive disability and suffering before death and who therefore would seem most likely to support having the option of assisted suicide.

Without recognizing the vast changes that will occur as they age, strong and capable young men may assume they will still both have and want control over their end-of-life care decisions. They appear to presume continuation of the decision-making authority they have enjoyed throughout most of their lives.

The situation changes as people experience the progressive declines that often accompany aging. As people approach death, they commonly have very few financial resources and often are profoundly dependent on the arrangements others make for their care. Which services are available largely reflects federal financing, including the coverage gaps when Medicare and Medicaid do not pay for services. Many people's poorest years are those nearest death, when income is low, care needs are high, and lack of community support for personal care during disability takes its largest toll. The prospect of increasing disability and eventual death is disheartening enough, but the added anxiety over the adequacy of savings and the "safety net" of government services is often terrifying.

For many, no reasonably desirable choices may exist. Then, physician-assisted suicide may not merely be a choice, one option among others; rather, it may become a coercive offer.[12] If physician-assisted suicide becomes a more popular choice, ending one's own life could come to be perceived as an obligation, that is, a societally endorsed course of action that is the only way to avoid suffering, indignity, and impoverishment. Physician-assisted suicide may not be what dying people would reasonably prefer if given a choice of reliable, comprehensive care, an option that is not now usually available. Thus rather than increasing the choices one has as death approaches, legalizing physician-assisted suicide may actually have the effect of constraining choices.

Personal circumstances and societal expectations do often shape individual desires, but what one believes he or she should do is not necessarily the same as what an individual really wants. Those confronted with limited resources, such as those who are poor, elderly, and frail, appear in general to oppose physician-assisted suicide. To claim that the public "wants physician-assisted suicide" is to ignore a significant, though under-recognized, portion of the population.

Does the public want physician-assisted suicide? Not when they understand other available options, and not those individuals most likely to be encouraged to use physician-assisted suicide.

2. Everyone Has a "Right to Die"

The debate has been influenced by claims of a "right to die," a slogan that suggests that physician-assisted suicide is a matter of individual choice between suffering and death. Framed in this way, physician-assisted suicide is a logical choice—sometimes, perhaps, the only reasonable choice. Proponents claim that a right to physician-assisted suicide arises out of the fundamental American right to liberty. Yet our liberty has always had limitations. When judging a particular restriction on liberty, one has to consider how fundamental a given freedom is to the concept of our basic inalienable rights and how detrimental the constraint is to that concept.

Moreover, the issue may not be well framed by claiming a right to die. More careful scholarship converts this claim to a right to noninterference, in that the government should not make it impossible for a person to take his or her own life. In a sense, law in the United States already allows this "right": no state makes suicide itself illegal. What is at stake is whether state law will allow physicians to assist. This is more complex. Some claim that the special skills of a physician are essential to prevent patient errors or failure. That claim is quite difficult to confirm. Physicians, at present, are not schooled in the art of ensuring death.

What seems to be in question is more the authority and social acceptability that having a physician involved would bring. If that is the case, then it is a social convenience to allow physicians to assist in suicide, rather than a personal right. Society bears no obligation to make a particular course of action easy or appealing. Some have claimed that patients have to engage physicians in suicide because only physicians have access to the lethal medications needed. Again, only a small class of potentially lethal agents is licensed exclusively to physicians. Having access to barbiturates and narcotics is not essential to physician-assisted suicide. Carbon monoxide, as an obvious example, is as readily available to a layperson. Personal freedom is not violated when society has merely made one course of action less attractive or convenient, especially since there are strong and independent reasons for having arranged availability of certain medications in this way.

The assistance of a physician in committing suicide cannot be constructed or defended as a right to die.

3. When Medicine Can Do "Nothing More," Physician-Assisted Suicide Is One Appropriate Response

Medical care often works to the detriment of those reaching life's inevitable and natural end. However, only rarely can "nothing more" be done, though current patterns of medical care may miss the opportunities to provide appropriate assistance.

Medicine has much to offer those who are dying. That many do not get what they need is not justification for physician-assisted suicide but an indictment of the current approach to end-of-life care. Appropriate health care could relieve overwhelming pain in those near death, support family caregivers, and provide reliable, trustworthy care. However, most patients cannot count on any of this. Currently, the only program for end-of-life care covered by Medicare is hospice. Yet hospice serves a very small population. In 1998, hospice provided benefits to 540,000 dying patients in their last few weeks of life.[13] The hospice benefit is limited to people who have a "terminal illness with a life expectancy of six months or less." Cancer and AIDS are virtually the only diseases that follow predictable courses of decline near death; thus, about 60 percent of hospice patients have cancer and many of the rest have AIDS.[14] Cancer patients are usually referred to hospice when the individual's functioning declines, usually three to six weeks before death.[15] By electing hospice, Medicare patients agree to forgo "life-prolonging" interventions and instead receive comprehensive medical and supportive services not otherwise covered by Medicare. In addition to this prognostic requirement, hospice effectively requires that the beneficiary have a home and a family or nursing home caregiver.

Medicare beneficiaries with diseases other than cancer or AIDS—the vast majority of older adults—generally do not have access to hospice care, primarily because their illnesses do not have "predictable" phases of decline at the end of life. This makes a determination of a "six-month" life expectancy difficult. Indeed, the usual person dying of heart failure still has a 50-50 or better chance to live six months when actually he or she lives only a week until death.[16] These patients are quite ill, but the timing of death is unpredictable.

In addition to the constraints of uncertain prognosis, many elderly people live alone, often in inadequate homes and without social support. Such patients are not generally eligible for hospice, though they desperately need hospicelike services, including advance planning, prescription medication, support services, symptom management, and coordinated care services—none of which are readily available. Providing comprehensive end-of-life care services to these individuals could significantly improve the quality of their remaining days. About one-fourth of Medicare funds are now spent on care at the end of life,[17] and payment is geared toward expensive high-technology interventions and "rescue" care. Studies show that almost 80 percent of Americans die in institutions.[18] Most dying patients and their physicians do not discuss death or routinely make advance plans for end-of-life care. The rates of pain and adverse symptoms near death are a national disgrace. Thus for many, physician-assisted suicide offers an opportunity to avoid dealing with this phase of life.

Consideration of the legalization of physician-assisted suicide should be taken as a challenge to improve end-of-life care and make it available to everyone. If dying is miserable and expensive, it is because we have allowed it to become that way. The last century has brought changes in how we die. In 1900, most people died before age fifty, of sudden illness. Now we are likely to die when we are more than seventy-five years old, having lived with chronic illness for months or years. Yet modern medicine and social arrangements are not prepared to handle the myriad needs of those approaching the end of life. The challenge lies not in figuring out how to do away with individuals when available resources become inadequate, but in improving the resources.

Claims that physician-assisted suicide is appropriate when medicine can do "nothing more" mistake the failings of our arrangements for services at the end of life for lack of possibilities altogether. Medicine in fact has a great deal to offer, right up to the end, and failure to do so demands reform, not physician-assisted suicide.

4. When a Patient Is Suffering Dreadfully and Requests Assistance in Bringing about a Desired Kind of Death, Legalized Physician-Assisted Suicide Would Be Appropriate

The common vision is that of a suffering patient who visits his or her physician to request a lethal prescription. The patient expects to leave the office with prescription in hand, heading home to place those pills on the counter so they are ready for use whenever the "right time" arrives.

A number of misperceptions plague this image, particularly with regard to alternatives at the end of life and the rapid access to physician-assisted suicide. First, physical suffering need not be a part of dying, and physician-assisted suicide is not the only remedy for suffering. Rates of intractable pain, even among cancer patients, are low; and if the patient is willing to accept sedation, pain can practically be eliminated.[19] Providing pain medication is already legal, even if it is perceived to have the side effect of hastening death. Other symptoms, such as nausea, depression, and shortness of breath, can also be medically relieved. Virtually all patients with serious illness can be physically comfortable.

Second, patients may bring about their deaths without physician-assisted suicide (e.g., by committing suicide unassisted, refusing life-sustaining treatment, or forgoing nutrition and fluids). Dehydration, for example, requires no assistance and is a generally comfortable way to die, especially for a very ill person who may have little interest in food and water or may actually be harmed by the imposition of feedings.[20] Contrary to public perception, forgoing artificial nutrition and hydration does not leave patients hungry or thirsty.[21] Furthermore, physician-assisted suicide does not provide an immediate solution. According to understandable safeguards built into virtually every proposed physician-assisted suicide statute as well as the law in effect in Oregon, a physician can act on a request for physician-assisted suicide only following a substantial waiting period, often at least two weeks. This is hardly the response envisioned by proponents' arguments and may even take longer than death by dehydration.

The argument that physician-assisted suicide is necessary to serve the needs of patients who are suffering terribly and who voluntarily request it quickly fails when we understand that patients do not have to suffer, there are already legally available medical alternatives, and access to physician-assisted suicide is too slow to count on.

5. The Right to Forgo Life-Sustaining Treatment Logically Includes Physician-Assisted Suicide

Many claim that no reasonable line can be drawn between acts of forgoing (withdrawing and withholding) life-sustaining treatment and acts of physician-assisted suicide. This argument holds that if forgoing life-sustaining treatment is ethically and legally acceptable, physician-assisted suicide is also justifiable. Physician-assisted suicide occurs "when a physician provides either equipment or medication, or informs the patient of the most efficacious use of already available means, for the sole purpose of assisting the patient to end his or her own life." Forgoing life-sustaining treatment by definition occurs when "medical intervention is either not given or the on-going use of the intervention is discontinued, allowing natural progression of the underlying disease state."[22] In each, death predictably results from the action taken. Therefore some claim that no cognizable difference exists between forgoing life-sustaining treatment and having physician-assisted suicide. In both, someone, usually a health care professional, acts to bring about death. The lower courts in the two physician-assisted suicide cases decided in 1997 found no justification for distinguishing physician-assisted suicide from withholding or withdrawing life-sustaining treatment.[23] Timothy Quill also argues that any purported difference is ethically irrelevant and that both methods ought to be available to physicians who desire to help their patients die comfortably.[24]

However, crucial distinctions do exist and have been serving medicine and patients well. Major American medical associations maintain distinctions between physician-assisted suicide and forgoing life-sustaining treatment.[25] Within the practice of medicine, physician-assisted suicide and withholding or withdrawing life-sustaining treatment may be distinguished according to practical and conceptual descriptions, legal ramifications for medical practice, and the procedural consequences of collapsing the distinction. Indeed, very few cases arise that would occasion any dispute as to which category was involved.

A consideration of the clinical setting also supports the lack of overlap between physician-assisted suicide and forgoing life-sustaining treatment. Descriptive differences involve the use of medical care, the effect of decisions, and the clinical intent. Patients wishing to forgo treatment are generally already receiving medical attention within the health care system, so decisions to withdraw care or withhold life-sustaining interventions occur in the context of a plan of care. This may not be the case for those seeking physician-assisted suicide, which may affect persons who do not have access to medical attention. Moreover, patients from whom life-sustaining treatment is withheld or withdrawn are usually very sick and close to death, regardless of aggressive intervention.

With physician-assisted suicide, an individual may be giving up an extended period of life, due to fear of suffering and other circumstances beyond an individual's control (including fear of incompetence itself).

When patients forgo life-sustaining treatment, the intent is not to bring about the patient's death but to respect the patient's wishes not to be subjected to undesired treatment. Medical treatment is withdrawn or withheld, and the underlying disease process then leads to the patient's death. Thus the patient is allowed to die following the natural course of his or her illness, but death is not artificially hastened. Although a physician may be active in removing life support, the physician's action is not a proximate cause of the death. If the particular life-sustaining technique had not been available, death would already have resulted. Additionally, the patient may continue to live, even when life support is removed. The physician would not proceed to suffocate a patient who resumes spontaneous respiration after a ventilator is withdrawn.

This scenario differs from physician-assisted suicide. In physician-assisted suicide, the intent is to bring about the patient's death. Certainly, a physician may be acting in accord with a patient's wishes and will eliminate the patient's suffering, but at the cost of explicitly and intentionally causing the patient's death in a manner distinct from the natural course to death. The physician is not preventing patient abuse nor alleviating pain, but actively abetting death. Death is the intended goal. If a first try at physician-assisted suicide does not succeed, the physician would have to proceed to help with another try.

The Supreme Court has established a right to forgo life-sustaining treatment based on a corollary to the common law requirement for a patient's consent to medical intervention.[26] The Court made clear that a patient's right to make a decision to forgo life-sustaining treatment does not fall under the purview of a right to die, but under a right to informed consent. The right to forgo life-sustaining treatment is a negative right or a right against bodily intrusion. Withdrawing or withholding treatment is not a matter of providing a patient with assistance in a quest to be dead but one of leaving that patient alone. A physician may not impose treatment on a patient who refuses an intervention, even if the physician believes the treatment will benefit the patient. The existence of such negative rights does not imply that one has a positive right to receive assistance in taking one's own life. Receiving a particular kind of medical intervention has no special authorization, while protection from battery is nearly absolute.

The procedural requirements of forgoing life-sustaining treatment and having physician-assisted suicide also have significant implications for public policy (see chapter 4). Decisions about life-sustaining treatment are similar to other medical treatment decisions. Proposals to legalize physician-assisted suicide, however, offer quite different restrictions. In all proposals, physician-assisted suicide is to be restricted to a certain category of patients—those who are terminally ill, competent, suffering, and acting without coercion—and its implementation is limited to particular methods. If physician-assisted suicide is truly analogous to forgoing life-sustaining treatment, it should be available to all patients, using whatever methods the physician and patient agree are most appropriate. Physician-assisted suicide is also to be available only for patients who are competent at the time of the request. No proposal to date allows for requests for physician-assisted suicide through advance directives or by surrogate decision makers. The same is not true of withholding or withdrawing life-sustaining treatment, which may be done in accord with an advance directive or at a surrogate's direction. The need for such restrictions suggests that distinctions between physician-assisted suicide and forgoing treatment are apparent even to those who advocate legalization of physician-assisted suicide.

The distinctions discussed surrounding the practical use of physician-assisted suicide and decisions to withhold or withdraw life-sustaining treatment suggest that the acts themselves are distinct. Patients in each scenario are not similarly situated in terms of clinical context, means to death, and law, and so need not be treated in a similar way. Patients in each situation share only the need for medical attention and the fact of eventual death.

Contrary to the arguments of proponents of physician-assisted suicide, distinctions between forgoing treatment and having physician-assisted suicide are widely endorsed, reasonably justified, and commonly used, in both medicine and law.

6. Allowing Use of Pain Medications That May Inadvertently Hasten Death Provides Support for Legalizing Physician-Assisted Suicide

Proponents of physician-assisted suicide also rely on an analogy to the provision of potentially life-shortening palliative care. The intent of a person providing palliative care is not to bring about the patient's death but to decrease the patient's pain and suffering. A recognized, but perhaps unavoidable, side effect may be the hastening of the patient's death. However, pain management techniques do not necessarily hasten death for a particular patient, nor is it clear that they actually often have that effect. As commonly used, pain medications rarely accelerate the patient's death. Patients using opioids chronically do not experience respiratory depressant side effects at doses that are effective in suppressing pain. Once the patient is habitually taking opioids, only a quite extraordinary dose would be lethal. Only for patients who have received no opioids is the respiratory depressant effect present at analgesic doses, and few dying patients are in this situation.

Even if a physician's act may hasten death, the physician is not acting to ensure an earlier death. The provision of "comfort care" also does not involve the exercise of a right to die, but instead is a matter of sound medical practice, aiming to relieve symptoms.

The use of pain medication can readily be distinguished from physician-assisted suicide on the basis of effect and intent.

7. Physicians Possess the Unique Expertise and Singular Ability to Bring About an Easy Suicide and So Are Necessarily Involved

Underlying claims about a right to physician-assisted suicide are fears of botched suicides and desires for ensured death. Physician involvement is thought to afford a guarantee of easy suicide. Only physicians are thought to have both the knowledge of pharmacology and the access to controlled substances believed necessary to facilitate successful suicides. To that end, proposals for legalized assisted suicide have required physician involvement.

Yet physician involvement guarantees neither an easy nor a successful suicide. Often physicians are not even taught effective symptom management; certainly, they are not schooled in how to take life. Indeed, expertise in how to ensure death is not commonly available in medical textbooks or journals. If advocates wish to ensure expertise, those who implement the death penalty may be more qualified than physicians generally.

Because of either patient condition or incorrect dosing, many patients will be unable to swallow or keep the pills down. This raises the probability that assistance beyond prescribing lethal medications will be essential and may even suggest that active euthanasia, or lethal injection, would be more effective and likely would seem more humane. Furthermore, the question of how to deal with a failed attempt remains, particularly if that act has rendered the patient worse off or unable to request or complete another attempt.

Even if physician-assisted suicide were legal, it might be difficult to find a physician willing to assist. Among those who favor physician-assisted suicide, only a minority is actually willing to participate.[27] The American Geriatrics Society spelled out the troubling and practical ethical conundrum that geriatricians and other health care practitioners face:

> Legalization of physician-assisted suicide would create a moral dilemma for geriatricians. Most elderly persons experience serious and progressive illness for extended periods before death and need significant social, financial and medical supports. These resources too often are not available, are of inadequate quality, are not covered by insurance, and are not provided by public entitlement programs. By collaborating in causing early deaths, when continuing to live has been made so difficult, geriatricians would become complicit in a social policy which effectively conserves community resources by eliminating those who need services. By refusing to assist with suicides because a patient's relative poverty and disadvantaged social situation is seen as coercive, geriatricians would condemn their patients, and themselves, to live through the patient's undesired difficulties for the time remaining.[28]

Evidence is thin, but it rules against physicians necessarily having the expertise, or the will, to assist a patient in committing suicide.

8. Currently Widespread but Clandestine Physician-Assisted Suicide Would Be Regulated Appropriately

Advocates frequently claim that physician-assisted suicide is practiced regularly. Their claims appear to be supported by studies in which physicians anonymously admit to having assisted in suicide or even to have euthanized a patient.[29] Most such studies have utilized quite inadequate methods. For example, these studies often do not provide an explicit definition of physician-assisted suicide.

For physician-assisted suicide to occur with regularity would require widespread complicity in illegal behaviors, since three-quarters or more of patients dying of serious illness are in hospitals and nursing homes. Widespread criminal activity could hardly go unnoticed by regulators and the general public.

According to one methodologically superior study of the rate of physician-assisted suicide,[30] about 3 percent of American physicians report that they have been party to physician-assisted suicide at least once. However, even with good definitions, many respondents confused physician-assisted suicide with euthanasia and with side effects of medications to relieve symptoms, so the actual rate is lower. While not an insignificant rate, it is hardly evidence of widespread violation of the law.

Furthermore, the fact that physician-assisted suicide may be occurring hardly provides a reason for making it legal. Although many in the United States now use illicit drugs and engage in underage drinking and agitate for the legalization of these activities, our society has decided that there are important reasons for maintaining their illegality. Foremost among these reasons is the protection of certain portions of society, both from their own bad decisions and from new societal expectations. The same may be true of physician-assisted suicide. Unless our society achieves a consensus on the value of life, works out the practical difficulties, and resolves the role conflict for physicians, any policy allowing physician-assisted suicide will continue to be problematic.

Contrary to the arguments of proponents, the current rates of physician-assisted suicide appear to be very low, and it is not clear that legalization would be beneficial, no matter what the actual rate of physician-assisted suicide.

9. The Law Can Protect People from Abuses of Physician-Assisted Suicide

Most proposed legislation requires that physician-assisted suicide be confined to patients who are terminally ill, suffering, and competent and who voluntarily and repeatedly request assistance from their physicians. Those who propose legalization of physician-assisted suicide contend that each of these conditions in part justifies legalization and that the needed categories can be clearly delineated. The legal constraints are thought to be sufficient to limit physician-assisted suicide to those who have made informed decisions to escape intolerable suffering in the final phase of life and to avoid subjecting others to abusive impositions. However, each of these conditions is problematic. Some are undefinable or unsustainable, or both, and undoubtedly each would lead to a number of contested cases. Even regulation of physician-assisted suicide does not guarantee that its practice will be limited according to the legal and clinical boundaries we create, nor can it ensure protection of those who may be most in need of protection.

Terminal illness and *terminal condition* have been "defined repeatedly ... in a model statute, the Uniform Rights of the Terminally Ill Act, and in over 40 state natural death statutes."[31] However, the terms are notoriously difficult to define, have uncertain criteria, and, as with any set of criteria, lead to myriad contentious cases. Despite the existence of what may be working definitions of *terminal illness,* a more rigorous definition seems necessary when its application may have such significant and irreversible consequences. Three general approaches might be used in attempting to define the category *terminally ill:* subjective judgment, statistical criteria, or disease severity threshold. However, none of these approaches yields the certainty and clarity necessary for implementing good public policy.

A subjective determination of who is "terminally ill" requires that some person or persons render a judgment that integrates an array of information about the patient's situation, prognosis, and appropriate care. Often patients, family, and professional caregivers negotiate the designation while discussing plans and making decisions that collectively mark a change from a strategy of correcting abnormalities with the expectation of long survival to a strategy focusing on function, comfort, and emotional and spiritual support with the expectation of death. In matters of routine patient care, various participants can arrive at the designation at somewhat different times, and the labeling can unfold differently with different participants in the conversation.

The obvious variation in this process would be troubling if physician-assisted suicide were available only for those categorized as "terminally ill." Availability of physician-assisted suicide contingent on this designation may result in pressure to accelerate the application of or resist the label. Thus this category would not describe an objectively determined status, independent of its effect. Rather, the possibility of physician-assisted suicide could alter the designation and the dynamics of its negotiation.

Regional and situational variation probably would be substantial and perceived as unfair, especially since no standards or assessment mechanisms exist. A rigorous or regularized process would sacrifice the personalization that commends this approach. Furthermore, no approach overcomes the problem that being labeled as terminally ill turns, in part, on the desirability of having physician-assisted suicide available. The variation, the inability to standardize, and the likelihood of significant litigation make this an unlikely determinant for defining the category of persons eligible for physician-assisted suicide.

Defining terminal illness with an explicit statistical threshold is more appealing because it seems to offer greater objectivity: a person is either below or above that threshold. A statistical threshold refers to a person's chance to live for a particular amount of time (e.g., a 50 percent chance to live for six months). However, this approach encounters serious difficulties.

First, the data needed to calculate estimates for individual patients that can be compared with a statistical threshold are not usually available. Very little research data exist to allow statistical prognoses of the timing of death. Various formulae have been reported for several limited populations.[32] However, most people will die after a course of illness that is not well described and that may not be predictable.[33] Even when reliable studies have been done, the estimates of time left to live are not precise. Uncertainty also arises in applying a research database to a more general population.

Second, the threshold is unavoidably arbitrary and likely to result in many borderline cases. Some categories reflect natural divisions of characteristics (e.g., gender). Some reflect arbitrary but administratively easy divides (e.g., the age of majority). Clearly, a statistical threshold for terminal illness is not a natural category like gender or a clear category like age. Any possible divide will separate persons who have quite similar situations and desires. The threshold then would roughly have to comport with relevant patient characteristics and also be administratively convenient. No effort has yet been made to articulate and defend such a threshold, and doing so will lead to several considerable, and probably intractable, problems.

No strategy can actually include only those who will die soon. Not only will any threshold include people who will live a long time, but the rate will increase with more inclusive thresholds.[34] For example, a population with exactly a 25 percent chance to live six months really would have one in four persons still alive at six months (unless assisted in suicide).

Furthermore, some diseases are just too unpredictable. A good threshold aims to include all those who will soon die of each serious chronic disease. Yet no strategy will optimize both specificity and sensitivity. Indeed, all available strategies perform badly in both arenas in a number of common illnesses.[35]

Public expectations will also foul up efforts to establish a specific threshold. Each possible threshold includes patients not now considered terminally ill, or excludes patients commonly considered to be terminally ill, or both. The popular conception of "terminal illness" primarily extends to patients with cancer, neurological degenerative diseases, and AIDS.

In general, we use *terminal illness* to refer to those patients for whom there is no available curative treatment, who are losing weight and function, and who are, or ought to be, psychologically "ready" to die. Any statistical threshold will include many persons who do not now merit this social label, or will exclude many who do, or both. For example, half of all persons who die of lung cancer today will have had a prognosis of better than 30 percent to live two months just one week ago,[36] so any more restrictive threshold will miss most persons dying of lung cancer. Yet such a threshold will include many persons with acute respiratory, cardiac, or liver failure, who usually are vigorously treated and qualify for transplantation only when seriously ill. If the category were expanded to include everyone with up to a 50 percent chance to live six months, most nursing home residents would qualify. If the category were restricted to those with a 1 percent chance to live two months, not only would one exclude virtually all cancer patients but those in the category would be so sick that they would, on average, die within a day.[37] Every option yields a mismatch between perceptions and achievable goals that renders the designation of terminal illness almost meaningless with regard to physician-assisted suicide.

Finally, the prognosis for survival can be affected by treatment, which can depend on patient and physician choice, availability of services, or the nature of the illness, or some combination of these. Treatment decisions that shape prognosis will be problematic. A person with diabetes could stop insulin, a person with a feeding tube could stop its use, or a person with heart disease could refuse a pacemaker. If, as a consequence, such a person becomes "terminally ill," then the category is dependent on volitional actions and not merely a patient's clinical status. So a statistical criterion does not eliminate manipulation. If people who choose to pursue life-sustaining treatment are denied classification as "terminally ill," they could be barred from access to physician-assisted suicide to which they would otherwise be entitled. The public debate has not delineated the effect on being qualified for physician-assisted suicide of a voluntary decision to pursue or not pursue treatment.

A very different way to define terminal illness is based on the extent of illness. While this approach is loosely tied to prognosis, it allows substantial uncertainty about an individual's expected survival time. The threshold could be linked to clinically significant and morally important events, such as the recurrence of cancer in a different site or the onset of fecal incontinence in a demented person. These events and thresholds could be understandable to patients, practitioners, and the public in a way that the statistical modeling is not. This would allow for the possibility of public accord on the general nature and some of the specifics of the thresholds.

However, there are problems with this approach. An individual's status is not well characterized by the extent of one serious disease. Rather, a person's future is shaped by the particular illness; reserve capacity of various body systems; social situation; personal orientation; and availability, use of, and response to treatment. Thus there unquestionably will be much variation. Additionally, many of the patients included will actually have long life spans. If one purpose of defining *terminal illness* is to restrict physician-assisted suicide to persons who have only a short time to live, this method of categorization will not succeed. This method is also afflicted with some of the problems already described: lack of data for groups of persons generally and for specific patients individually, inability to arbitrate the effects of inducing "terminal illness" through treatment choices, and incompatibility with existing social construction of the category.

In addition to the requirement for terminal illness, physician-assisted suicide proposals and law limit access to persons who are competent to make such a decision at the time it is implemented. Thus there is a need to determine who is and is not competent for this purpose. As with categorizing the terminally ill, identifying competence is a difficult and perhaps impossible task, especially as there are difficulties with both legal and clinical considerations.

While competence is formally a legal construct determined by the courts, in practice, physicians and families often decide whether the patient is still capable of making important decisions. Some statutes specifically set forth a procedure that allows nonjudicial determinations of competence, usually requiring concurrence among health professionals. However, statutes and other legal sources provide little guidance as to what should be measured and what standard should be applied. This is left to the evaluating physician, or mental health professional, who is expected to assess the patient's capabilities and gauge them against the demands of the situation.

Public sentiments also affect the amount of decision-making capacity required. Generally, a very low standard of mental performance is required in order to write a will for disposition of one's personal property, since there is a strong public interest in having estates settled. However, a person is usually required to show a higher level of mental abilities in order to forgo life-saving treatment. Appropriate competence standards for physician-assisted suicide have not been determined. There is not even a professional consensus as to what components of cognitive and emotional functioning should be measured, much less how capable the person must be in order to qualify for physician-assisted suicide. Physician determinations of competence inevitably will be subjective, complex, and different among physicians. The resulting variation will be random and perhaps unfair.

It may be possible to rely on a specified set of tests and create a threshold for performance to determine competence. However, the multifactorial character of competence and the inadequacy of measures will make this endeavor difficult. Furthermore, the illnesses and treatments that are commonplace among very seriously ill patients characteristically limit various components of competence. The adverse effects of illness and treatment also vary over time.

As another option, measurement and performance requirements for physician-assisted suicide could be established. Competence is a multifactorial concept, which includes, for example, ability to learn and recall information, consider likely outcomes, assess desirability of outcomes, communicate about the situation and the choices, and reach a decision. An individual can lack capacity to make some decisions but not others. A person also can be generally confused but clear about a particular situation. Since the combinations and complications are legion, using a specific threshold in one or in just a few domains oversimplifies what actually is a complex task. That simplification could mean that a fixed threshold will find some persons to be competent despite obvious and relevant disabilities while others could actually handle this choice well despite a determination of incompetence.

A special problem with lengthy dying is fear of the indignity associated with incompetence. If policy is to allow physician assistance in suicide for only those with contemporaneous competence, then those who have conditions likely to lead to incompetence may feel pressure to undertake preemptive suicide. This is a special risk in early dementia, when patients retain the ability to understand but have failing memory. At this stage, a patient may have nonprogressive memory loss or a very slow rate of progression, and thus the chance for additional comfortable and capable years. However, a patient also may rapidly progress to cognitive disability. Persons in this situation might seek to avoid the dreaded outcomes by pre-emptive physician-assisted suicide. This pattern could create substantial pressures for allowing some forms of advance direction by which a person could specify the degree of disability that would trigger lethal actions. Once a person is no longer competent or capable of acting himself or herself, assisted suicide is no longer an option. Thus policy may be forced to move beyond assisted suicide to considerations of euthanasia.

Not only must an individual be terminally ill and competent to make decisions to have access to physician-assisted suicide, but also he or she must be acting voluntarily or without undue influence. Yet the experience of illness appears inherently coercive: dying persons are very sick and usually experience a welter of strong emotions, such as anger, fear, exhilaration, and self-disparagement. They are generally vulnerable to the suggestions, expectations, and guidance of others. In this context, pressure or encouragement from family, friends, and caregivers or even general societal expectations may become inappropriately coercive.

How the care system expects dying persons and their families to act may be the most important factor influencing the actual care provided. Large variations in whether people die at home or in a hospital in various regions of the country are strongly related to hospital bed supply and regional hospice investment, and not to preferences, wealth, family presence, or other patient characteristics.[38] Patients may assume they are making independent, informed decisions, when really their choices are guided by the usual course of care undertaken by the institution and health care professionals providing the care.[39]

While it is easy enough to bar decisions made under threat of violence, gentle coercion of the very sick is hard to discern or to prevent. Would we count it as undue influence if we found that most persons in certain nursing homes, or certain capitated managed care systems, were "freely choosing" to commit suicide? Would we count it as undue influence if heirs encouraged physician-assisted suicide? What if an elderly, terminally ill grandfather felt that he had become unreasonably burdensome for his aging adult child?

Persons nearing death are generally quite disabled, and their care is costly. Many people at that stage need assistance in tasks of daily living, hygiene, supply and medication procurement, maintenance of an abode, and management of symptoms as well as support for emotional and spiritual needs. These services are costly and require either private payment or Medicaid, for many of the services needed are not provided by health insurance or Medicare. Thus persons approaching death are often severely pressured by financial concerns. Is financial concern to count as undue influence or not? This is a particular dilemma for those who serve frail, disabled, and poor patients. The availability of physician-assisted suicide may itself become coercive in a society where health care services are not a right but a privilege that is circumscribed by individual situation, location, and finances.

Even with various pressures, of course, the patient could still be making his or her own decisions. It would be troubling to bar the patient from accessing physician-assisted suicide because of the perception of undue influence, even if the decision is not the result of the undue influence. In fact, if coercion barred physician-assisted suicide, a family member who really wanted to thwart the patient's choice for assisted suicide could deliberately set out to create the appearance of undue pressure on the patient and thus preclude legal access to physician-assisted suicide.

Some proposals for physician-assisted suicide also require that the patient be "suffering," "in pain," or "acting rationally." The nature and measurement of these conditions have not been articulated and justified. The interaction with treatment is again important, since sedation can always eliminate physical symptoms. This course is available at present, without any change in the law. Then again, most patients can be made physically comfortable without sedation. Perhaps many would be eligible for physician-assisted suicide only if they turned down these available treatments and therefore had severe symptoms.

Some symptoms, such as emotional suffering, weariness, and weakness, are not easily assuaged. Relief through counseling and medications is usual but not reliable. Perhaps this is in part because physicians and society generally are reluctant to consider sedation as a response to emotional distress. If this is so, then one must question the implication that physician-assisted suicide might be an acceptable response. If society is not willing to sedate a person in order to relieve anguish, it may not be appropriate to make that person's suicide easier.

Given the possibilities of suffering, physician-assisted suicide may appear to be a "rational" option. Indeed, many advocates see rationality as a necessary and worthy attribute. Suicide may often be understandable, but weighing the outcome of nonexistence against other outcomes requires some distinctly nonrational considerations. Furthermore, any decision of this import should not be wholly rational but should include a nonrational emotional commitment. One would find it quite incomprehensible to advocate merely "rational" choices for most major life choices—having children, for example.

In sum, no aspect of the proposed definitions of terminal illness that are invoked in safeguards for physician-assisted suicide admits ready categorization. Both conceptual and empirical difficulties afflict each element, making them tenuous limits at best. Definitions and limits have not been delineated. Even the experience of physician-assisted suicide in Oregon and the Netherlands has not yielded clear, consistent, readily understandable guidelines. Without such guidelines, public policy is limited to guesswork and many patients will be subject to arbitrary, possibly discriminatory decisions. Possibilities abound for manipulation so that physician-assisted suicide is effectively easier for those who are elderly, poor, or frail, and for other vulnerable populations. Clearly, legislated guidelines will not be enough to protect everyone, no matter how well intentioned.

The categories of "terminal illness," "competence," and "voluntariness" are not readily defined or enforced, which leaves eligibility for physician-assisted suicide unclear. Lacking clear guidance, policy would allow a serious risk of abuse.

Conclusion

The most powerful calls for physician-assisted suicide come from individuals experiencing suffering we would all prefer to avoid. But for every tragic case of individual suffering spotlighted in the media, whole categories of people suffer without similar attention. Certainly, in some particular situations, physician-assisted suicide may seem appropriate, even necessary. However, justifying an individual act does not mean that a widespread practice can or should be justified. What is good for one person may not be good for groups of people and may be harmful to several groups of people—as physician-assisted suicide appears likely to be. In developing policy, we must remember that physician-assisted suicide is about more than individual rights and distressing situations. Oliver Wendell Holmes reminded us, "Hard cases make bad law." Now we need a corollary about population well-being and policy: Hard individual situations make bad public policy.

The calls for legalizing physician-assisted suicide arise in a social system that is inattentive to the complex physical, emotional, and spiritual needs of people as they near the end of life. Additionally, abuse is a real risk, especially among those who are elderly, frail, disabled, and economically disadvantaged. Resolving a patient's suffering should not rely on assisting that patient's suicide. Rather, providing comfort care, especially when cure is no longer possible, is an important task for health care professionals. Making good palliative care a real option involves developing a new research agenda, enhancing medical education, and changing priorities in health care delivery and funding. With a priority on palliative care, physician assistance in dying could come to mean supportive and comfort care rather than a lethal prescription.

Ultimately, arguments for physician-assisted suicide can be effectively countered by data as well as principles. Not only are all extant proposals for legalization unworkable or hazardous to vulnerable persons, but the community would be better off keeping physician-assisted suicide illegal while learning how to provide reliable, good care to all with serious, eventually fatal illnesses.

Depression and the Will to Live in the Psychological Landscape of Terminally Ill Patients

*Harvey M. Chochinov, M.D., Ph.D., and
Leonard Schwartz, LL.B., LL.M., M.D.*

In 1995 and more recently in February 2000, I (H.M.C.) testified before Canada's Special Senate Committee on Euthanasia and Assisted Suicide. For more than a decade, our clinical work and research has focused on trying to understand the emotional issues faced by patients nearing death. Not surprisingly, depression, and the role it plays in undermining dying patients' wish to carry on living, has been a particular focus of our work. As such, we have attempted to establish the prevalence of depression among patients nearing death, examined screening strategies to help clinicians identify depression more readily, and looked carefully at the relationship between depression and various other factors that might undermine a dying patient's wish to go on living in the face of his or her approaching death. If these factors, which range from the physical and psychological to the spiritual and existential, are not understood then vulnerable individuals will be at risk of having their lives ended rather than having their problems addressed. And if the relationship between depression and the wish to die were the whole story or merely a matter of cause and effect, then my job as a witness—and the job of the senators deliberating about Canada's position on euthanasia and assisted suicide—would have been simpler.

In a 5-4 split decision, the Senate Committee ultimately chose not to recommend changes to the current laws prohibiting euthanasia and assisted suicide. Perhaps the closeness of their vote is reflective of the deep societal divisions that exist regarding policies that allow death to be hastened, as well as the intrinsic complexity of these issues. No request for hastened death can be understood, however, without first attempting to understand the psychological landscape within which that request arises. This chapter attempts to outline some of the critical psychological considerations and the research literature that inform our current understanding of the difference among a wish to die, the waning of will to live, and depression in patients nearing death.

Depression and the Dying

Care of the terminally ill patient is emerging as one of the most important issues in health care today. Recent initiatives, such as the American Medical Association's Education for Physicians on End-of-Life Care project, the Open Society Institute's Project on Death in America, and the Robert Wood Johnson Foundation's Last Acts Campaign, are designed to improve the quality of care for these patients.[1] Achieving better care requires not only a good understanding of the physical domains of care and patient concern, but also an extension of this inquiry that includes psychological, spiritual, and existential considerations. After all, every patient whose death is imminent will at some point ponder the question, Is life still meaningful and worth living? Depression can influence a patient's answer. It is thus essential that those who care for terminally ill patients are aware of depression and its influence on one's sense of meaning and the wish to go on living, even in the face of death. Those providing care also need to be aware of therapeutic strategies to address depression, ways to improve quality of life, and how to assist the dying patient in the search for meaning as life comes to a close.

All patients with a terminal prognosis will understandably experience some periods of profound sadness. Such a reaction is part of what it is to be human and face vulnerability, loss, and ultimately death. However, clinical depression—or depressive syndrome, as it is sometimes referred to—may also present in the later stages of a patient's illness. Clinical depression is a condition marked by a persistent, prominent sad mood; loss of interest in almost all activities; an overwhelming sense of helplessness, hopelessness, and worthlessness; and preoccupation with thoughts of death. In addition to these psychological symptoms, people with major depression will also experience a variety of physical symptoms, including fatigue, poor concentration, anorexia, weight loss, and insomnia.

Not surprisingly, clinical depression may lead some patients to a heightened desire to hasten death. Studies of terminally ill patients and ambulatory AIDS patients have demonstrated that the most significant predictor of support for physician-assisted suicide was depression and psychological distress. One study of 378 ambulatory HIV patients in New York City found that 63 percent of respondents favored physician-assisted suicide, and 55 percent acknowledged considering such an option for themselves.[2] Two-thirds of the severely depressed patients in the study, and 72 percent of those who expressed suicidal ideation, expressed interest in physician-assisted suicide. Patients with cancer or other terminal illnesses are at increased risk of suicide, compared to the general population.[3] Suicide risk factors include pain, depression, delirium, and various disabilities resulting from having an advanced illness. In one study of psychiatric disorders among suicidal cancer patients, 39 percent were thought to have a major depression; 54 percent were diagnosed with an adjustment disorder with anxious and/or depressed features; and 20 percent were delirious.[4] While a severely confused state may render some patients unable to carry out self-destructive acts, mild delirium can place patients at higher risk for completed suicide due to its disinhibiting effects.[5]

Elderly persons are at greater risk for depression as well as for suicide. The older cancer patient has not only lost his or her prior state of good health, but often is confronting a variety of other challenges, including loss of physical abilities, loss of financial stability, death of spouse/partner/friends, and loss of self-esteem (retirement, change in social standing). While depression can sometimes present as it does in younger patients, elderly depressed patients frequently do not endorse having a prominent depressed mood and instead may complain of loss of interest in most activities, as well as cognitive complaints, such as poor memory or concentration. Careful history taking will demonstrate that depressive features often antedate these changes.[6]

Depression plays a significant role in cancer suicide. It is thought that these patients, depending on the nature of their malignancy, are at up to twenty-five times greater risk of successful suicide than the general population. Depressive symptoms may occur in many patients with advanced cancer, with 10 percent to 20 percent of patients meeting diagnostic criteria for major depression.[7] One study suggested that the more physically compromised the patient as a result of advancing illness, the more likely he or she was to present with significant depressive symptoms.[8]

Physicians must therefore be aware of the possible existence of a depression in seriously ill patients and the effect this may have on their desire for death. A patient who appears ambivalent or apathetic about continued treatment may in fact be suffering from depression. These patients are in danger of receiving less than optimal care, or of suffering from a potentially treatable illness, if depression is misperceived as "a normal reaction" to serious physical illness. It is essential for physicians to screen for and treat depression among those who are terminally ill, not to dismiss this illness as an inevitable and natural event.

Depression also appears to influence patients' choices for medical treatment, especially in geriatric populations. In one recent study of elderly depressed patients, the desire for life-sustaining medical treatment increased following treatment of depression.[9] Those patients who had initially been severely depressed or hopeless were also more likely to overestimate the risks and underestimate the benefits of treatment. Thus in severely depressed patients (especially those who are hopeless) advance treatment directives should be deferred until the depression has been treated.

Assessment of Depression and the Wish to Die

Only within the last fifteen to twenty years have doctors begun to consider both the issue of depression in terminally ill patients and the appropriate measures for assessment and treatment of this condition. A seminal article published by James Brown and colleagues in the mid-1980s was one of the first to broach the topic of whether it was ever "normal" for dying patients to covet an early death. They found that in one group of forty-four terminally ill patients selected from a palliative care unit, three of the patients were or had been suicidal and seven more had expressed a desire for early death. All ten of the patients who desired early death were found to be clinically depressed based on the *DSM–III* criteria for major depression, or a significantly high score using the Beck Depression Inventory (BDI, a standard self-report instrument used in psychiatric research).[10] The authors noted that limitations of the study included the lack of a brief and effective interview suitable for very ill patients, and the lack of special criteria for depression that exclude fatigue, poor concentration, anorexia, weight loss, and insomnia.

Commentators have noted that the *DSM* criteria for major depression are not based on studies of patients with significant physical illnesses. One of the difficulties with the standard diagnostic criteria, particularly the physical criteria, is that they may be present among terminally ill patients not as a result of depression but rather simply due to the underlying advanced disease. The physical criteria thus lack what clinicians refer to as diagnostic specificity. As a result, at least four major approaches for diagnosing depression have been developed:

1. *Inclusive approach:* This approach uses the Schedule for Affective Disorders and Schizophrenia (SADS) and Research Diagnostic Criteria (RDC). All symptoms of depression, even those that might be due to a physical illness, are included.

2. *Etiologic approach:* The patient's symptoms are counted only if they are not caused by a physical illness; one difficulty for this is to distinguish between symptoms that are caused by an underlying physical illness as opposed to a depression.

3. *Substitutive approach:* This approach suggests that the diagnostic criteria for depression should be altered in medically ill patients. For example, decreased energy is a poor discriminator for depression in those who are medically ill, whereas "indecisiveness" may be a better discriminator of depression. Some commentators suggest substituting physical symptoms of depression (change in weight or appetite, sleep disturbance, loss of energy or fatigue, and difficulty in thinking or concentrating) with nonphysical or psychological symptoms, such as brooding, self-pity, pessimism, or reactivity, as criteria for the diagnosis of depression in the severely ill patient.[11]

4. *Exclusive approach:* Anorexia and fatigue are eliminated from the criteria for depression, as all too often they may be present on the basis of the underlying advanced illness itself.

After reviewing these approaches, Stephen Cohen-Cole and Alan Stoudemire suggested that the inclusive approach might be the most appropriate for seriously medically ill patients.[12] Although this method has a risk of false positives (i.e., high sensitivity and low specificity for the detection of depression), this risk is preferable to the alternative: lack of treatment for depression in those patients who desperately require it.

Brown and colleagues emphasized the need for a brief and effective screening interview to detect depression in severely ill patients.[13] One recent study compared four brief screening measures for depression in terminally ill patients.[14] These were a single-item interview, a two-item interview, and two self-report instruments (the BDI and a visual mood scale). The single-item screening approach essentially asked patients if they felt depressed most of the time. One hundred and ninety-seven patients receiving palliative care for advanced cancer were assessed using a complete standardized diagnostic interview including the four screening measures referred to above. The results from the four screening measures were then compared to the results from the diagnostic interviews. The researchers found that the single-item interview correctly identified the eventual diagnostic outcome of every patient and was superior to both of the self-report measures. They also noted that inclusion of questions concerning loss of interest or pleasure in activities did not improve diagnostic accuracy but might be appropriate in a brief screening interview. Inclusion of these questions provides for complete coverage of core depressive symptoms and reduces the possibility of missing the diagnosis in patients suffering from depression. Thus it appears that simply asking patients if they are feeling depressed most of the time is a very simple and effective way to screen for clinical depression in this patient population.

In addition to depression, clinicians must also be aware of the possibility of organic mental disorders, which are prevalent in patients with advanced disease. The presence of these syndromes in patients who request death by assisted suicide or euthanasia calls into question the patients' capacity to make such a request. Syndromes to be aware of include organic mood and anxiety disorders. Unfortunately, it is easy to overlook the diagnosis of an organic mental syndrome, because symptoms of dementia are often mistaken for a psychiatric disturbance. Feelings of disbelief, denial, numbness, irritability, hopelessness, and suicidal ideation can all occur in severely ill patients. These symptoms are also found in major depression, anxiety disorders, and adjustment disorders. However, as dementia progresses, the organic nature of the presenting symptoms becomes more obvious. Neuropsychological testing may help distinguish dementia from a depression or an adjustment disorder. It may also be difficult to assess whether the organic mental syndrome is transient or long lasting, whether it affects competence, and whether the desire to die expressed by the patient is similar to the view he or she held prior to the development of the cognitive problem. When faced with a request for euthanasia or assisted suicide, a thorough assessment should be completed, specifically looking for the presence of dementia or delirium. When one considers that approximately 25 percent of hospitalized medical and surgical patients suffer from dementia and that the prevalence of delirium in dying patients approaches 80 percent, the importance of this issue is clear.[15]

When a terminally ill patient expresses a desire to die, caregivers often reach in one of two directions. The expression of a desire for death may be regarded as a normal result of the debilitating effect of illness and suffering. There may be instances in which a waning will to live is a natural consequence of nearing the end of life. Relatively less is known about patients whose decreasing desire for life is part of a natural or normal expression of the desire to "let go" as they approach their final days.

Alternatively, the expression of a desire to die may be viewed as clear evidence of a major depression, which may affect the competence of the patient to make such decisions. As we shall see, for patients who are fixated by a desire to die, depression is often a major causative factor. Furthermore, the absence of clinical depression does not mean that the patient's reaction to terminal illness is unimportant, or that it can safely be ignored. In fact, both views may be correct, in that suffering can lead to a desire for death, and depression can negatively affect the will to live. The use of brief and effective screening measures for depression, a thorough assessment designed to rule out an organic mental syndrome, and measures to assuage suffering or relieve symptoms is an important initial response to the severely ill patient's wish for death.

The Will to Live and the Desire for Death

The "will to live" of dying patients is not static; it may fluctuate according to patients' clinical status and subjective experience of their symptoms. One recent study among terminally ill patients used a series of visual analogue scales to assess pain, anxiety, depression, well-being, dyspnea, nausea, activity, drowsiness, appetite, and the will to live; it found that will to live in patients nearing death fluctuated substantially.[16] The four main predictors of the will to live scores—depression, anxiety, dyspnea, and sense of well-being—also fluctuated significantly over time. Initially, anxiety was the most significant predictor of fluctuation in will to live, but later depression, and finally shortness of breath was the most important determinant of the patients' endorsement of their will to live. If patients' will to live is dependent on their symptoms, it may well be that appropriate symptom management, together with reassurance and fostering of a good patient-physician relationship, will significantly affect a patient's will to live or corresponding desire for death.

One might assume that all patients who are dying would be overwhelmed by hopelessness. Yet that simply does not appear to be the case. Even among patients whose medical prognosis is hopeless, pervasive hopelessness is usually found only among patients who are suffering from depressive syndrome. This of course raises the intriguing question, What is hope and can it persist when not based on the expectation of a prolonged life ahead? In a recent study of almost two hundred patients with advanced terminal cancer, each patient underwent an interview to assess hopelessness and suicidal ideation, and also completed the BDI— Short Form.[17] A correlation was found between measures of suicidal ideation and depression, but the correlation between suicidal ideation and hopelessness was even stronger. The study hypothesis, that suicidal ideation would correlate more highly with hopelessness than with depression, was confirmed in subsequent analysis. This finding has important implications for the evaluation of suicidality in patients with advanced disease. The simple existence of a depression may not be as significant as the existence of hopelessness in attempting to predict suicidal ideation and intent in severely ill patients.

This being said, depression remains an important factor in understanding and predicting a patient's desire for death. Significant numbers of terminally ill patients in palliative care facilities experience or will express at least a fleeting or occasional desire to die. In most cases, these episodes are brief and do not reflect a sustained or committed desire that one might associate with a request to hasten death. However, almost 10 percent of patients in one study reported an unequivocal desire for death to come soon and indicated that this desire was consistent over time.[18] A strong association was found between desire-for-death ratings and clinical depression, based on interviews from the SADS. About 60 percent of patients who had a genuine desire for death met criteria for clinical depression. However, among patients who did not endorse a genuine, consistent desire for early death, the prevalence of clinical depression was about 7 percent. Depression was a more important factor than either pain or low family support in estimating the desire for death. It is possible that prolonged pain may increase the risk for depression, while family support may offer protection against it. However, once depression has developed, the emergence of a desire for death may be a more direct step. Clearly, while pain and social support are important in evaluating a request for hastened death, understanding the psychological underpinnings of these requests is pivotal to appreciating the nature of a patient's wish to die.

Evaluating suicidal ideation in a palliative care setting requires the consideration of several issues. Numerous risk factors for suicide have been identified among patients with advanced disease, including physical problems, such as pain, delirium, and fatigue; social factors, such as the extent of emotional or family support; and prior psychopathology and psychiatric history. However, depression is the one factor that has the most empirical support. Studies of oncology outpatients have found that depression, not pain, was related to hoarding drugs in preparation for a possible future suicide attempt.[19] However, treatment of pain and other physical symptoms can have a significant effect on the expressed suicidal intent or desire to die. In one recent study of patients who requested lethal prescriptions from doctors in Oregon (after the passage of the state's Death with Dignity Act made physician-assisted suicide legal in certain circumstances), it was found that 46 percent of patients who made such a request *changed their minds* after significant interventions (such as relief of pain or other physical symptoms) were initiated by their attending physicians, while only 15 percent of patients who did not receive such significant interventions changed their minds concerning the desire to die.[20]

As noted above, hopelessness is a good clinical marker for suicidal ideation. When hopelessness becomes the focus of a patient's psychological response to issues of death and dying, then in some cases he or she may see suicide as a rational and appropriate alternative, as compared to the decline toward a natural death. Thus the assessment of hopelessness is an important tool in understanding suicidal intent among those who are terminally ill. The meaning of hope and its preservation even in the face of impending death are thus important issues to be addressed in the care of dying patients.

Therapeutic Considerations

A recent study asked patients with severe or terminal illness for their views on end-of-life issues. Patients identified five domains of care affecting quality of life: receiving adequate pain and symptom management, avoiding inappropriate prolongation of dying, achieving a sense of control, relieving the burden on those they love, and strengthening relationships with them.[21] The undermining of care in any of these domains may see the patient become more vulnerable to a preference that death be hastened.

The physician-patient relationship is seldom more important than in the context of treating a terminally ill patient. The greatest fear of dying patients is the process itself: "dying" is usually feared more than death. The patient may have concerns about being abandoned or left helpless or dependent on others for even management of basic bodily functions or daily care, or fears of being left untreated or undertreated. Symptoms such as pain, depression, nausea, anxiety, and fatigue can significantly lessen quality of life and should be aggressively treated. A young woman referred to our service with metastatic breast cancer indicated a wish to die. It soon became apparent that her wish to see her life end stemmed directly from her as yet poorly controlled pain. Once good pain relief was achieved, she was able to live out her final days on her family's ranch near the horses she loved.

However, not all the concerns of the dying patient are physical in nature. Longstanding disputes and grudges, family conflicts, and concerns about the meaning of one's life may be significant issues faced by the patient in the last days of his or her life. It may be helpful for patients to focus on some meaningful life goals. In some instances this might include feeling well enough to attend a wedding or other special event, completing a writing project, or endowing a personally meaningful cause. More modest but equally meaningful for many patients is the sharing of important memories, the reinforcement of personal beliefs, or the expression of wishes for family and friends. These activities can bring a sense of resolution, inner peace, and completeness to the patient with a terminal illness. Many patients can find comfort within their religious traditions; therefore, it is important to understand the patient's system of beliefs and relationship to a community of believers. Furthermore, all patients have existential concerns, such as the meaning or significance of life goals achieved or abandoned, regrets about past events, or concern about the future welfare of family members. These existential issues can provide the foundation for further therapeutic interventions.

It would be unrealistic to think that all sadness in the face of terminal illness could be eliminated. Clinical depression, however, is a highly treatable source of suffering among those who are dying. Patients who are treated for their depression often recover the ability to enjoy social discourse and may rekindle some prior interests. Successful treatment can often normalize physical symptoms of depression, such as lack of energy, loss of sleep, and low appetite. Perhaps most critical is the renewed ability to find meaning in life, in spite of impending death. For example, an elderly gentleman with metastatic lung cancer recently presented to our service with a request to die. During the course of his illness he had become wheelchair bound and had incurred many losses that saw him no longer being able to take part in many previously pleasurable and meaningful activities. In spite of having always been somewhat emotionally constricted and "always in control," he now found himself constantly crying, and perseverating about the futility of living and a wish for death. He indicated that he was no longer able to experience any pleasure whatsoever and that he had a pervasive sense of hopelessness and feelings of guilt—specifically related to his sense that he had become a burden to his family and care providers. With three weeks of antidepressant therapy and supportive counseling, his depressive symptoms remitted entirely, allowing him to enjoy spending time with his wife, who helped nurse him throughout his final three months of life on the palliative care ward.

A number of studies have shown that in patients with cancer, appropriate antidepressant therapy results in improvement of mood and overall quality of life.[22] Many other studies have shown individual psychotherapy, structured cognitive therapy, or behavioral therapy to be often effective approaches to depression in the cancer setting.[23] Most psychotherapeutic approaches in patients who are terminally ill combine promoting active coping strategies to maintain the level of functioning, and assisting patients to understand, manage, and work through their feelings related to their disease. Active coping and regaining a sense of mastery and control can sometimes be achieved with group or mutual supportive therapy. These modalities offer the ability to share common experiences with others similarly afflicted, thus reducing the sense of emotional isolation that often accompanies illness.

Existential psychotherapy is an intervention that involves the evaluation and re-evaluation of one's relationship to life, with the goal of helping patients live more fully in each moment. It is an appropriate intervention for some persons facing a terminal illness, because they are confronted daily with choices affecting their quality of life and often have questions concerning the meaning, purpose, and value of their life. How seriously ill patients cope influences both their emotional state and their ability to adjust. It has been demonstrated that avoidance of feelings, denial of concerns, feelings of helplessness or a stance of passive compliance, and social isolation will result in decreased quality of life and possibly increase risk of disease or mortality. However, open and honest expression of both feelings and thoughts corresponds to a higher quality of life and may bolster one's physical health. For example, David Spiegel and colleagues utilized an existential approach to group psychotherapy with patients suffering from recurrent breast cancer.[24] This group met weekly for an entire year, utilizing a traditionally interactive, emotionally supportive therapeutic style. The treatment group lived almost twice as long as the control group. Although some have questioned these results, large duplication trials are currently under way. The effect of this approach on group members' quality of life was also notable: patients in the treatment group had less mood and psychosocial distress than those in the control group.

Existential considerations provide the broadest of perspectives from which to understand the quality-of-life issues that challenge those who are terminally ill. One such challenge is the issue of pain, which needs to be understood in terms of its physical, psychological, social, and existential dimensions. Some authors distinguish pain from suffering, noting that suffering is often described as the reaction to or consequence of physical pain. As Cassell indicated, "suffering is experienced by persons, not merely by bodies, and has its source in challenges that threaten the intactness of the person as a complex social and psychological entity. Suffering can include physical pain but is by no means limited to it."[25] Thus suffering reaches beyond the domain of the physical and can be seen as a reaction to loss of function, hope, and the fracturing of relationships. To reduce suffering, existential psychotherapy emphasizes the use of strategies to develop meaningful actions in the patient's life, and assists patients to acknowledge and to the extent possible accept their suffering and impending death. The value of a patient's own life experiences, knowledge, and memories and the capacity for teaching others is emphasized. Central to this approach is the nature of the relationship between the therapist and the patient, and between the patient and others, including family members. Group existential psychotherapy is one approach that allows the patient to hear about the experience of others, thereby providing "lateral experience" from which the patient may consider alternative ways of understanding and action. As well, the exposure to the perspectives of other patients can help break down the patient's own assumptions about life, facilitate an adjustment to his or her current circumstances, and assist in choosing actions that are truly meaningful. The group has the potential to facilitate the sharing of experiences, which may help the patient realize that he or she is not alone and that others have different perspectives that may bear consideration.[26] One woman participating in our local group for patients with advanced breast cancer spoke of the comfort she felt knowing her example provided comfort to others and that even after her death, her memory would be preserved.

Another intervention that has evolved for patients who are physically ill is the psychodynamic life narrative. It is particularly useful for patients whose previously successful adaptation has been disrupted by a crisis or a specific life event, such as a physical illness, that has led to anxiety, depression, or demoralization. The life narrative allows patients to give their current experience meaning in the context of their life histories and to view their current reaction as the logical product of their previous experience, rather than as an arbitrary or inevitable response to their illness. It offers coherence, order, and logic in a situation that is largely chaotic, unpredictable, and beyond the patient's individual control. Engaging in a psychodynamic life narrative also provides the patient with a protective therapist-physician. Such a benevolent and committed figure will often provide reassurance, reminiscent of a good parent. The therapist attempts to capture the life narrative, and over time the process assumes the quality of a shared experience.[27] Our service recently saw an elderly gentleman with an advanced oral malignancy. This patient gained considerable comfort in being able to review his life as a successful actor and found that the therapeutic task of sharing this history both provided a context within which to understand his current existential distress ("Why bother living?") and helped give his life a much-needed sense of meaning and purpose.

However, doing therapeutic life narrative goes beyond benevolence and good intentions. These assurances are helpful only if directed to the real source of the patient's concern and anxiety. Patients' reactions to illness, either simple or serious, not only reside in their personality characteristics and attitudes, but reflect the particular meaning of the experience in the context of their present and past life. It is important to convey an understanding of the implication of the illness for the patient. The goal is to have the patient examine his or her life in an effort to contextualize the illness and give it meaning that will permit its integration with previous life experience. Patient distress may not be directly related to the fear of death itself but to concerns regarding missed opportunities, loss of autonomy and control, and regret for decisions not taken. All these may be examined through use of the psychodynamic life narrative.

The existentialist Viktor Frankl suggested that suffering may be a catalyst both for having a need for meaning and for finding meaning. The diagnosis of a terminal illness may thus be both a cause for distress and an opportunity for growth and meaning. Suddenly having to prioritize, spending more time with loved ones and in turn experiencing personal growth, may be the direct result of having to cope with a foreshortened life expectancy. Thus the ability to find meaning within traumatic events has also been associated with an increased ability to adapt to them. Frankl suggested that meaning can derive from three sources: creative, experiential, and attitudinal.[28] The first refers to creative values, including artistic work or pursuits, or causes in which one could be active. The second source of meaning concerns valued experiences, such as the experience of love for others. Thus as noted earlier, some studies have found that social support is one of the most important variables associated with a good adjustment to cancer.[29] Another example of meaning through experience is the ability to appreciate beauty. This could be beauty in nature, or simply experiencing kindness from another person. Humor also plays an important role in helping patients to adjust to their difficult circumstances. Humor requires looking at one's situation from a distance and separating oneself from it. It therefore helps foster a safe environment in which very difficult topics can be discussed. Finally, the third source of meaning is the attitude with which one bears unavoidable suffering. Even if the situation cannot be changed, or is for the most part not subject to modification, the individual can exert some sense of control by adapting his or her attitude to the new reality. Thus Frankl suggests that the one freedom left is the freedom to choose one's attitude in bearing one's suffering.

Irvin Yalom, in his years of work with cancer patients facing death, noted two powerful and common methods of alleviating fears about death. These methods are essentially beliefs or "delusions" that are important in providing a sense of safety. The first is belief in one's personal specialness; this is a feeling that the individual is above and beyond the ordinary laws of human biology and destiny. It provides a sense of safety from within. The second common delusion is the belief in an ultimate rescuer, which allows the patient to feel forever watched over and protected by an outside force. Though patients may grow ill and arrive at the very end of their lives, they believe there is an omnipotent force that will always bring them back. Yet when death approaches, patients are faced with the chilling truth: they are born alone and must die alone. Yalom observes that many dying patients remark that the most awful thing about dying is that it must be done alone. Yet even at the point of death, the willingness of another to be fully present can be of tremendous comfort. As one of Yalom's patients stated, "Even though you're alone in your boat, it's always comforting to see the lights of the other boats bobbing near by."[30]

The common existential problems for patients with advanced cancer include feelings of hopelessness, futility, meaningless, remorse, death anxiety, and disruption of personal identity. Distress may be related to past, present, or future concerns. For example, concerns regarding the past can result in a sense of disappointment related to unfulfilled aspirations, or a devaluing of previous achievements. Present concerns may revolve around changes in body image or intellectual, social, and professional functioning. If the future is perceived to offer only continuing physical and emotional distress until death, the patient may see no value in continuing to live. While treating depression might certainly alter a wish to hasten death, other interventions that bolster one's sense of purpose and meaning must also be invoked. For example, therapeutic approaches that address concerns about current personal integrity, disappointment about perceived past failures, death anxiety, and issues of hopelessness and meaninglessness can be of great help.

Cognitive therapies can help the patients and their families to reappraise their lives to decrease distress and to enhance a sense of positivity. Cognitive restructuring can also help a patient identify meaningful and achievable short-term goals and thus preserve a sense of self-worth and self-efficacy. Life review techniques that focus on positive feelings stemming from positive recollections, while acknowledging but not minimizing negative recollections, can help with the reappraisal of life events commonly used by cancer patients in the search for meaning.

Insight-oriented therapy can help the patient to realize that meaningful and fulfilling aspects of life may lie ahead—joys to be experienced, things to be said, tasks to be completed, and relationships to be enjoyed. The use of simple measures, such as appropriately fitted clothes, cosmetic prostheses, and assistive or orthotic devices, can help to increase the patient's level of social function. Finally, for existential distress that is truly refractory in the sense that it cannot be adequately controlled despite aggressive efforts to identify an appropriate therapy, the option of controlled sedation remains. While this method would obviously interfere with the methods of therapy discussed previously, at the end of life, the goals of care may change such that the relief of suffering takes precedence over all other considerations.[31]

Conclusion

In social policy considerations regarding euthanasia and assisted suicide, it would be tempting to see the issue of depression as leading to simple and specific directives. However, life—and in this instance the clinical and empirical data—are rarely so straightforward. As was reported to Canada's Special Senate Committee on Euthanasia and Assisted Suicide, not all patients making requests that their death be hastened are clinically depressed, and sometimes the waning of one's will to live in the face of death may be part of a natural process of accepting and preparing for death. However, our understanding of the psychology of these issues is in its early days. Vulnerable, depressed individuals are clearly at risk for seeing their health care provider acquiesce to a request for hastened death without necessarily having a clear understanding of the physical, psychological, spiritual, and existential factors that underpin the very request itself. Feeling overwhelmed in the face of suffering—and a sense of impotence and therapeutic failure—may lead some health care providers to eliminate, rather then engage and grapple with, the problem of patients requesting a hastened death.

Few palliative care services provide expert psychiatric consultation or ongoing psychiatric care for those that might benefit. There is also relatively little research being conducted on the psychological complexities of patients nearing death, and even less work that specifically targets the issue of a wish for hastened death. Least of all is interventional research that attempts, through pharmacological or psychotherapeutic methods, or both, to influence the will to live of patients nearing death. Clearly, psychiatrists and experts in mental health care are best situated to understand and explore the psychological underpinnings of a dying patient's request that death be hastened. Although these requests may appear straightforward and eminently understandable, appreciating the depth of their complexity offers a real opportunity to respond more empathically and to be more therapeutically effective for this vulnerable group of patients.

While depression should always be considered in the evaluation of a dying patient's request to hasten death, the issues of meaning and hope provide a broader context informing a therapeutic approach. Relief of pain, and treatment of depression and reversible causes of a desire to die, are vital. It is the patient's global quality of life and the meaning he or she ascribes to it, however, that will truly determine the emotional texture and course of the last stage of life. The assessment of a terminally ill patient who appears depressed may begin with a simple screening question that asks if he or she is depressed most of the time. Understanding the complex internal world of the patient nearing death who no longer wishes to live, requires that our questions probe further. Beyond depression and its complexities, meaning and purpose provide a broader framework within which the patient's suffering can be witnessed, explored, and empathically responded to.

A Better Way

A Hospice Perspective

Cicely Saunders, O.M., F.R.C.P.

The interchange between advocates of voluntary euthanasia and physician-assisted suicide and proponents of the hospice and palliative care movement is of long standing and began at a personal level. At the end of 1959, Dr. Leonard Colebrook, the chair of the Voluntary Euthanasia Society, visited with me and forty-five patients with terminal malignant disease at St. Joseph's Hospice, Hackney, East London. He wrote afterward, "The visit did help me very much to try and get this difficult problem in perspective. I still feel that there would be little or no problem of euthanasia if all the terminal disease folks could end their lives in that atmosphere you have done so much to create—but alas that can hardly be for many a long year and meanwhile, how many thousands will end their lives in very different circumstances? You will raise the standard of terminal care throughout the profession—more power to you."[1]

St. Joseph's Hospice opened in the East End of London (a deeply deprived area) in 1905. It was founded by the Irish Sisters of Charity, who had opened a Hospice for the Dying in Dublin in 1879, taking the word *hospice* from the early Christian era. The word had then been used to describe a place where hospitality was offered to pilgrims and other travelers as well as the sick and destitute. These early hospices had no particular concern to admit the dying, although many guests must have ended their days in their care. The word had then been first used for an institution specifically for the incurably sick and dying by Mme. Jeanne Garnier in Lyons, France, in 1842, but the Sisters of Charity do not appear to have known this and chose this name for the last journey quite independently.

The lonely dying of a Jewish man of forty from Warsaw, Poland, in 1948 was the focus for a new, research-based approach in this field. During his inpatient care at both a teaching and later a county hospital, as his social worker and friend, I discussed with him what facility could have met his needs better than a busy surgical ward. In referring to a proposed legacy of £500 he said to me, "I'll be a window in your home." On another occasion, he asked "only for what is in your mind and in your heart." With these two phrases he posed a challenge to openness of all kinds: to the world, to all who would come, and to all future demands. On thinking over his second request, I came to realize that our patients would ask much skill of us, including research and study to establish a sound scientific basis for care and knowledge of family dynamics and of political acumen, matched with a closer personal relationship than seen in most acute care. After his peaceful death came an assurance that he had made his final journey in a freedom of the spirit that we should also work to make possible. It took nineteen years to build the "home" around the window, including my training in medicine and seven years of clinical research.

By the time St. Christopher's Hospice opened in South East London in 1967, there was already an as yet unnamed "hospice movement."[2] Links with pain researchers, social workers, psychologists, and sociologists, and with earlier institutions, such as Calvary Hospital, New York, had grown from 1958 on as part of a project on the "Nature and Management of Terminal Pain." The foundation of the field of later research was based on the experience of seven years analyzing the notes of 1,100 patients with far advanced cancer and their "total pain."[3] This was summed up concisely by one patient who said, "It was all pain," and by another response to the simple question, "Mrs. H, tell me about your pain." She replied, without further prompting: "Well, doctor, it began in my back but now it seems that all of me is wrong. I could have cried for the pills and the injections but I knew that I mustn't. No one seemed to understand how I felt and it seemed as if all the world was against me. My husband and son were marvelous but they would have to stay off work and lose their pay. But it's wonderful to feel safe again."

This described a whole experience for Mrs. H, comprising physical, psychological, family, and spiritual needs. The regular giving of oral morphine or diamorphine, which I observed first as a volunteer nurse in St. Luke's Hospital (founded in 1893 as St. Luke's Home for the Dying Poor in London), had changed the patients in St. Joseph's Hospice from "pain full to pain free," as one of the sisters later wrote. Before then, as elsewhere, it was "4 hourly p.r.n." with patients having to "earn" their relief by having pain first. What this was like for those with severe pain was described to me in a conversation with another patient tape recorded in 1961:

> *Patient:* Well, it was ever so bad. It used to be just like a vise gripping my spine—going like that and would then let go again—and I didn't get my injections regularly—they used to leave me as long as they could and, if I asked for them sometimes, they used to say, "No, wait a bit longer." They didn't want me to rely on the drugs that were there, you see. They used to try and see how long I could go without an injection. . . . I used to be pouring with sweat, you know, because of the pain. . . . And I was having crying fits—I mean, I think I haven't cried lately—I think I've only cried once since I have been here, that's all—well over a week. And I was crying every other day at the other hospital. I was very depressed, ever so depressed; But I'm not at all depressed here, not like I was there.
>
> *C.S.:* Since you've been here and I put you onto regular injections, what's the difference?
>
> *Patient:* Well, the biggest difference is, of course, this feeling so calm. I don't get worked up, I don't get upset, I don't cry, I don't get very depressed—because I was getting awfully depressed—you know, really black thoughts were going through me mind, and no matter how kind people were—and people were ever so kind—nothing would console me, you see. But since I've been here I feel more hopeful, as well. I feel that I'm going to get better and I'm going to go home. Whereas there I didn't, you see. And no one would tell me that I was either. I kept asking various people, and nobody would give me a clear answer. But since I've been here, I don't feel that desperate need to ask, "Am I going to get better, am I . . . I mean, I want to know."
>
> *C.S.:* But you don't feel desperation?
>
> *Patient:* No, I don't feel the hopelessness.

This was indeed a problem of drugs and medical care, but there was much more to it than that. The patient was in the hospice for nine months with multiple metastases and paraplegia. She did a great deal to solve her difficult family situation (she was only forty), she entertained innumerable visitors, and she was busy all the time. Her family, her own vicar, all the nurses, and, above all, the sister of the ward herself had very demanding parts to play as the patient gradually came to understanding and acceptance and a greatly deepened faith. The work was that of St. Joseph's Hospice as a whole, but the victory and the final peace were her own. That is the kind of success that means most to us.[4]

Sadly, there are still stories in which fears of drug dependence inhibit effective pain relief. How hospice development was concurrent with clinical pain research was summed up in 1986 by Patrick Wall:

> Up to the 19th century, most medical care related to the amelioration of symptoms while the natural history of the disease took its course toward recovery or death. By 1900, doctors and patients alike had turned to a search for root cause and ultimate cure. In the course of this new direction, symptoms were placed on one side as signposts along a highway which was being driven toward the intended destination. Therapy directed at the signposts was denigrated and dismissed as merely symptomatic. By the second half of this century a reaction set in as seen by such remarkable developments as the hospice movement. The immediate origins of misery and suffering need immediate attention while the long-term search for basic cure proceeds. The old methods of care and caring had to be rediscovered and the best of modern medicine had to be turned to the task of new study and therapy specifically directed at pain.[5]

This was the perspective recognized by Colebrook in 1959 and from which those involved in the hospice movement maintained a dialogue with those advocating the legalization of voluntary euthanasia and, later, physician-assisted suicide. Colebrook himself became a personal friend and modified his views considerably and encouraged me in my efforts to establish scientific hospice care. The original focus on the multifaceted pain of terminal malignant disease enabled research among a homogenous group of patients and showed that given oral medications in individually optimized doses with the increasing number of adjuvants available, patients could be free of pain and still alert with normal affect, able to find new physical ease, deepened relationships, and a more confident search for meaning in the life remaining. Following this, Dr. Robert Twycross was invited to carry out a double-blind, controlled trial of heroin and morphine. The trial concluded that morphine is a satisfactory substitute for orally administered heroin. This was an important finding because heroin is not available in most of the world. The study showed that it is not so much the drug that is used as the way it is used: given regularly by mouth in individualized optimized doses with other analgesics as necessary.[6] Twycross also showed, as in the original St. Joseph's Hospice study, that tolerance was not a clinical problem, nor was drug dependence an issue.[7]

The spread of the hospice movement since then has been remarkable in its diversity, yet each team has shared recognizably similar aims. There are now hospices all around the world. A sample from some twenty-one countries contributed to *Hospice Care on the International Scene*.[8] The Hospice Information Service at St. Christopher's Hospice works together with other international organizations now involved in the field, including the World Health Organization.[9] To my knowledge, the alternative of physician-assisted suicide is rarely, if ever, mentioned in reports from developing countries. From a personal perspective, I would not judge a patient who took his or her own life. We often give patients living at home supplies of medication to control their symptoms that they could use in this way, but we never suggest, directly or indirectly, that they should take this step. Notably, we have cared for some twenty thousand patients, but only three inpatients and two home care patients have taken their own lives, and none used medication supplied by St. Christopher's Hospice. Some have asked us to hasten their deaths; far more have asked us to let them die, meaning not to use any life-prolonging treatments. Those who have said "I want to die" have almost always been referring to symptoms that were not previously relieved or to poor communication.[10]

Increasingly, the original concentration on cancer has broadened to look at the wider range of end-of-life care as research has revealed both the need for and the prospects of relief and support. Much of the well-documented knowledge gained from cancer care has been shown to be relevant to the wider scene. It is possible and rewarding to live well to the end of life and to find unexpected insights and strengths both in dependence and in its support. By no means has this possibility reached all in need, but that it could be made available must surely give the perspective recognized by Colebrook so many years ago that the old methods of care and caring must be rediscovered. Even before meeting him, I had written the following: "This is not to deny that patients do suffer in this country but to claim that the great majority need not do so. Those of us who think that euthanasia is wrong have the right to say so, but also the responsibility to help to bring this relief of suffering about."[11]

The need to promote all currently available and legal means of alleviating suffering at the end of life is powerfully presented by a group with "convergent views." Coming from different standpoints, the authors of *Hospice Care on the International Scene* point out the responsibility of physicians "to give comprehensive palliative care to terminally ill patients and to make every effort to explore, understand and address suffering that persists despite their best efforts."[12]

"Humane" care presupposes an awareness of the impact of dependence and deterioration, and a recognition that hopes of cure and longer life are now illusory and partings inevitable. A whole field of death education studies has focused down to an individual's need to end life in a way suited to character and to develop personal stratagems for coping. The Polish Jew who left such creative principles in his brief statements and quiet end gave the rule of listening to the person who is facing his or her "moment of truth." This analogy to the bullfight sets the person in need in the center; everything else flows from the challenge of that human experience, common to all who do not die with catastrophic suddenness.[13] But can anyone not yet facing that moment be truly aware of the anguish of dependence and parting? Another patient, also Polish, answered my question, "What do you need most from someone who is caring for you?" Although he hesitated, saying that because English was his eighth language he was not sure he could answer adequately, I persisted. His reply was "For someone to look as if they are trying to understand me." This still seems relevant to anyone facing a personal crisis and encourages us to understand that our patients do not really ask for success here, only for the willingness to try. That remains the position of the vast majority of hospice workers who believe that the legalization of euthanasia or physician-assisted suicide would gravely undermine the humanity of society.

Physicians, others on the multiprofessional team, family members, and other intimate caregivers are not the only ones who should feel the responsibility to give comprehensive palliative care that seeks to understand and address the many needs dying patients have; society as a whole should feel that responsibility. The strength of the whole hospice and palliative care movement has been its roots in the societies from which it has originated.

Hospice Care on the International Scene vividly describes how cultures in developed and developing countries have very different possibilities and pressures, yet suffering at the end of life has called forth programs in response that bring with them the same basic principles of operation. As the foreword states, "The presentations have an archival value. They will serve as a record of how the international hospice movement functioned during the critical early period [and] . . . have an immediate value to all who are concerned with the humane and effective care of terminally ill people and their families."[14] Much of the growth in programs of terminal care has been in home care and hospital teams that developed first in the United States and Canada soon after the opening of St. Christopher's Hospice in 1967 and its own home care service in 1969.

In the United Kingdom, the specialty of palliative medicine has developed from and continues to flourish within the separate hospices as well as within units and teams of the National Health Service. From early days it seemed important that the newly developing skills should be employed at an earlier, more appropriate point in the course of illness; referral to hospice could mean that "futile" treatments were avoided and patients given time and opportunity for completing important personal tasks of reconciliation, forgiveness, and farewell, always recognizing that some will wish to enter clinical trials until life's end.

Hospice is a complex set of attitudes and skills, not a building. Much of this care and treatment can be accomplished at home with the support of teams so well developed in the United States, as well as from the original foundation of St. Christopher's Hospice. Funded by the Department of Health as a "research and development project," this original team set out in 1969. It currently serves around five hundred patients at home at any one time and has the backup of a fifty-bed inpatient unit and twenty day center places, offering respite and end-of-life admission as part of total continuity of care. This in itself has meant that few, if any, patients or families raise the possibility of physician-assisted suicide. In his extensive and detailed study of seventy-seven patients referred originally for home care, Hinton found that physician-assisted suicide was not a salient concern for patients or families.[15] Around 50 percent of U.K. hospice admissions end in discharge home; a similar number of hospice patients will end their days there.

Only three of the other twenty countries contributing to *Hospice Care on the International Scene* discuss the subject of physician-assisted suicide.[16] The position in the United States has been mentioned above, and while hospice care at home has been the option of many thousands of patients, the growth of palliative care consultants and teams within general hospitals would seem to have the potential for a major impact on mainstream medicine. In both cases the duty to learn more accurate prognostic skills remains a major challenge. Nicholas Christakis ends his book *Death Foretold* tellingly:

A Duty to Prognosticate

The role of prognostication in medicine is thus multifarious. Like prophecy, prognostication affects what people feel, think and do, and what happens as a result. Like prophecy, it addresses issues of meaning and explanation: it seeks order in apparent randomness, good in seeming evil, and hope in inevitable death. The uncertainty and gravity of the future in patients who are suffering from life-threatening illness heighten the need for prognosis, but have on balance militated toward its avoidance. The balance might beneficially be shifted. For although physicians avoid prognostication, they are nevertheless called to it.[17]

People need time to evaluate their lives, repair their relationships, and plan for others. They may also find new depth of enjoyment in a transient world. "I've had it all out with my wife. Now I can relax and talk about something else," a hospice patient said to me many years ago.

Chapters in *Hospice Care on the International Scene* from both France and China refer to public and professional discussions of physician-assisted suicide that have stimulated attention to better end-of-life care. Neither considers assisted suicide a part of such a specialty.[18] It does not seem possible that the change of gear from active treatment to the hospice or palliative care approach should include this option.

The ethical principles of care have to balance patient autonomy or control with the justice owed to society as a whole. Our choices are not made in a purely individual setting, and the change in society's attitude when a hastened death is available is illustrated by the changes that have taken place in the Netherlands (described in chapters 5 and 6). After a visit to that country by members of the House of Lords Select Committee on Medical Ethics, its chairman Lord Walton, a neurologist, summed up their disquiet: "We concluded that it would be virtually impossible to ensure that all acts of euthanasia were truly voluntary. . . . We were also concerned that vulnerable people—the elderly, lonely, sick or distressed—would feel pressure, whether real or imagined, to request early death."[19] The Select Committee's conclusion was that the law against euthanasia should not be changed, and its members recommended that the practice of palliative care should be more widely researched and taught.

In the Netherlands, a small hospice described in chapter 6 has been successful in doing that. Using widespread consultation among family doctors it finds that nearly all the patients who initially propose assisted suicide change their minds at a later date when reassured by the demonstration of effective care and the promise of nonabandonment. The very small number who still opt for euthanasia are transferred to hospitals for which this remains a policy. The hospice staff do not carry this out themselves, believing it to be contrary to their philosophy and practice.[20] The hospice avoids confrontation with physician advocates of euthanasia and instead maintains an educational program in palliative care that is helpful to doctors and patients.

In the United Kingdom the hospice movement strongly opposes the intrusion of law into clinical practice at the end of life. Continually seeking better ways to help patients at the end of life, I believe, best respects patients' and families' true needs.[21] Autonomy must be seen in the context of a society that emphasizes youth and active achievement and so cannot be trusted not to bring pressure on those it considers an emotional or economic burden. I remain committed to helping people find meaning in the end of life and not to helping them to a hastened death. It is my hope that the hospice movement will stand firm in this and that hospice professionals will never give up working to improve practice and support the patients who come to hospice seeking truly comprehensive care.

However, if the hospice mantra, "You matter because you are you and you matter to the last moment of your life and we will do all we can not only to help you die peacefully but to live until you die,"[22] is to be maintained and recognized ever more widely, we must not be complacent. There must be a continuing search for better practice with a firm scientific basis, widespread undergraduate and graduate teaching, and skillful education of the public and political figures involved in health care. The potential for creative living, repairing of relationships, and the discovery or reinforcement of personal values and sense of worth are the aims of exemplary end-of-life care. The hospice and palliative care movement worldwide exists to maintain them in the face of all arguments for a legalized premature ending of life.

In all its varied manifestations, hospice care has encouraged open communication, ongoing and led by the patients in their own way and time, often as they struggle with unfamiliar and conflicting emotions.

Stark confrontations, which reimbursement programs have sometimes made almost inevitable, are not common where continuity of care throughout a deteriorating illness is maintained as a priority. Consultations by hospice doctors and nurses in the wards and clinics of local acute hospitals facilitates this and adds satisfaction to both professional teams as well as easing the journey of patient and family, who can be involved in decisions on a continuing basis. Establishing a compassionate, engaged relationship at the outset is essential.

In its turn, such cooperation between hospice professionals and other caregivers will ensure that symptoms are skillfully controlled from an early stage, not left to become a crisis in the terminal stage of a patient's care. Fewer difficulties will arise with patients who have learned to expect relief rather than unacknowledged pain. Hospice and palliative care units have a responsibility for ongoing research and education. The *Oxford Textbook of Palliative Medicine*[23] stands at the end of decades of evidence-based development and many publications. General textbooks have long included chapters on dealing with a variety of problems at the end of life as this expertise has increasingly been recognized.

Acknowledgment of such skills led to the recognition of palliative care as a clinical specialty in the United Kingdom, Australia, and New Zealand, all in 1987. Other countries are working to follow suit, and while much writing now often comes from a wide spectrum of contributors, most of the early work arose from within the hospice movement.

As noted above, this expertise goes far beyond addressing mainly physical distress; rather, it approaches the whole experience of pain, including psychological, family, and spiritual pain.[24] Emotional support may be given as part of the general approach of a professional with time to listen but may call for skillful involvement from psychiatrists, psychologists, and social workers. Simple, even routine care is given, but again, expertise of experience and depth may be needed to remain beside deep existential anguish.[25] Such demands call for a team approach, which in its turn gives support to its own members. Overextension or overinvolvement and the consequent danger of "burnout" can be largely avoided by teamwork, a sense of common purpose, and good management. Part-time workers and volunteers in many hospice teams bring important perspectives. In many early programs, volunteers (who were often professionals working in off-duty time) brought their commitment to the beginnings of a new enterprise. Carefully selected, trained, and supervised volunteers have remained the mainstay of many of the bereavement programs that form part of most hospices. At least an equal commitment may be made to a dysfunctional and conflicted family facing the loss of a member as well as an ongoing befriending or counseling after the patient's death.

The balance of openness of all kinds with ever-developing skills has been matched in hospice and palliative care with personal concern. With time for listening and less pressure for acute assessment and treatment, the staff have met their patients and families in a more measured way than they have been accustomed to in acute services. Intensive personal care is given time—"His spirit revived when he came here," a widowed volunteer told me recently. After years she has returned to help day center patients with gardening, her own hobby. Time spent immersing themselves in the good earth, albeit in wheelchairs, has rejuvenated the patients' spirits. Relationships and the beauty of growing things have nurtured feelings of self-worth and a sense of meaning. The offer of such creative possibilities at the end of life is an alternative that hospice teams around the world are bringing to those in their care. This can be made possible only by appropriate treatment over which the recipient has some control.

Conclusion

Assertions of common humanity and personal importance at the end of life may seem to many a utopian dream, impossible to replicate in the modern acute hospital ward. However, consulting hospital teams have repeatedly shown how much confidence and peace can be given to the patients they meet in often surprisingly brief encounters. Witnessing their skills and attitudes offers important educational opportunities to the regular staff. This has been of major importance in translating hospice expertise to the milieu in which a majority of patients are likely to die. Similarly, visits by home care teams to the many who die in nursing homes may offer more appropriate end-of-life care than an emergency transfer to the hospital.

Hospice and family care has spread worldwide in the last three decades. Family commitment in many developing countries has been enhanced by comparatively simple input, largely from nursing teams with appropriate medical support. Hospital teams have proliferated on several continents. Regional meetings offer professional learning and support, with the World Health Organization and other international bodies supporting educational programs.

These teams have interpreted basic principles to suit the resources of their own settings. A group in St. Christopher's Hospice drew up the following definition of those principles: "Hospice and palliative care starts from the understanding that each human being is a person, a single bodily and spiritual whole and that the proper response to a person is respect. Respect means being so open to each man, woman and child, not as simply an individual, but as someone with a story and a culture, with beliefs and relationships, that we give them the value that is uniquely theirs."[26]

This aim may often be only partially realized but stands as a philosophy that offers a more truly humane attitude to a person than the offer of physician-assisted suicide. While acknowledging that some people will still desire assisted suicide even in the kind of setting I have described, most hospice workers believe that the enactment of laws enabling such a step would undermine the right for respect and care for a great many vulnerable, already disadvantaged, people.

Compassionate Care, Not Assisted Suicide

Kathleen Foley, M.D.

T he physician-assisted suicide debate in the United States has called attention to a crisis in our health care system: the profound inadequacy of the care of chronically ill and dying patients. In a 1997 report entitled *Approaching Death*, the Institute of Medicine of the National Academy of Sciences reviewed the medical, social, economic, and institutional factors preventing Americans from receiving appropriate, humane, compassionate care at the end of life.[1] The report outlines the barriers and deficiencies in care and offers recommendations to various stakeholders. It emphasizes the need for public discussion about the care of the dying but points out that in our current culture of death avoidance and denial such "death talk" is one of the last societal taboos.

International Palliative Care Initiatives

The efforts of the Institute of Medicine follow on earlier recommendations by the World Health Organization (WHO) in its monograph *Cancer Pain Relief and Palliative Care.*[2] The WHO identified the inadequate care of patients with incurable cancer as well as other diseases as a serious national and international public health problem requiring the development of programs in palliative care. An international panel defined palliative care as "the active total care of patients whose disease is not responsive to curative therapies." Control of pain, psychosocial distress, and existential, religious, and cultural issues is the focus of care emphasizing the patient's quality of life not quantity of life. This approach is patient- and family-centered and should be part of any primary care health system. The term *palliative* was chosen to be inclusive of hospice and supportive care programs, and to describe a broad health care delivery system that could be either hospital- or home-based and widely applicable to all patients with incurable diseases.

Moreover, the WHO expert panel clearly distinguished palliative care from physician-assisted suicide and euthanasia and included as one of its major recommendations that "member states not consider legislation allowing for physician assisted suicide or euthanasia until they had assured for their citizens the availability of services for pain relief and palliative care."[3]

In 1999 the Council of Europe issued recommendations on the care of the dying, fully supporting the WHO recommendations and arguing strongly that palliative care programs are needed. The Council cited the European Convention on Human Rights, Article 2, which states that "no one shall be deprived of his life intentionally."[4] Of note, all of these documents conceptualize the care of those who are dying as a societal issue, not merely a medical issue, and all have called for broad participation of all members of society in addressing the care of the dying as a public health issue. Thus discussion on the legalization of physician-assisted suicide needs to address the quality, availability, and acceptability of the current options of care for patients with serious life-threatening illness.

Factors in the Physician-Assisted Suicide Debate

In framing this discussion, it is important to remember that there has been a century-long history of advocacy in the United States for physician-assisted suicide and euthanasia (discussed in introduction). In the 1980s and 1990s, this issue has emerged in arguments for legalization of physician-assisted suicide and euthanasia by a series of professional and public advocacy groups. The various factions and factors driving many aspects of this debate include the physician advocates—for example, Drs. Jack Kevorkian, Timothy Quill, Sidney Wanzer, and Marcia Angell—and public advocacy groups, such as the Hemlock Society and Compassion in Dying.

The multiple social, medical, and economic factors include the profound changes in the trajectory of dying as large numbers of patients live with cancer and AIDS for months and years following the diagnosis of an incurable illness; an increasingly aging population; advancements in high-technology medical support systems for patients with respiratory and cardiac failure; and deeply contested limitations in health care resources, particularly for patients with chronic, incurable illness. At the heart of the debate has been the issue of patient autonomy and the focus on the patient's right to choose a dignified death.

What has emerged in this debate in the last ten years is that physician-assisted suicide, and care at the end of life, are complex social and medical problems. Physician-assisted suicide was initially pictured as a compassionate response to the need for "balancing a reverence for life with the belief that death should come with dignity."[5] In the last five years, perceptions have shifted, and many now view physician-assisted suicide as a potentially cost-effective way to limit care to a marginalized, chronically ill population of patients.

The portrayal of this debate in the public press was initially galvanized by Kevorkian, who portrayed end-of-life symptoms, such as pain, as untreatable and unbearable, and physician-assisted suicide as the only option for patients who were suffering needlessly. This clearly encouraged a public perception that death is always painful and that individuals need to control their own dying because medical institutions and health care professionals will either keep them alive too long or let them die without control of pain or other symptoms. When Kevorkian administered a lethal drug dose to a disabled patient with amyotrophic lateral sclerosis (ALS) and shared the videotape of this experience with the American public on *60 Minutes,* the media focused on the fact that the simple way to address suffering in those who are disabled or who have incurable disease is to kill the sufferer. Little media attention was given to the options for care of patients with ALS to improve the quality of their living as they are dying.

Similarly, decisions by the Second and Ninth Circuit Courts of Appeals that reversed state bans (in New York and Washington) on assisted suicide used language that showed little respect for the vulnerability and dependence of dying patients. Judge Stephen Reinhardt, ruling for the Ninth Circuit, applied "the liberty interest clause" of the Fourteenth Amendment and advocated a constitutional right to assisted suicide. He stated that "the competent terminally ill adult having lived nearly the full measure of his life has a strong interest in choosing a dignified and humane death rather than being reduced to a state of helplessness, diapered, sedated, and incompetent."[6] This statement enraged disabled persons, who argued that even in their helpless, diapered, and incompetent state, they were both dignified and humane. Judge Roger J. Miner, writing for the Second Circuit Court of Appeals, applied the equal rights clause of the Fourteenth Amendment and went on to emphasize that the state has no interest in prolonging a life that is ending.[7] This statement is more than legal jargon; it serves as a chilling reminder of the low priority given to the dying when it comes to state resources and protection.

Public advocacy and legal cases involving physician-assisted suicide have provided a unique opportunity to engage the public, health care professionals, and the government in a national discussion on how American medicine and society should address the needs of dying patients and their families. Such a discussion is critical if we are to understand the process of dying from the point of view of patients and their families and identify existing barriers to appropriate, humane, compassionate care at the end of life. Rational discourse needs to replace the polarized debate over physician-assisted suicide and euthanasia, and facts, not anecdotes, are necessary to establish a common ground and frame a system of health care for the terminally ill that provides the best possible quality of living for those who are dying.

Epidemiology and Ethnography of Dying

What are the facts? In the United States, approximately 2.5 million people die each year. We have almost no information on how they die and only general information on where they die: 71 percent die in hospitals, 17 percent die in nursing homes, and the remainder (10 percent to 14 percent of whom are receiving hospice care) die at home. There is wide variation in the place of death: Oregon reports that only 31 percent of patients die in hospitals, while in New York State 71 percent die in hospitals.

We have little understanding of what accounts for this variability, but data from SUPPORT (Study to Understand Prognoses and Preferences for Outcomes and Risks of Treatment) suggests that it is not necessarily the individual choice of the patient that determines the place of death but rather the number of hospitals in the region.[8] Similarly, data on Medicare expenditures in the last six months of life show enormous variation around the country, with a twofold to threefold variation in costs among states suggesting disparity in care services that are available to patients and families. Moreover, one-third of the Medicare budget is spent in the care of patients during their last six months of life, leading to concern about the appropriateness and adequacy of costly care.[9]

With the majority of adults in the United States now dying in hospitals, it has become all too evident that both hospitals and physicians are not equipped or trained to handle the medical and psychosocial problems that face those who are dying and their caregivers. Several studies have categorized the barriers to adequate palliative care programs, ranging from the lack of professional knowledge and skills in palliative care to significant financial and structural barriers in the health care delivery system.[10] Increasing attention has focused on the need to identify the opportunities to improve the delivery of palliative care at the end of life as a first step toward developing corrective approaches and preventing needless suffering.[11] It has been strongly argued that palliative care must become an integral component of primary medical care.

The Goals of Palliative Care

The goals of palliative care include the alleviation of suffering, the optimization of quality of life until death ensues, and the provision of comfort in death. Persistent suffering that is inadequately relieved undermines the value of life for the sufferer. Without hope that this situation will be relieved, patients, their families, and professional caregivers may see euthanasia and assisted suicide as their only alternatives.

Alleviation of suffering is universally acknowledged as a cardinal goal of medical care.[12] Yet to formulate a response to the challenge of suffering, clinicians require a clinically relevant understanding of the nature of the problem. We have proposed a taxonomy of the factors that contribute to suffering in patients with advanced disease[13] and have developed a clinical paradigm that tries to acknowledge the interrelated distress of the patient, the family, and health care providers as they face a terminal disease. Using the cancer patient as an example, an encounter with advanced cancer is a cause of great distress to patients, their families, and professional caregivers attending them. Two-thirds of patients with advanced disease have significant pain; numerous other physical symptoms diminish such patients' quality of life; and many patients endure enormous psychological distress. From an existential perspective, even without pain or other physical symptoms, continued life is without meaning for some patients. For the families and loved ones of patients, there is similar great distress in this process—from anticipating loss, standing witness to the patient's physical and emotional distress, and bearing the burdens of care. Professional caregivers as well may be stressed by the suffering that they witness and that challenges their clinical and emotional resources. On this model, the suffering of each of these groups is highly interrelated, since the perceived distress of any one of these three groups may amplify the distress of the others.

The goal of palliative care is to address the complex issues of suffering from the perspective of the patient and the family and define a system of care appropriate to the needs of the individual patient. This formulation of the therapeutic response requires an understanding of the phenomenon of suffering and the factors that contribute to it. Failure to appreciate or effectively address the full diversity of contributing factors may confound effective therapeutic strategies. The available data suggest that health care professionals—specifically physicians and nurses—are not adequately trained to assess and manage the multifactorial symptoms commonly associated with patients at the end of life and lack training in all aspects of palliative care.[14]

Factors Associated with Suffering in Patients

Three major factors contribute to patients' suffering: pain or other physical symptoms, psychological distress, and existential distress.

Pain Symptoms

Pain is the most common symptom in dying patients; according to recent data from U.S.-based studies, 56 percent of outpatients with cancer, 82 percent of outpatients with AIDS, 50 percent of hospitalized patients with various diagnoses, 36 percent of nursing home residents with cancer, and 89 percent of children dying of cancer have inadequate management of suffering during the course of their terminal illness.[15] Members of minority groups and women, both those with cancer and those with AIDS, as well as the elderly, receive less pain treatment than other groups of patients. In a survey of 1,177 physicians who treated a total of more than 70,000 patients with cancer in the previous six months, 76 percent of the physician respondents reported that lack of knowledge was a barrier to their ability to control pain.[16] Fifty-six percent of these physicians' patients reported moderate to severe pain. Severe pain that is not adequately controlled interferes with patients' quality of life, including activities of daily living, sleep, and social interactions.

Other physical symptoms are prevalent among those who are dying. Studies of patients with advanced cancer, patients with AIDS, and the elderly in the year before death show that they have numerous symptoms that diminish the quality of life, such as fatigue, difficulty breathing, delirium, nausea, and vomiting.[17] Studies in children with cancer demonstrated a comparable number of symptoms.[18]

Psychological Symptoms

Concurrent with these physical symptoms, patients have a variety of well-described psychological symptoms, with a high prevalence of anxiety and depression in elderly patients and those with cancer or AIDS. For example, studies in elderly patients demonstrate that depressive symptoms interfere with their ability to make decisions about resuscitation.[19] More than 60 percent of patients with advanced cancer have psychiatric problems, with adjustment disorders, depression, anxiety, and delirium reported most frequently.[20]

The diagnosis of depression is often difficult to make in medically ill patients, yet recent studies demonstrated that patients' response to the simple question "Are you depressed?" serves as a reliable indicator of whether psychological distress is present.[21] Numerous studies have reported underdiagnosis and undertreatment of depression in those who are medically ill. Conwell and Caine reported that depression was underdiagnosed by primary care physicians in a cohort of elderly patients who subsequently committed suicide: 75 percent of the patients had seen a primary care physician during the last month of life but had not been diagnosed or treated for depression.[22]

Data provided by Dr. Harvey Chochinov and colleagues (see chapter 12) show a relationship between depression and patients' desire for death.[23] Hopelessness is a common component of the patients' wish to die and is more evident than depression alone. We know that this desire is highly unstable and influenced by a number of other factors.

Attention has also focused on the interaction between uncontrolled physical symptoms and the vulnerability to suicide of patients with cancer or AIDS.[24] Suicide is the eighth leading cause of death in the United States. Various factors indicating vulnerability to suicide have been identified in cancer and AIDS patients that can help to identify patients' potential risk for suicide. In a cohort of cancer patients receiving treatment for pain and epidural spinal cord compression, 17 percent reported suicidal ideation, with 8 percent reporting a well-developed plan for action.[25] Data from both cancer and AIDS patients suggest that uncontrolled pain contributes to depression and that persistent pain interferes with patients' ability to receive support from their families and others. Specific studies in patients with AIDS identify them to have a high risk of suicide independent of physical symptoms.[26] Among New York City residents with AIDS, the relative risk of suicide in men between the ages of twenty and fifty-nine was 36 percent higher than the risk among men without AIDS in the same age group and 66 percent higher than the risk among the general population. Patients with AIDS who committed suicide generally did so within nine months of receiving their diagnosis; 25 percent had made a previous suicide attempt; 50 percent reported severe depression; and 40 percent had seen a psychiatrist within four days of committing suicide. In short, suicide risk is higher in patients with cancer and AIDS than in the general population.

From our experience in caring for a population of dying patients in the Supportive Care Program at Memorial Sloan-Kettering Cancer Center, patients' concern about suicide was openly discussed by over 25 percent of our patients.[27] All of the patients who expressed the potential of suicide had progressive disease with accumulating debility. They had hope of neither prolonged survival nor the return of normal function. Although the nature of our data does not allow detailed group comparisons, there was no significant difference in demographics, medical complications, social supports, or most symptoms between those who endorsed suicide as an option and others who rejected it. Only a particularly severe degree of overall fatigue appeared to distinguish the former patients.

Patients appeared to use their discussions of suicide as a means to ensure that the listener understood the depth of their suffering. When such discussions took place, clinicians and nurse practitioners would ask patients to describe the circumstances that would induce them to act on this option. Patients were usually very forthright and relieved by such discussion, commonly naming such things as excruciating pain, becoming a burden on their family, losing the ability to think, being demeaned by loss of bowel and bladder function, and becoming paraplegic. In some cases, giving permission to speak about these actual or potential losses in the context of suicide appears to serve a useful function, giving patients a sense of having communicated what these losses meant to them. In these discussions, the practitioner addressed each of the fears, reassuring the patient that every event could be managed. It is noteworthy that several patients subsequently developed a complication that they had previously described as one of the most feared, such as paraplegia or loss of bowel and bladder function, yet none committed suicide. Adaptation appeared to be the norm even in these highly distressed patients as long as sufficient support was provided in the home, suffering was acknowledged, and close communication and monitoring were continued.

This experience with this patient population has pointed out how much the ethical and medical discussions about physician-assisted suicide and euthanasia have neglected the potential role played by unrelieved symptoms and profound fatigue experienced by patients and their caregivers. It also pointed out how little data we have to evaluate whether patients have been offered appropriate symptom management and families have received appropriate support and to what extent such support systems might radically alter the issue. Our experience has been that such efforts dramatically alter the patient's perspective on suicide. As noted in chapter 8, recent data published from an anonymous physician survey about patients' request for assistance in death in Oregon, palliative care interventions did lead 46 percent of patients to change their minds about the request for assistance in death.[28]

Existential Distress

A third category of suffering that compounds the multiple physical and psychological symptoms terminally ill patients experience is their degree of existential distress. Increasing attention has focused on the need to understand the spiritual, religious, and cultural dimensions of patients' dying experience. A recent survey on spiritual beliefs in the dying process that elicited patients' concerns about not having the opportunity to say goodbye, or being in a vegetative state for a long period of time, or being a burden to their family provides some information about their perspectives on these issues.[29] In a recent focus group study about what was important in care at the end of life, patients cited a variety of concerns, including freedom from pain and the opportunity to choose their place of death. They also pointed out two other factors that had not previously been well identified: their desire to be cared for as "whole persons," with attention to their spiritual, religious, and cultural beliefs, and their wish to be identified as contributing to and maintaining a role in society.[30] No longer having a social role is often described by patients as a major reason they view themselves as a burden not only to their families but to themselves.

We need to better understand such existential distress in patients and families. An indirect evaluation of the degree to which patients report existential distress has been summarized in a report by Dr. Anthony Back and colleagues, who interviewed Washington State physicians whose patients requested assistance in dying. The physicians summarized their perception of why patients requested assistance, citing fear of future loss of control, fear of future loss of dignity, and concern about being a burden as the major reasons.[31] Similar data from physician reports of patients requesting physician-assisted suicide in Oregon identified these concerns as well.[32] Although many of these patients had significant medical symptoms, we have little information on how these symptoms may have influenced their degree of existential distress. Existential concerns are ones physicians may be least able to address with medical therapies.

Factors Associated with Caregivers' Suffering

Recent attention has focused on caregivers as well, demonstrating that increased burden of disease in the patient leads to increased stress for the caregiver, with associated physical and psychological distress. To what degree caregivers' physical fatigue and psychological distress affect their ability to sustain and care for a family member with advanced disease remains poorly defined. Caregiver burden falls most heavily on women with low income, who often must leave their jobs to provide care for family members at home.[33]

Health care professionals also suffer, with increasing reports of "burnout" among physicians—who are increasingly being forced to see large number of patients in short periods of time and lack knowledge and training in palliative care. In a recent membership survey of the American Society of Clinical Oncology (ASCO) on issues in end-of-life care, oncologists clearly acknowledged the fact that their inability to provide and to find services to care for their patients at the end of life is a contributing factor in their willingness to aid patients in death.[34] Other studies have shown that training and knowledge of palliative care are major reasons health care professionals do not support the legalization of physician-assisted suicide.[35]

Health Care Professionals' Lack of Education

Inadequate response to the complex suffering of dying patients—physical, psychological, and existential—in part results from health care providers' lack of knowledge and education.[36] According to the American Medical Association's report on medical education, only 5 of 126 medical schools in the United States require a separate course in the care of the dying.[37] Of 7,048 residency programs, only 26 percent offer a course on the medical and legal aspects of care at the end of life. In a survey of 1,068 accredited residency programs in family medicine, internal medicine, and pediatrics, and fellowship programs in geriatrics, each resident or fellow coordinated the care of ten or fewer dying patients annually.[38] Almost 15 percent of these programs offer no formal training in end-of-life care. Despite the availability of hospice programs, only 17 percent of the training programs offer hospice rotation, and only half of these programs require a hospice rotation. In a survey of 55 residency programs and more than 1,400 residents conducted by the American Board of Internal Medicine, the residents were asked to rate their perception of adequate training in care at the end of life.[39] Only 62 percent reported that they had received adequate training in telling patients that they are dying, only 38 percent in describing what the process would be like, and only 32 percent in talking to patients who request assistance in dying or hastened death. Medical textbooks devote less than 1 percent of their content to addressing the care of dying patients.[40] Nurses and social workers are similarly poorly educated.

Health Care Professionals' Lack of Knowledge

This lack of training in the care of the dying is further evidenced in practice. Physicians' lack of knowledge about national guidelines for such care and their lack of knowledge about the control of symptoms are obvious barriers to the provision of good care at the end of life. Poor communication between physicians and patients, as evidenced in the SUPPORT study, directly affects decisions about care at the end of life.[41] In the ASCO survey, participating oncologists reported that they had difficulty telling patients bad news and that this led them, at times, to overtreat patients with ineffective therapies.[42] Similarly, a study of patients' understanding of their prognosis demonstrated that when patients were not aware of their prognosis they often chose therapies that they would not have chosen if they had had a full, clear understanding of their illness.[43]

Physicians' lack of knowledge about national guidelines on withholding and withdrawing care and the use of palliative care approaches has led to confusion about the difference between forgoing life-sustaining therapy (the legal right of every competent patient) and active euthanasia. Because of the wide use of life-support technologies in dying patients, many medical professionals incorrectly believe that a decision to forgo life-sustaining treatment may be equivalent to active euthanasia. And health care professionals remain unsure of the distinction between euthanasia and the administration of sufficient medication to treat suffering in dying patients.

In a study by Dr. Mildred Solomon and colleagues, physicians and nurses in five institutions were surveyed about their knowledge about and attitudes toward a range of issues, from ethical guidelines to institutional guidelines and the specific topic of pain control in patients at the end of life.[44] Of note, 89 percent of those surveyed agreed that sometimes it is appropriate to give pain medication to relieve suffering even if it may hasten a patient's death, with 87 percent believing that pain treatment is effective and 81 percent considering undertreatment the most common form of abuse of patients. But as many as one-third of the medical and surgical attending physicians agreed with 44 percent of nurses that the fear of hastening a patient's death is why clinicians give inadequate pain medication. This survey points out the dissonance between what clinicians agree is appropriate for dying patients and what their clinical behaviors actually are. In end-of-life care of patients, belief and behavior continue to conflict and have an enormous impact on institutionalizing appropriate care for the dying. Such uncertainty, which comes from health care professionals' lack of knowledge of palliative care, results in inadequate control of distressing symptoms in terminally ill patients.

A recent survey of the members of the American Academy of Neurology demonstrated that 40 percent of neurologists worry that to give morphine to a dying ALS patient is a form of active euthanasia.[45] This lack of knowledge and confusion on the part of physicians has been fueled by the fact that the circuit courts and their legal discussions supporting physician-assisted suicide have asserted that physicians are already assisting in patients' death when they withdraw life-sustaining treatments, such as respirators, or administer high doses of pain medications that secondarily hasten death. This judicial reasoning that eliminates the distinction between letting a patient die and killing clearly runs counter to most thinking in bioethics and to physicians' standards of palliative care. In the real world in which physicians care for dying patients, withdrawing treatment and aggressively treating pain are acts that respect patients' autonomous decisions not to be battered by medical technology and to be relieved of their suffering. In these settings, the physician's intent is to provide care, not to cause death.

Some clinicians have argued that morphine drips are "slow euthanasia."[46] This perspective led to a series of compelling papers clearly distinguishing the intent of palliative care physicians, whose goal is to prevent and treat suffering, from that of physicians who intend to hasten the death of patients. Yet physicians often struggle with doubts about their own intentions. The court arguments fuel physicians' ambivalence about withdrawing life-sustaining treatments or using opioids and sedatives to treat intractable symptoms in dying patients. Physicians are trained and socialized to preserve life; saying that they struggle with doubts about their own intentions in performing these acts is not the same as saying that their intention is to kill. In palliative care the goal is to relieve suffering, and the quality of life, not the quantity, is most important. Specialists in palliative care therefore do not think they practice physician-assisted suicide or euthanasia, but have developed guidelines for aggressive pharmacological management of intractable symptoms in dying patients, including sedation for those near death. Palliative care experts believe that in order to restore the balance between a physician's obligation to prolong life and obligation to relieve suffering, a peaceful death must be acknowledged as a legitimate goal of medicine and as an integral part of a physician's responsibility.

In the Supreme Court's decision on physician-assisted suicide, the Court clearly distinguished physician-assisted suicide and euthanasia from the aggressive use of palliative care therapies for symptom management even if they might shorten the patient's life.[47]

Increasingly, there is a preponderance of evidence demonstrating that the proper use of pain medications, such as morphine, in patients with chronic pain as well as patients at the end of life does not hasten their death. There are accumulating data to suggest that the proper use of opioids may in fact prolong patients' lives. Studies by Dr. Frank Brescia and colleagues at Calvary Hospital in New York City show that there is no correlation between the dose of opioids a patient receives in the last weeks of life and the timing of his or her death.[48] Studies of dying patients demonstrated that those patients who received morphine lived longer than those who did not receive morphine.[49] Studies recently published from a series of hospices show no difference in the time to death between those patients who were sedated to control their symptoms and those patients who were not sedated.[50] Finally, the doses of opioids that are often used to treat patients at the end of life are highly variable. The great majority of dying patients are receiving doses in a range equivalent to what is commonly considered part of postoperative pain management. These doses are safe and effective and commonly used in patients who have not been previously exposed to opioids. In short, health care professionals' lack of knowledge, coupled with a lack of understanding of the appropriate use of opioids and other sedative drugs in patients in palliative care settings, has created a mythology that is not based on scientific evidence.

The Public's Lack of Knowledge and Education

This lack of knowledge is not just limited to health care professionals but includes patients and families who are not fully aware of their options for care. Surveys reveal that fewer than 10 percent of the public know what hospice care is. Fewer than 20 percent have completed advanced directives or have talked with their caregivers or health care proxies about what kind of care they wish to receive if they become incompetent.[51] In studies of patient-related barriers to symptom control, patients report that they are reticent to complain to their physicians because they do not want to be identified as complainers, and that physicians have inadequate time during visits with patients. At the same time, patients' fear of addiction leads them to tolerate pain rather than take a pain reliever. Yet pain is the symptom patients fear most commonly, and 69 percent of patients report that uncontrolled pain would be a reason to commit suicide.[52] Patients are also unaware of their right to refuse treatment or to have burdensome therapy stopped and often continue on treatment for cancer, as an example, because of fear of abandonment by their treating physician.

There is an enormous need for public education programs to address this lack of knowledge about the options for care. Yet in actuality patients' options for care have been affected significantly by the changes in the health care delivery system that have occurred over the last five years as patients' choice of hospital, doctor, prescription plan, and home care service have been markedly limited by what health maintenance organization they participate in. This rearrangement of health care services has negatively affected the care of patients with serious life-threatening illness; clearly, with such limitations on their options for care, patients are not able to make autonomous decisions.

Other Barriers to Palliative Care

A wide range of institutional, regulatory, and financial barriers to end-of-life care have also been identified, ranging from the lack of a palliative care team or units in hospitals, to excessive regulatory control of the use of pain medications, to the lack of adequate funding in Medicare and private insurance programs for prescription medications critical to symptom control.

For patients dying in hospitals, there is a major effort to discharge them to alternative systems of care—either to home or to a nursing home. Yet these alternatives lack the expert support required to address the needs of this patient population, thus putting enormous burdens on patients and families in both home care agencies and nursing homes. SUPPORT demonstrated that one-third of families exhausted their financial resources in caring for a dying elderly family member at home.[53] Conversely, patients dying in hospitals who do not have advanced directives and family proxies may receive aggressive intensive care that is costly and unwanted.

Fewer than 20 percent of all dying patients receive hospice care in the United States, with cancer patients making up more than 50 percent of those who do; 93 percent of hospice patients are white. The Medicare hospice benefit requires that patients be terminally ill with a prognosis of six months or less and willing to give up access to other medical therapies. This capitated benefit forces patients to shift care from their traditional system and often leads to discontinuity and concern about abandonment by their longtime physician. Yet hospice care provides a high level of expertise in pain management and symptom control and provides a team of health professionals trained in palliative care to address patients' physical and psychosocial needs. Increasingly, hospices are being audited because their patients live "too long," raising the specter of fraud and abuse of the hospice benefit.[54] Yet prognostication is fraught with problems. The unintended consequence of this government oversight has been to force hospices into admitting patients often on "the brink of death," limiting their ability to provide their comprehensive care to patients and families early in the dying process.

These are only a few of the barriers that currently limit patients and families from receiving adequate care. Moreover, there is enormous variation in hospice care across the country. The hospice model is predominantly a nurse-centered one, with physician medical directors who see patients infrequently and rely heavily on nursing expertise. Quality standards for hospice and outcomes practice are not established, making it difficult to assure patients and families that they are receiving quality end-of-life care. Hospices vary widely in their services, with some providing care to certain patients that other hospices will not accept. For example, some hospices will not use intravenous fluids in a patient who is unable to take fluids by mouth, and others will not accept patients on patient-controlled analgesic pumps for continuous administration of their pain medicines. Psychological and psychiatric services to hospice patients often require extra consultation that may not be widely available in the region in which a patient lives, even though social workers are an important part of the hospice team.

Dr. Susan Tolle has argued that Oregon provides excellent palliative care, using criteria like morphine consumption and the number of patients dying in nursing homes who do not return to hospitals for care as indicators of such quality palliative care.[55] These indirect and general indicators should not be considered real surrogates for identifying clearly what is quality care. Such assessment requires data from patients and family that we do not yet have, despite some studies, such as the recent Oregon survey by Tolle and colleagues of families of patients who died, which showed that patients did not receive optimal pain control.[56] In fairness, Oregon is not alone in its lack of data. There are no state or national standards to assure patients and families that they are receiving quality end-of-life care appropriate to the individual needs of the patients.

Conclusion

We have a long way to go to improve end-of-life care for patients and to integrate high-quality palliative care and hospice programs into our system of health care delivery. Our current culture marginalizes those who are dying and creates needless suffering. There is now a unique opportunity to improve the care for this population and to address how we should show true respect for their autonomy. Physicians play a unique role in changing the system of care. Communicating effectively with patients, providing psychosocial support, managing symptoms well, and making timely referrals to hospice will improve care and support for patients and families.

Numerous efforts are under way to meet the challenge of institutionalizing humane, compassionate care for the dying. Over the last five years, major educational initiatives for health care professionals and the public, coupled with a broad advocacy effort to change institutional and economic barriers, have allowed for the public discussion so necessary to improve the quality of living for those who are in the process of dying. These programmatic and educational efforts, outlined in the conclusion, mark the beginning of a process that holds the promise of revolutionizing the care of patients at the end of life.

Conclusion:
Changing the Culture

Kathleen Foley, M.D., and Herbert Hendin, M.D.

Leon Kass, Edmund Pellegrino, Daniel Callahan, and Yale Kamisar began *The Case against Assisted Suicide* by presenting ethical, philosophical, and legal arguments as to why neither autonomy nor compassion—the major justifications for assisted suicide—provides an adequate basis for legalizing the practice. We would add that patient autonomy is an illusion when physicians do not know how to assess and treat patient suffering and the choice for patients becomes either continued agony or a hastened death. It is not surprising that studies show that the more physicians know about palliative care, the less they favor assisted suicide or euthanasia, while the less they know, the more they favor it.[1]

Strong empirical evidence derived from the experience with legally sanctioned assisted suicide and euthanasia in the Netherlands, in Oregon, and in Australia (chapters 5–9) supports the conclusion that legalization, ironically, increases the power and control not of patients but of physicians, who can suggest it, not provide suitable alternatives, not understand or ignore patient ambivalence, and even put to death patients who have not requested it. Zbigniew Zylicz's experience in the Netherlands indicates that the easier expedient of assisted suicide or euthanasia also undermines the incentive for physicians to learn to provide the quality of palliative care that should be available to terminally ill patients. In Oregon, when given any palliative care options, patients were far less likely to choose physician-assisted suicide.

Who is most endangered by the absence of good palliative care? As Cicely Saunders and Kathleen Foley make clear, their numerous physical and psychological symptoms coupled with their fragile economic status clearly define those who are seriously ill as vulnerable to pressure to hasten death. Recent studies of the dying experience of patients and families have demonstrated this vulnerability as expressed by patients' concerns of being a burden both socially and economically, while their caregivers experience high levels of emotional distress.

When, assisted suicide or euthanasia is sanctioned, however, those who are depressed, disabled, economically disadvantaged, or elderly are especially vulnerable, as the chapters by Harvey Chochinov and Leonard Schwartz, Diane Coleman, and Felicia Cohen and Joanne Lynn make clear. Before addressing what needs to be done if we are to provide palliative care for all who are terminally ill, it is best to examine what must change if we are to see to it that these particularly vulnerable patients are included in any plans to provide adequate care at the end of life.

Depression, Anxiety, and the Wish to Die

As Chochinov and Schwartz have pointed out, psychological distress characterized by anxiety and depression is common in patients with serious life-threatening illness. Yet patients with far advanced disease in the United States rarely have access to specialized psychological consultation. Serious limitations in knowledge restrict the ability of primary care physicians to diagnose and treat the emotional distress of anxiety and depression. Whether such patients are cared for at home or enrolled in hospice programs, they have inadequate access to psychological and psychiatric assessment and treatment.

The presence of clinical depression *per se* is not regarded in Oregon or the Netherlands as evidence of diminished ability to make an informed decision. A recent ruling in the Netherlands led to the acquittal of a doctor who had given a lethal drug cocktail to an eighty-six-year-old former patient and politician who had suffered from severe depression. This same patient had attempted suicide two years earlier. In agreeing with experts who argued that assisted suicide was warranted because suffering need not be only unrelenting physical pain, the court reinforced the opinion reached in earlier Dutch cases.[2] Even when there is other evidence of inability to give informed consent, as in the case of Kate Cheney in Oregon, we have seen how it can be circumvented when the family, or an advocacy organization, finds a consultant known to favor assisted suicide.

The prevalence of depression in seriously ill patients who want to hasten death and the ways in which it is expressed suggest that patients who request assisted suicide have much in common with suicidal patients who are not physically ill.[3] Both patients who attempt suicide and those who request assisted suicide may test the affection and care of others, confiding feelings like "I don't want to be a burden to my family" or "My family would be better off without me." Such expressions often reflect depressed feelings of worthlessness or guilt or may be a plea for reassurance. Not surprisingly, they are also classic indicators of suicidal depression in people who are in good physical health. Whether physically healthy or terminally ill, these patients need assurance that they are still wanted; they also need treatment for depression.

We know that factors in addition to depression play a role in determining the likelihood of suicide. Anxiety and hopelessness, for example, are predictors of suicide, distinguishing depressed patients who are likely to kill themselves from those who are not.[4] The patient's affective state can often best be described as one of desperation, a mixture of anguish, anxiety, and urgency over obtaining relief.[5] Anxiety, and anxiety about dying in particular, is an important but relatively unstudied factor among patients who request assisted suicide. Death anxiety is often displaced onto other symptoms or concerns so that it is harder to recognize.

Not all patients who want to die, with or without assistance, are clinically depressed. Yet whether or not they are depressed, patients who request assisted suicide are similar to other suicidal patients in that they are usually ambivalent about their desire to die and are often expressing an anguished wish for help. When this ambivalence is not heard and such requests to die are taken literally and concretely, an assisted suicide can occur with the patient in a state of unrecognized terror.[6]

Patients who respond to fatal illnesses with a desire to hasten death have more than depression or ambivalence in common with suicidal patients in general. It is not surprising that Zylicz, in his informal motivational classification of these patients (chapter 6), describes a group of those requesting physician-assisted suicide as having inordinate needs for control. Excessive needs for control are frequent among suicidal patients. They tend to set conditions under which they will continue to live. Serious illness and approaching death make such control impossible. Determining how and when they die provides an illusory sense of regaining control. The knowledge that they are going to end their lives or will be helped to do so can have a calming influence on these patients that masks their depression and anxiety.

Frightened and misinformed patients who request assisted suicide present a different problem. Zylicz as well as Chochinov and Schwartz give examples of patients whose desire for an expedited death disappeared when their fears and misinformation were addressed. In most cases in Oregon and the Netherlands about which we know the details, such relief does not seem to have been provided.

Words like *probably* and *seem* or *may* are required in discussing the psychological features of dying patients because much of what clinicians report has not been tested by formal research. There has as yet been no study comparing suicidal patients in general with those requesting physician-assisted suicide. Only recently are a relatively small number of researchers doing studies that will give us more psychological information about terminally ill patients. Recently published data showed that patients have a wide range of adaptations and that information about their prognosis and knowledge of their impending death is not necessarily associated with despair or hopelessness.[7]

In the past decade we have begun to learn how to treat effectively different types of suicidal patients, from those who have attempted suicide to those who are preoccupied with a desire for death. Even more recently we have begun to evaluate these treatments scientifically to establish their relative efficacy. Similar research among patients who request physician-assisted suicide has barely begun.

The vast majority of those who request assisted suicide or euthanasia are not primarily motivated by current pain or suffering but by dread of what will happen to them in the future; they fear future pain, dependency on others, loss of dignity, the side effects of medical treatment, and, of course, death itself. Their fears of death are often displaced onto these other concerns. Patients do not know what to expect and cannot foresee how their conditions will unfold as they decline toward death. Facing this uncertainty, they fill the vacuum with their fantasies and fears. When these fears are dealt with by a caring and knowledgeable physician, the request for an expedited death usually disappears.

Anxiety about death has been observed to center around fears of separation as well as fears of disintegration and loss of either physical or emotional control. Suicidal patients give a variety of meanings to death that serve to reduce these anxieties: death can be pictured by them not as a separation but as a reunion or rebirth; not as a loss of control but as a means to gain the power of revenge or retaliatory abandonment through being able to determine when and how they die. Or they can see death as a punishment and thus relieve guilty anxiety for real or imagined sins.[8]

The ancient world was aware of the relationship between guilty fear and suicide. The Greek hero Hercules, whose assisted suicide was discussed in the introduction to this volume, had earlier in his life wished to kill himself after he killed his first wife and their children in a "fit of madness." The fit was visited on him by the goddess Hera, who bore him a lifelong grudge for being the illegitimate son of her husband, Zeus. Overwhelmed by remorse, Hercules was persuaded to accept his twelve labors instead of suicide as an atonement. As the son of a god, however, Hercules showed no anxiety about death. Fearless in combat, he had won a battle with death to bring back to life Alcestis, the wife of his friend Admetis. And after his own death and fiery immolation on a funeral pyre, Hercules went to Olympus as an immortal, where he was reconciled with Hera and married her daughter Hebe.

For all who are not immortal, however, death anxiety is a fact of life, repressed most of the time but close to consciousness when one is threatened with death or must deal with others who are dying. Doctors who want to help patients who ask for a hastened death must be able to understand how deciding on suicide or assisted suicide serves to relieve the death anxieties of patients. They must be able to address and help relieve those anxieties in some other way.

Requests for assisted suicide usually express a desperate need for help and an ambivalent wish to die. They must be met with a compassionate attempt to understand and relieve the desperation that underlies the requests. Why is it that physicians often become paralyzed in such cases, suspend their usual processes of inquiry, and simply treat the patient as a dying person whose last wish should be granted? Such behavior appears to be related to anxieties that physicians share with patients about their inability to control death.

Lewis Thomas, one of the deans of modern American medicine, wrote insightfully about the sense of failure and helplessness that physicians may experience in the face of death.[9] Such feelings may explain why physicians have such difficulty discussing terminal illness with patients.

A majority of physicians avoid such discussions, while most patients would prefer frank talk. This phenomenon was identified in the American Society of Clinical Oncology's survey of oncologists' attitudes and behaviors with regard to end-of-life care. Clinicians who found it difficult to manage dying patients reported that they avoided frank discussions about prognoses with patients and offered continued active therapy despite its ineffectiveness. Up to 25 percent of clinicians reported that they did not like or want to care for dying patients.[10]

These feelings may also explain both the doctors' tendency to use excessive measures to maintain life and their need to make life—and death—a physician's decision. Physicians who unwisely prolong the dying process and those who practice euthanasia may have more in common than they realize.

By deciding when patients die, by making death a medical decision, the physician preserves the illusion of mastery over the disease and over the feelings of helplessness that lack of control induces. The physician, not the illness, is responsible for the death. Assisting suicide and performing euthanasia become ways of dealing with the frustration of being unable to cure the disease.

Contemporary anxieties about death seem to have led to an increasing need for individuals to feel some control over death by determining how and when it occurs. The attraction of assisted suicide and euthanasia may in part be understood in the context of an increasingly widely shared need to achieve an illusory control over our fears of death.

What about Those Who Are Disabled?

Physicians consistently underestimate the quality of life of patients who have disabilities. Such underestimation leads physicians to make statements to disabled individuals and their families that may have a traumatic influence on treatment decisions to withhold or withdraw care, even when all medical factors are otherwise equal.

There is also evidence that health care providers are inconsistent in following advance directives and anecdotal evidence that people with disabilities are viewed as less worthy of health care resources. They must often use advocates and lawyers to press for health care; this is most evident in the disability community with pressures to sign "do not resuscitate" orders and the imposition of such orders in the absence of patient or family permission.

We need more knowledge about end-of-life decision making among people with disabilities. Little of the systematically obtained evidence has considered such factors as health insurance coverage, economic resources of patient or family, or managed care influences. Few data are available on physician education and expertise in the care of the dying and disabled patient. What is the role and availability of hospice care for those patients with disability, and what are the indicators of quality of care, particularly for these patients attempting to live independently at home? What about the presence or absence of suicidal factors and personal losses in the lives of these individuals?

In the absence of meaningful evidence concerning these and other factors relevant to assessing the extent of abuse and coercion for this population of patients, Diane Coleman believes that it is irresponsible to argue for dramatically increasing their risk by legalizing active measures to cause death. As she points out (chapter 10), anyone who depends on health care to live faces the potential of being denied health care despite his or her wishes by an insurance company or family decision. Coleman urges strongly that society work to ensure that this risk is minimized and that the factors that influence these decisions be studied and evaluated and the problem areas addressed. To make assisted suicide a solution for the problems of those who have incurable conditions before these steps have been taken is unconscionable.

People with disabilities clearly deserve equal protection of the law. Yet laws and social policies that provide suicide intervention to healthy and nondisabled people while providing suicide assistance and even euthanasia to people with illnesses and disabilities are fundamentally discriminatory—resulting in the deaths of members of the devalued minority group. Those who are disabled have allied themselves most closely with dying patients, seeing themselves as equally devalued and without a voice in the current medical health care system. During the U.S. Supreme Court hearings on the Oregon and New York assisted suicide cases, people with disabilities protested on the steps of the Court, led by Coleman and the organization she heads, Not Dead Yet.

There is no question that as we address the care of patients with disability it is both cheaper and easier to provide physician-assisted suicide than round-the-clock nursing care, high-technology physical and respiratory support systems, and financial and psychological support to the caregivers. In the Oscar-winning documentary *Breathing Lessons*, Mark O'Brien, quadriplegic from polio and living in an iron lung, poignantly states that the state of California does not seem to care about him and would prefer to see him dead. Mark fought valiantly to live independently at home but received no state support for home services, such as companions to monitor his care. The state would have paid for his care had he lived in an institution.[11] Mark O'Brien died from pneumonia at the age of forty-nine, two years after the making of the documentary.

State Legislation and Voter Initiatives

Elderly people, many of whom have outlived their family members and spouses, have complex multiple illnesses, significant cognitive failure, and limited resources. There is ample evidence to demonstrate that patients without insurance have less access to care and fewer end-of-life care services available to them. Patients who are socioeconomically deprived have higher rates of medical illness, including cancer, cardiovascular disease, and diabetes. They often present with advanced, incurable disease, and if they are minorities or elderly, they are inadequately treated for their pain. Disparities in care associated with patients' economic status have made us conscious of the vulnerability of those who are poor when physician-assisted suicide is sanctioned.

Variations in Medicaid coverage for hospice care for those patients who are not receiving Medicare, coupled with the large percentage of such patients having no insurance at all (such as the homeless), make them identified as "charity cases" for end-of-life care. Although there are several small efforts throughout the country to provide care for such patients in halfway houses, in homes, and in some hospice programs, recent evidence demonstrates that patients, families, and even providers find the care that is now provided to be often inappropriate, at times unwanted, and commonly inadequate.[12] Dying elderly patients and their families are increasingly dissatisfied with the fragmentation, compartmentalization, inefficiency, unreliability, and insensitivity of the care system.

Reforming Medicare

The current Medicare payment system continues to create serious financial disincentives and disadvantages for providers who wish to deliver good care. About three-fifths of Medicare beneficiaries have supplemental insurance to help them meet deductibles, co-insurance, and certain uncovered services. Medicaid pays the Medicare premiums and cost sharing for the one-sixth of Medicare recipients who are poor enough to qualify, but this reimbursement structure does not pay for an interdisciplinary care team, outpatient prescription medications, on-call services, or continuity across time and delivery settings. Medicare also does not pay for self-administered medications or for a case coordinator. At the present time, fee-for-service Medicare pays for medical treatments but not for long-term continuity or palliative services. This is just the reverse of what many dying elderly patients need and prefer.

Although hospice programs have demonstrated effective care for people in the last phase of life, they serve only about 20 percent of the dying, for about a month on average, with cancer patients accounting for 70 percent of the admitting diagnoses. The current Medicare hospice benefit does not really provide the care needed by patients with chronic medical illnesses, such as congestive heart failure or chronic neurologic disorders. These patients most typically have a course that is characterized by a slow decline in function punctuated by periodic life-threatening crises with widely variable and unpredictable survival times.

There is a need to revise the Medicare system to assure elderly persons of continuous good-quality care at the end of life. The current system was created to provide a system of acute care for the elderly. It is inadequately designed to meet the chronic care needs of the seriously ill patient for symptom control, for caregiver assistance, and for home care.

A program called Medicaring has been suggested to replace the current hospice benefit to allow functional disability and severity of illness to be the indicators for eligibility for hospice care, in contrast to the current criterion of the patient having a prognosis of six months or less.[13] The current Medicare system needs to be readjusted as soon as possible to meet the needs of the threefold increase in the aged population expected in the next ten years.

Legal Approaches

Although state task forces, community programs, groups of health care professionals, and private foundations are now focusing on improving the care of those who are terminally ill in ways that we discuss further below, their efforts are set against a backdrop of an ongoing struggle over legalization of assisted suicide. Efforts by proponents to legalize physician-assisted suicide, which they see as at least a partial solution to the problems of caring for those who are terminally ill, did not end when the U.S. Supreme Court in 1997 rejected the notion of a constitutional right to assisted suicide. Although the Court specified that it was not ruling one way or the other on the constitutionality of the Oregon assisted suicide law, legalization advocates claimed that the Court decision was a partial victory since it left them free to persuade states to legislate permission rather than prohibition of assisted suicide. As Yale Kamisar has pointed out (chapter 4), this was a right they always had. It was the fact that such persuasion had not been successful that had led proponents to the judicial route, and eventually to the Supreme Court.

State Legislation and Voter Initiatives

Advocates have taken the struggle over legalizing assisted suicide back to state legislatures, where a number of states considered but did not pass measures to legalize physician-assisted suicide. Bills explicitly prohibiting assisted suicide have been passed in three states that did not previously have them, while four other states added civil penalties to existing laws prohibiting assisted suicide. At the present time, thirty-eight states now have laws explicitly prohibiting assisted suicide, in seven the practice is implicitly prohibited by common law, in several the law is unclear, and only in Oregon does a law exist to permit physician-assisted suicide in limited circumstances.

Before the Oregon referendum, legalization initiatives had been turned down in Washington and California. Those initiatives included euthanasia as well as assisted suicide. Learning from that experience, Oregon proponents restricted their proposal to physician-assisted suicide. In 1998 Michigan considered an initiative modeled after the one in Oregon, but it was also voted down. And in November 2000 Maine joined California, Washington, and Michigan in turning down physician-assisted suicide.[14] Notably, in Maine the proponents of physician-assisted suicide had raised $1.6 million, in contrast to the $950,000 raised by those opposing the legislation. Also different from Oregon, where the medical associations had remained neutral on the topic, the Maine Medical Association and Maine Hospital Association strongly opposed the legislation. Both sides claimed that the other used controversial ads, some of which were pulled in the final days of the debate. Although several months before the vote polls indicated almost two-to-one support for assisted suicide, the actual vote was 51.7 percent against versus 48.3 percent in favor. Such a reversal was the pattern in Michigan and California as well. As voters learn the details of the proposed law and the problems it would create, their attitudes change.

Although having such initiatives that rely on a popular vote may seem a reasonable way to resolve social problems, as David Broder, Pulitzer Prize–winning journalist of the *Washington Post*, documented in a recent book, the referendum process is easily manipulated by moneyed interests and works against the checks and balances of the republican form of government envisioned by the Constitution.[15] In discussing the use of the referendum to decide the question of assisted suicide, the distinguished legal ethicist and health law expert George Annas makes the following point: "On relatively simple questions this method is reasonable. But neither euthanasia nor physician-assisted suicide is a simple question, and legalizing either requires not only carefully worded legislation but a thorough and detailed public debate and discussion. Contemporary initiative petitions tend to degenerate into televised sloganeering, and permit neither of these."[16]

State Courts and Physician-Assisted Suicide

Proponents continue to use the courts as a potential ally. They have turned their attention from the U.S. Constitution to the constitutions of a handful of states, such as California, Florida, and Alaska, that contain strong privacy provisions, and they have contended that these states' laws prohibiting assisted suicide violate state constitutions. In all three states the courts found that those states' assisted suicide laws are in accord with their constitutions and that the right to privacy does not include a right to assisted suicide. The Florida Supreme Court, in reversing a ruling by a lower court, declared that three compelling interests outweighed the petitioner's desire for assistance in committing suicide: the preservation of life, the prevention of suicide, and the maintenance of the ethical integrity of the medical profession. In Alaska, Judge Eric Sanders, presiding over a case brought before the Alaska Superior Court, came to a similar conclusion, pointing out that the state's obligation to "the preservation of human life and the protection of vulnerable individuals outweighs any individual's decision to end his or her own life." Judge Sanders also wrote that "conduct which can be characterized as personal and private is not necessarily protected on some inherent personal autonomy right. Privacy rights are not monolithic. . . . When a matter does affect the public, directly or indirectly, it loses its wholly private character, and can be made to yield when an appropriate public need is demonstrated."[17] Compassion in Dying, the organization that brought the case, appealed to the Alaska Supreme Court, but the court unanimously supported the earlier decision.

A more idiosyncratic challenge to a state assisted suicide law was raised in Colorado when an eighty-one-year-old man contended that the state's ban on assisted suicide violated his federal constitutional right to "free exercise of religion"; the Colorado Court of Appeals rejected his claim.

Federal Legislation and Physician-Assisted Suicide

Opponents of assisted suicide have also attempted to use federal legislation to prevail. In 1997 Congress passed a law prohibiting the use of federal funds and health programs for assisted suicide, an act that has relevance to Oregon, which subsequently had to return some Medicare funds to the federal government.[18] Opponents have also urged the Drug Enforcement Administration (DEA) and Congress to use the 1970 Controlled Substances Act, which gave the DEA responsibility for regulating substances such as barbiturates and narcotics, to prevent use of these drugs for assisted suicide in Oregon. The act specifies that controlled substances can be used only for a "legitimate medical purpose" approved by the federal government. Since physician-assisted suicide is not such an approved use, the DEA had presumed that it could prohibit the use of controlled substances for assisted suicide. Attorney General Janet Reno ruled, however, that since the act was written before there was any consideration of assisted suicide, it should not be used to prohibit the use of controlled substances for assisted suicide when a state has authorized such use. (As discussed below, Reno's successor, John Ashcroft, disagreed.) Attorney General Reno indicated that if Congress wanted the act to cover assisted suicide, it would need to pass authorizing legislation.

A bill was introduced in Congress in 1998 for that purpose.[19] Revised in 1999 to meet the concerns of the American Medical Association (AMA), which now supports it, the Pain Relief Promotion Act (PRPA) *precludes* the use of controlled substances for euthanasia or assisted suicide but stipulates that the use of controlled substances to alleviate pain or discomfort, even if they increase the risk of death, is an approved use that is in the public interest. The act provides for minimal funding of palliative care research and education and authorizes a program to educate local, state, and federal law enforcement personnel in the legitimate use of controlled substances in pain management and palliative care.

It is the assisted suicide provision of the act that is the subject of controversy and has divided opponents of physician-assisted suicide. The PRPA does not prohibit physician-assisted suicide, only the use of controlled substances for the purpose. But while there are many drugs that are not controlled substances that could be used for that purpose, most physicians would not be inclined to use them.

Opponents of the act have argued that the legislation violates the state's traditional right to regulate medical practice and the physician's right to prescribe drug therapies. Supporters of the legislation saw Reno's ruling as interfering with congressional authority and a contradiction of the principle that state law is subordinate to federal law.

While the AMA, the National Hospice and Palliative Care Organization, the American Academy of Pain Management, the Pain Care Coalition, the American Society of Anesthesiologists, Physicians for Compassionate Care, the Hospice Association of America, and other major medical groups have supported the proposed legislation and believe it will encourage palliative care, the American Cancer Society, the American Academy of Neurology, and the American Pain Foundation, which also are against physician-assisted suicide, are opposed to this legislation, believing it will have the opposite effect. They fear the PRPA will expand the role of the DEA, encouraging the agency to investigate unnecessarily palliative care decisions made by physicians caring for terminally ill patients. Many physicians have had bad prior experiences with the DEA and do not believe that the provisions of law will be sufficient to protect them from overzealous or ill-informed DEA investigators. Moreover, they argue that the patient with pain is being used as a pawn in legislation aimed at restricting physician-assisted suicide in Oregon by preventing physicians from prescribing controlled substances for that purpose.

It is hard to be sure which view is correct, since much would depend on the attitude of those who administer the law. Opponents of the PRPA do not want to take a chance on what the attitude will be. Those in favor of PRPA believe the impact of having Congress send a message to the country indicating its opposition to assisted suicide while supporting palliative care more than justifies PRPA's enactment. In 2000 the bill was approved by the House of Representatives and subsequently by the Senate Judiciary Committee, but it was not taken up by the full Senate before the end of the congressional session. Senator Orrin Hatch of Utah, however, was successful in attaching to the Violence against Women Act language that declared 2001–2010 as the decade of pain and pain control to implement this initiative. Unfortunately, no funds were provided.

A recent ruling by the Bush administration's attorney general, John Ashcroft, may have broken the PRPA legislative stalemate.[20] In the fall of 2001, the new attorney general overturned his predecessor's 1998 ruling and reinstated the DEA's determination that the Controlled Substances Act prohibits the use of narcotics and other dangerous drugs controlled by federal law to assist suicide. Attorney General Ashcroft observed that unlike pain management, which has long been recognized as a good reason for using drugs, "assisting suicide is not a 'legitimate medical purpose.'" He emphasized that there are "important medical, ethical, and legal distinctions between intentionally causing a patient's death and providing sufficient dosages of pain medication necessary to eliminate or alleviate pain."

In concluding that the DEA's original reading of the Controlled Substances Act was correct (not Attorney General Reno's), Ashcroft relied on a May 2001 decision of the U.S. Supreme Court (*United States v. Oakland Cannabis Buyers' Cooperative*) that medical use of marijuana is no defense to a violation of the Controlled Substances Act even in a state that has approved the use of medical marijuana by voter initiative.[21] Ashcroft's reading of the Controlled Substances Act will not go unchallenged. Indeed, the day after Ashcroft issued his directive, Oregon Attorney General Hardy Myers and several terminally ill patients asked a federal court to impose a stay on it. Plaintiffs maintained that the U.S. attorney general had exceeded his authority under federal drug laws and was improperly interfering with Oregon's authority to regulate medicine. However, in light of the Supreme Court's recent medical marijuana ruling, which emphasized the need to apply the Controlled Substances Act uniformly, there is a good chance that Attorney General Ashcroft's reading of the act will ultimately prevail. Some opponents of assisted suicide fear that regardless of the outcome, the legal struggle will create a distracting shift from a debate on palliative care to one on states' rights.

Some of those who have long argued for legalizing physician-assisted suicide, like Thomas Preston, now suggest that legalization may not be necessary. Preston maintains that the Supreme Court opinion in *Washington v. Glucksberg* confirming that sedation in the imminently dying is acceptable medical care provides a basis to avoid the social divisiveness of the struggle over legalization by permitting us to forge a consensus that concentrates instead on providing adequate end-of-life care.[22]

Although this might seem to be a reasonable proposal, it may be the product of political expediency since it is coupled with the proposition that Congress do nothing to interfere with the Oregon assisted suicide law. Advocates have long been afraid that understanding and acceptance of sedation as a therapeutic approach, which would essentially mean that no dying person must suffer pain, would undercut the basis for legalization of assisted suicide and euthanasia. They have alternately attempted to describe such sedation, as Preston himself has done, as a disguised or unacknowledged form of euthanasia or demonized the procedure.

The latter approach was an integral part of the brief in *Vacco v. Quill* filed with the Supreme Court by advocates of legalization. The brief contained disturbing and distorted descriptions of patients who might request sedation when they were close to death because their suffering could not be relieved in any other way. Patients were described as being put into a "deathlike" state, in the "monstrous" condition of having their "minds chemically shut down" while they were "imprisoned in their decaying bodies." If these patients had chosen to forgo medically administered nutrition, the brief described them as "deliberately starved to death."[23] The reality is that dying patients are sleepy or delirious from the multiple medical factors related to their dying, and they are not able to eat or drink. Nutrition and hydration therapies are not necessarily discontinued, depending on the patient's and families' perspective on withholding and withdrawing such support systems.

Had the Court accepted the frightening and misrepresentative picture of sedation presented in the brief, it would have been hard for physicians to recommend and patients to seek what is at times necessary. The Court furthered hospice and palliative care by accepting such sedation for those who are imminently dying as an essential and beneficial aspect of the medical care that may be needed to help dying patients and as an integral component of palliative care.

The Court made clear that sedation for imminently dying patients is acceptable when based on the principle of informed consent and double effect, that is, when the sedation is necessary to relieve suffering, the physician's intention is to relieve suffering, and the patient and his or her surrogate accept that the patient is dying and have consented to sedation. As we have noted earlier, the majority of justices went further in embracing what could be seen as the right of patients to palliative care.

Social Transformation

The legal battles and public debate about physician-assisted suicide have provided a forum for a national discussion on how we care for our dying in the United States. They have clearly raised awareness of the inadequacy of care and have helped to allow the public to articulate their fears and concerns and to call attention to the existing barriers to humane, competent, compassionate care for the dying.

Although the topic of end-of-life care has been the interest of a small number of health care professionals and health care policy experts over the last twenty-five years, nothing could have predicted the intense attention that has focused on dying and the development of a series of wide-ranging initiatives by communities, states, the federal government, nongovernmental organizations, and health care system foundations and organizations. Clearly, the time has come for an open public discussion of what we as a society can do to promote improved care of patients with serious life-threatening illness. There is no question, however, that history will view this time as one in which both public and professional attention was focused on this topic in part by the physician-assisted suicide debate, Jack Kevorkian, an aging population, limitations in health care resources, and contemporary anxieties about dying. Public attention to the care of the dying has shifted from the *60 Minutes* videotape of Kevorkian euthanizing a patient with amyotrophic lateral sclerosis, for which he was convicted of second-degree murder, to Bill Moyer's four-part Public Broadcasting System (PBS) program entitled *On Our Own Terms*. Watched by 19 million Americans, the program described how palliative care and hospice care are provided and that they should be an integral part of the care of all patients facing death. This PBS program was associated with a national outreach effort and a *Time* magazine cover story.[24] With a goal of demonstrating hospice and palliative care approaches, the program provided for the American public the opportunity to better understand their options for care at the end of life and encouragement for them to talk with their families about what they would want for care when they face death.

Building up to this broad public educational effort has been the Robert Wood Johnson Foundation's network of organizations focused on improving end-of-life care. This effort, entitled Last Acts, has an expansive Web site and over 500 groups and organizations around the country that work through daily e-mails, educational programs, newsletters, as well as task forces addressing issues that include pain management, psychological matters, existential distress, spirituality, financing, and caregiver needs. These national public educational efforts have been coupled with a wide variety of state-based efforts.

State Initiatives

Over twenty states have developed initiatives on end-of-life care focused on identifying the barriers to good-quality care at the end of life within each state and developing strategies to overcome such obstacles. For example, New York Attorney General Dennis Vacco created a task force to address the barriers in New York State to appropriate end-of-life care. Based on the recommendations of this task force,[25] the fourteen deans of New York State medical schools agreed to develop educational programs in palliative care within their curricula. At the same time, the New York State Department of Health created a task force to address the health-related barriers. The task force recommended a change in the regulations governing triplicate prescriptions for controlled substances identifying such laws as impeding physician prescribing of opioid drugs for pain management. The New York State legislature passed into law a duplicate prescription process with electronic monitoring as an approach to facilitate opioid prescribing practices by physicians. Similar types of legislative changes for advanced directives and surrogate decision making have occurred in West Virginia and New Jersey.

Community Programs

At the local level, community groups have formed to look at how particular localities care for their dying. Perhaps the most extensive of these is the Missoula Demonstration Project, which is lead by Dr. Ira Byock, a hospice physician, in Missoula, Montana, and national program office director of the Robert Wood Johnson Foundation's Promoting Excellence in End of Life Care. The demonstration project is a community-based endeavor to grapple with end-of-life care issues. In various initiatives, people from many walks of life work to improve the quality of life. There are health care professional task forces to raise awareness and teach skills related to pain management and advanced care planning. Public health task forces focus on the realities of dying, caregiving, and grief within the life of faith communities and workplace communities, schools, clubs, and neighborhoods. Missoula has created a Life Stories Task Force dedicated to helping people review and record their personal histories. Through this task force, Missoulians have learned to use such histories to create memorial books with loved ones who are dying. Similar efforts on a smaller scale are developing in communities throughout the country, again hoping to focus attention on the specific needs of the community and the development of creative efforts to meet the needs of patients and families.

Various grassroots advocacy organizations have developed, including the Partnership for Caring (www.partnershipforcaring.org) and Americans for Better Care of the Dying (www.abcd-caring.org). Both focus attention on and coordinate grassroots efforts for change. They serve as advocates for national and local initiatives to improve care through education and policy programs, networking, newsletters, and conferences.

Health Care Professional Initiatives

To the credit of health care professionals, they were the first to acknowledge clearly their lack of leadership in addressing the needs of dying patients. This is well exemplified in the 1997 report of the Institute of Medicine (IOM), which set the tone for the type of reform needed to improve the care of the dying.[26] This prestigious academic group acknowledged the failure of medicine in the care of the dying and made seven different recommendations to different caregivers for improving the care of the dying. The seven recommendations range from support for public education, professional education, research, and policy initiatives to a call to action for the profession of medicine to take the lead in improving end-of-life care. The IOM report has had a major impact on creating an agenda for medicine in addressing this important issue. In response to its admitted failure in leadership, the AMA has developed a highly professional broad educational program called EPEC, Educational Program in End of Life Care, to train practicing clinicians around the country in the principles and practice of palliative care.

Several faculty development programs have been created. These include the Veterans Administration Faculty Leaders Project, which is a two-year initiative in which faculty leaders develop end-of-life care and palliative care curricula to be used in training resident physicians specializing in general internal medicine and its subspecialties (http://www.va.gov/oaa/flp). The Project on Death in America has provided funding to sixty-eight physicians and nurses identified as outstanding clinical faculty committed to improving end-of-life care. The fifty-nine awards granted represent thirty-eight medical schools in the United States, four medical schools in Canada, and three schools of nursing. The program aims to promote the visibility and prestige of clinicians committed to this area and to enhance their effectiveness as academic leaders, role models, and mentors for future generations (http://www.soros.org/death/index.htm).

Since 1997 a significant number of specialty societies as well as the Joint Commission on Accreditation of Healthcare Organizations have endorsed or adopted a consistent set of core principles for end-of-life care. These organizations concur that the medical community needs to strengthen clinical competency and specialty skills to ensure good-quality care at the end of life, and they have made a commitment both to raise awareness and to provide educational endeavors within their specialty groups.

The American College of Physicians and the American Board of Internal Medicine have developed initiatives to enhance competency and testing of physicians in end-of-life care. The American Association of Medical Colleges, in collaboration with the New York Academy of Medicine, has agreed to address end-of-life care in undergraduate medical education through new initiatives. At each level there is a need to institutionalize palliative care in health care professionals' training in medical school, in residency and training, in fellowship training, and in clinical practice. It does appear that the building blocks for these programs have been laid and that over the next five to ten years general training for all practitioners as well as specific training for palliative care specialists will be established.

At the same time, a continuing medical education program for practicing nurses entitled End of Life Nursing Education Consortium

(ELNEC) provides train-the-trainer programs on end-of-life care. A Social Work Leadership Award Program supported by the Project on Death in America at the Open Society Institute has to date provided awards to twenty social workers with a focus on emphasizing the critical role social workers play in helping patients and families address the complexities of death, grief, and bereavement.

The training of psychiatrists in the psychological dimensions of palliative care will have to be a critical part of these efforts. Few psychiatrists are trained to recognize depression in those who are terminally ill, a group in which the diagnosis is particularly difficult to make. Psychologists and psychiatrists, except those trained in psycho-oncology, are not formally educated in hospice and palliative care. There are no existing national quality standards for the evaluation of patients with psychological distress with serious, life-threatening illness, although, as we noted in chapter 7, the National Comprehensive Cancer Network recently developed a set of consensus guidelines to evaluate psychological symptoms in patients with cancer.

The focus on efforts to legalize assisted suicide and euthanasia has also served to obscure the positive role mental health professionals can play in end-of-life care. Psychiatrists have been assigned and have accepted the role of gatekeepers who can be consulted to determine whether patients are capable of making an informed decision—in short, whether patients are competent. When consulted as a gatekeeper, the psychiatrist is placed in the position of standing in the way of a patient's getting what he or she wants, a role not conducive to the communication needed if the patient is to be helped.

The psychiatrist in most cases will not be called to help unless the patient's physician makes a referral. This is not as simple as it sounds for the referring physician or the patient. In addition to the subtle prejudice that a depressed mood is normal in a dying patient, both patients and families want to avoid what they perceive of as the stigma of a psychiatric evaluation at this time of life. This is less likely if the referring physician understands the request for assisted suicide as a symptom of the distress that accompanies terminal illness and makes the referral on that basis. To transform the culture of end-of-life care, we need to make help in coping with the emotional distress of terminal illness as much a part of our psychiatric/medical culture as is managing physical symptoms.

Foundation Initiatives

The philanthropic commitment to the development and improvement of end-of-life care has been commendable. The Robert Wood Johnson Foundation has committed almost $90 million to these efforts, the Soros Foundation's Project on Death in America has committed $45 million, and numerous other foundations, including the Commonwealth Fund, the Nathan Cummings Foundation, and the Fetzer Foundation, have committed significant resources to address these issues. The American Foundation for Suicide Prevention has begun to fund research into the psychological aspects of terminal illness as well as treatment research aimed at reducing anxiety and depression in dying patients and making their remaining time more meaningful. To encourage broader philanthropic funding in these areas, several foundations joined together to create Grantmakers Concerned with Care at the End of Life (GCCEL). This initiative is looking to expand funding coalitions in end-of-life care and serve as a resource to foundations about opportunities for funding in end-of-life care (http://www.gccel@sorosny.org).

The debate over assisted suicide has helped to stimulate the medical community, and palliative care specialists in particular, into accepting the challenge to provide better care at the end of life. What we have learned from the Netherlands, Australia, and Oregon, however, indicates that legal sanction for assisted suicide and euthanasia complicates, distracts, and interferes with the effort to improve end-of-life care. Defeating attempts to legalize assisted suicide, however, should not be our central objective. In Maine, for example, the debate over the assisted suicide referendum highlighted the fact that hospice care is not available to poor people in the state. Maine is only one of six states where there is no Medicaid hospice benefit, and the state ranks last in the use of hospice. During the referendum battle, the Maine Medical Association pledged to work to change this situation.[27] If this can be done in Maine and we take advantage of our many other current opportunities at the community, state, and federal levels to move to address the needs of patients at the end of life, assisted suicide will cease to seem an option that is truly needed, and the question of legalization may become irrelevant.

The challenge we face is to create a culture that identifies the care of the seriously ill and dying as a public health issue. Reframing the Medicare benefit to better address the needs of this patient population; expanding and underwriting professional educational initiatives in palliative care at the undergraduate, graduate, and continuing education level; and experimenting with demonstration projects that identify and promote new models of health care delivery for patients are some of the ways to improve care for patients and families facing serious life-threatening illness. Coupled with these initiatives must be the nurturing and development of broad public educational initiatives and support for advocacy groups such as Americans for Better Care of the Dying and Partnership for Caring. At the same time, we need to develop process measures and outcome measures to track the changes and improvements in care to define better what is quality care and to facilitate the institutionalization of these programs into health care policy and reform. For this to occur, there needs to be a strong social commitment to both respecting the individuality and dignity of dying patients and their families, and providing them with real choices for real care at the end of life.

Notes

Introduction

1. *Washington v. Glucksberg*, 521 U.S. 702, 737 (1997) (O'Connor, J., concurring), and *Vacco v. Quill*, 521 U.S. 793 (1997).

2. T. Preston, "Whither Peace in Dying?" Paper given at Andrews University conference, The End of Life: Assisted Suicide and the Hospice Movement, 6 April 2000, Berrien Springs, Michigan, 2.

3. R. K. Portenoy, N. Coyle, K. M. Kash, et al., "Determination of the Willingness to Endorse Assisted Suicide: A Survey of Physicians, Nurses, and Social Workers," *Psychosomatics* 38 (1997):277–87.

4. H. Hendin and G. Klerman, "Physician-Assisted Suicide: The Dangers of Legalization," *American Journal of Psychiatry* 150 (1993):143–45.

5. *Compassion in Dying v. Washington*, 79 F.3d 790, 824 (9th Cir. 1996) (en banc).

6. R. Dworkin, *Life's Dominion: An Argument about Abortion, Euthanasia, and Individual Freedom* (New York: Vintage Books, 1994).

7. E. Hamilton, *Mythology* (Boston: Little Brown, 1942), 224–43.

8. F. Kennedy, "The Problem of Social Control of the Congenital Defective," *American Journal of Psychiatry* 99 (1942):13–16; Y. Kamisar, "Some Non-Religious Views against Proposed 'Mercy-Killing' Legislation," *Minnesota Law Review* 42 (1958):969–1042, 994.

9. H. G. Gallagher, *By Trust Betrayed: Physicians, Patients, and the License to Kill in the Third Reich* (Arlington, Va.: Vandamere Press, 1995), 56.

10. Ibid., 43–64.

11. E. Slater, "Choosing the Time to Die," in *Suicide: The Philosophical Issues*, ed. M. P. Battin and D. May (New York: St. Martin's Press, 1980), 199–204, 202.

12. D. Humphry and M. Clement, *Freedom to Die: People, Politics and the Right-to-Die Movement* (New York: St. Martin's Press, 1998), 313.

13. H. Hendin, *Seduced by Death: Doctors, Patients, and Assisted Suicide* (New York: Norton, 1998).

14. C. Gomez, *Regulating Death: Euthanasia and the Case of the Netherlands* (New York: Free Press, 1991); H. Hendin, "Seduced by Death: Doctors, Patients and the Dutch Cure," *Issues in Laws and Medicine* 10 (1994):123–68; J. Keown, "Euthanasia in the Netherlands: Sliding down the Slippery Slope," in *Euthanasia Examined:*

Ethical, Legal, and Clinical Perspectives, ed. J. Keown (New York: Cambridge University Press, 1995), 261–96.

15. P. J. van der Maas, J. J. M. van Delden, and L. Pijnenborg, *Euthanasia and Other Medical Decisions Concerning the End of Life* (New York: Elsevier, 1992); P. J. van der Maas, G. van der Wal, I. Haverkate, et al., "Euthanasia, Physician-Assisted Suicide, and Other Medical Practices Involving the End of Life in the Netherlands, 1990–1995," *New England Journal of Medicine* 335 (1996):1699–1705.

16. H. Kuhse and P. Singer, "Doctors' Practices and Attitudes Regarding Voluntary Euthanasia," *Medical Journal of Australia* 148 (1988):623–27.

17. D. W. Kissane, A. Street, and P. Nitschke, "Seven Deaths in Darwin: Case Studies under the Rights of the Terminally Ill Act, Northern Territory, Australia," *Lancet* 352 (1998):1097–1102.

Chapter 1: "I Will Give No Deadly Drug"

1. Of course, any physician with personal scruples against one or another of these practices may "write" the relevant exclusions into the service contract he offers his customers.

2. L. R. Kass, *Toward a More Natural Science: Biology and Human Affairs* (New York: Free Press, 1985). See chapters 6–9.

3. L. R. Kass, "Death with Dignity and the Sanctity of Life," *Commentary,* March 1990, 33–43. Regarding the alleged "right to die," see L. R. Kass, "Is There a Right to Die?" *Hastings Center Report* 23, no. 1 (1993):34–43. On the question of legalizing physician-assisted suicide and euthanasia, see also L. R. Kass and N. Lund, "Courting Death: Assisted Suicide, Doctors, and the Law," *Commentary,* December 1996, 17–29.

4. Y. Kamisar, "Some Non-Religious Views against Proposed 'Mercy-Killing' Legislation," *Minnesota Law Review* 42 (1958):969–1042.

5. The inexplicable failure of many physicians to provide the proper—and available—relief of pain is surely part of the reason why some people now insist that physicians (instead) should give them death.

6. See n. 4, Kamisar 1958, 990.

7. J. Keown, "Some Reflections on Euthanasia in the Netherlands," in *Euthanasia, Clinical Practice, and the Law,* ed. L. Gormally (London: Linacre Centre for Health Care Ethics, 1994), 193–218, 209. Keown is citing F. C. B. van Wijmen, *Artsen en het Zelfgekozen Levenseinde* [Doctors and the Self-Chosen Termination of Life] (Maastricht: Vaakgroep Gezondheidrecht Rijksuniversiteit Limburg, 1989), 24 (table 18).

8. Data are from P. J. van der Maas, J. J. M. van Delden, and L. Pijnenborg, *Euthanasia and Other Medical Decisions Concerning the End of Life* (New York: Elsevier Science, 1992), as reported in J. Keown, "Further Reflections on Euthanasia in the Netherlands in the Light of the Remmelink Report and the Van Der Maas Survey," in Gormally 1994 (see n. 7), 219–40, 224.

9. G. van der Wal, P. J. van der Maas, J. M. Bosma, et al., "Evaluation of the Notification Procedure for Physician-Assisted Death in the Netherlands," *New England Journal of Medicine* 335 (1996):1706–11.

10. H. Hendin, C. Rutenfrans, and Z. Zylicz, "Physician-Assisted Suicide and Euthanasia in the Netherlands," *Journal of the American Medical Association* 277 (1997):1720–22. For a fuller and chilling account of the Dutch practice, see H. Hendin, *Seduced by Death: Doctors, Patients, and the Dutch Cure* (New York: Norton, 1996).

11. See n. 8, Keown 1994, 230.

12. Analogous pressures now operate in the matter of abortion. Even obstetricians opposed to abortion are often compelled to discuss it, if only to avoid later lawsuits should the child be born with abnormalities.

13. See my essay on the Hippocratic Oath, Kass 1985 (see n. 2), chapter 9, esp. 232–40. See also, in the same volume, chapter 8, "Professing Medically: The Place of Ethics in Defining Medicine," esp. 217–23.

14. The ancient Hippocratic physicians' refusal to assist in suicide was not part of an aggressive, so-called vitalist approach to dying patients or an unwillingness to accept mortality. On the contrary, understanding well the limits of the medical art, they refused to intervene aggressively when the patient was deemed incurable, and they regarded it as inappropriate to prolong the natural process of dying when death was unavoidable. Insisting on the moral importance of distinguishing between letting die (often not only permissible but also laudable) and actively causing death (impermissible), they protected themselves and their patients from their own possible weaknesses and folly, thereby preserving the moral integrity ("the purity and holiness") of their art and profession.

This view of the matter has been preserved in Western medical ethics down to the present day. The proscription of medical killing has been reaffirmed in numerous medical codes and statements of principle. The American Medical Association's current Code of Medical Ethics, for example, very explicitly rules out physician-assisted suicide on the ground, among others, that it is "fundamentally incompatible with the physician's role as healer"—a point I develop in the next section of this chapter (Opinions of the Council on Ethical and Judicial Affairs, American Medical Association, Opinion 2.211).

15. See the "Profession: Intrinsically Ethical" section of this chapter, where, in discussing the fragility of the goal of health, I distinguish between serving the goal of health and "ministering to the needs and relieving the sufferings of the frail and particular patient." I also include the need to care for the patient's self-concern—that is, for what people call the patient as "person," not just as human organism. *Essentialism* and *essentialist* often function as terms of abuse—in medical ethics and philosophy, they function not unlike like *racist* and *fascist* in political discourse—and even where they are given a definite meaning, the name calling often serves in lieu of a refutation. Is it wrong to say that the medical profession is, at its center, the healing profession?

16. F. G. Miller and H. Brody, "Professional Integrity and Physician-Assisted Death," *Hastings Center Report* 25, no. 3 (1995):8–17, 12. Miller and Brody are among the few writers who take seriously the need for preserving the intrinsic moral integrity of the medical profession and who share my view that medicine may violate the body only to serve a valid medical goal, not merely to satisfy the patient's requests. We differ because, as I argue in the next paragraph, they regard "achieving a peaceful death" as a legitimate medical goal and, further, because they accept a dualism of person-body that I criticized a few paragraphs earlier: "Respect for the person, who finds his or her continued existence intolerable, takes precedence over the person's embodied life" (13).

17. Quoted in A. M. Capron, "Euthanasia in the Netherlands: American Observations," *Hastings Center Report* 22, no. 2 (1992):30–33.

18. See R. J. Lifton, *The Nazi Doctors: Medical Killing and the Psychology of Genocide* (New York: Basic Books, 1986), 32–48.

19. The result of the Quinlan case shows that the right to discontinue treatment cannot be part of some larger "right to die" or right "to determine the time and manner of one's own death." Indeed, it is both naive and thoughtless to believe that we can exercise such a "right" short of killing ourselves or arranging to be killed on schedule. The whole notion of the so-called right to die exposes the shallowness of our exaggerated belief in mastery over nature and fortune, a belief that informs our entire technological approach to death.

Chapter 2: Compassion Is Not Enough

1. D. Hume, *An Enquiry Concerning the Principles of Morals: A Critical Edition*, ed. T. L. Beauchamp (Oxford: Clarendon Press, 1998); M. Scheler, *The Nature of Sympathy*, trans. P. Heath (Hamden, Conn.: Archon Books, 1970). See also J. V. Welie, *In the Face of Suffering* (Omaha, Neb.: Creighton University Press, 1998); A. Schopenhauer, *On the Basis of Morality*, trans. E. F. J. Payne (Providence, R.I.: Berghahn Books, 1995); A. Schopenhauer, *The World As Will and Representation*, vol. 2, trans. E. F. J. Payne (Clinton, Mass.: Falcon's Wing Press, 1958), 106–10; Edith Stein, *On the Problem of Empathy*, trans. W. Stein (Washington, D.C.: ICS Publications, 1989); M. de Unamuno, *The Tragic Sense of Life in Men and Nations*, Bollingen Series LXXXV (Princeton, N.J.: Princeton University Press, 1972), 150; T. E. Quill, C. K. Cassell, and D. E. Meier, "Care of the Hopelessly Ill: Proposed Clinical Criteria for Assisted Suicide," *New England Journal of Medicine* 327 (1992):1380–84.

2. See n. 1, Hume 1998; F. Hutcheson, *On Human Nature: Reflections on Our Common Systems of Morality on the Social Nature of Man*, ed. T. Mautner (Cambridge: Cambridge University Press, 1993); A. Smith, *The Theory of Moral Sentiments* (Edinburgh: Bell and Bradfute, 1808).

3. See n. 1, Hume 1998.

4. M. P. Battin, "Is a Physician Ever Obligated to Help a Patient Die?" in *Regulating How We Die: The Ethical, Medical, and Legal Issues Surrounding Physician-Assisted Suicide*, ed. L. L. Emanuel (Cambridge, Mass.: Harvard University Press, 1998), 21–47.

5. D. Brock, *Life and Death* (Boston: Cambridge University Press, 1993); H. Brody, "Assisted Death: A Compassionate Response to Medical Failure," *New England Journal of Medicine* 327 (1992):1384–88; T. E. Quill, *Death and Dignity: Making Choices and Taking Charge* (New York: W. W. Norton, 1993); S. H. Wanzer, S. J. Adelsstein, and R. E. Cranford, "The Physician's Responsibility toward the Hopelessly Ill," *New England Journal of Medicine* 310 (1984):955–59; S. H. Wanzer, D. D. Federman, S. J. Adelstein, et al., "The Physician's Responsibility toward Hopelessly Ill Patients: A Second Look," *New England Journal of Medicine* 320 (1989):844–49.

6. J. C. Edwards, *Ethics without Philosophy: Wittgenstein and the Moral Life* (Tampa, Fla.: University Presses of Florida, 1982).

7. H. Jonas, M. Donhoff, and R. Merkel, "Not Compassion Alone: Interview with Hans Jonas, Marion Donhoff, and Reinhard Merkel" (trans. H. Hannum and H. Hannum), *Hastings Center Report* 25, no. 7 (1995):48.

8. T. Engberg-Pederion, *Aristotle's Theory of Moral Insight* (Oxford: Clarendon Press, 1984), 140–41; L. A. Kosman, "Being Properly Affected: Virtues and Feelings in Aristotle's Ethics," in *Essays on Aristotle's Ethics*, ed. A. O. Rorty (Berkeley: University of California Press, 1980), 109–15.

9. J. F. Tuohey, "Euthanasia and Assisted Suicide: Is Mercy Sufficient?" *Linacre Quarterly*, November 1993, 45–49.

10. See n. 4, Battin 1998.

11. J. H. van den Berg, *Medical Power and Medical Ethics* (New York: Norton, 1978), 63.

12. F. Degnon, "Levinas and the Hippocratic Oath: A Discussion of Physician-Assisted Suicide," *Journal of Philosophy and Medicine* 22 (1997):99–123.

13. L. W. Doob, *Panorama of Evil* (Westport, Conn.: Greenwood, 1978).

14. Netherlands Ministry of Welfare, Health, and Cultural Affairs, *Medical Practice with Regard to Euthanasia and Related Medical Decisions in the Netherlands: Results of an Inquiry and the Government View* [Remmelink Commission Report] (The Hague: Ministry of Welfare, Health, and Cultural Affairs, 1991); T. E. Quill, "Doctor, I Want to Die, Will You Help Me?" *Journal of the American Medical Association* 270 (1993): 870–73; see n. 1, Quill et al. 1992; see n. 5, Wanzer et al. 1984, 1989.

15. D. Callahan, "When Self-determination Runs Amok," *Hastings Center Report* 22, no. 2 (1992):52–55; T. Salem, "Physician-Assisted Suicide: Promoting Autonomy or Medicalizing Suicide?" *Hastings Center Report* 29, no. 3 (1999):30–36; E. D. Pellegrino, "The False Promise of Beneficent Killing," in Emanuel 1998 (see n. 4), 71–91.

16. R. Dworkin, T. Nagel, R. Nozick, et al., "Assisted Suicide: The Philosopher's Brief," *New York Review of Books*, 27 March 1994, 41–47; J. Rachels, "Active and Passive Euthanasia," in *Ethical Issues in Death and Dying*, ed. T. L. Beauchamp and S. Perkin (Englewood Cliffs, N.J.: Prentice-Hall, 1978), 241–42.

17. T. E. Quill, "Death and Dignity: A Case of Individualized Decision-Making," *New England Journal of Medicine* 324 (1991):691–94.

18. E. D. Pellegrino, "Compassion Needs Reason Too," *Journal of the American Medical Association* 270 (1993):874–75.

19. W. Osler, *Aequanimitas, with Other Addresses to Medical Students, Nurses and Practitioners of Medicine*, 3rd ed. (Philadelphia: Blakiston, 1932).

Chapter 3: Reason, Self-determination, and Physician-Assisted Suicide

This chapter draws on two previous articles of mine: "Reasons, Rationality, and Ways of Life," in *Contemporary Perspectives on Rational Suicide*, ed. J. L. Werth, Jr. (Philadelphia: Taylor & Francis, 1999), 22–28; and "Self-Extinction: The Morality of the Helping Hand," in *Physician-Assisted Suicide*, ed. R. F. Weir (Bloomington: Indiana University Press, 1997), 69–85.

Chapter 4: The Rise and Fall of the "Right" to Assisted Suicide

In writing this chapter, I have relied on two earlier articles I wrote on the general subject: "The 'Right to Die': On Drawing (and Erasing) Lines," *Duquesne Law Review* 35 (1996):481–521; and "On the Meaning and Impact of the Physician-Assisted Suicide Cases," *Minnesota Law Review* 82 (1998):895–922.

1. See Y. Kamisar, "Some Non-Religious Views against Proposed 'Mercy-Killing' Legislation," *Minnesota Law Review* 42 (1958):969–1042.

2. C. E. Schneider, "Making Biomedical Policy through Constitutional Adjudication: The Example of Physician-Assisted Suicide," in *Law at the End of Life: The*

Supreme Court and Assisted Suicide, ed. C. E. Schneider (Ann Arbor, Mich.: University of Michigan Press, 2000), 164–217, 164.

3. 410 U.S. 113 (1973).

4. 497 U.S. 261 (1990).

5. See *Griswold v. Connecticut,* 381 U.S. 479 (1965); *Eisenstadt v. Baird,* 405 U.S. 438 (1972).

6. 410 U.S. at 152–53.

7. 410 U.S. at 157–58.

8. See, e.g., R. A. Sedler, "Are Absolute Bans on Assisted Suicide Constitutional? I Say No," *University of Detroit Mercy Law Review* 72 (1995):725–33, 728–33.

9. 505 U.S. 833 (1992).

10. 505 U.S. at 851, second emphasis added.

11. See n. 8, Sedler 1995, 728.

12. D. Callahan, *The Troubled Dream of Life* (New York: Simon & Schuster, 1993), 107–8.

13. R. B. Ginsburg, "Speaking in a Judicial Voice," *N.Y.U. Law Review* 67 (1992):1185–1202, 1199.

14. L. H. Tribe, *Abortion: The Clash of Absolutes* (New York: W. W. Norton, 1990), 105.

15. 521 U.S. 702 (1997).

16. 521 U.S. 793 (1997).

17. New York State Task Force on Life and the Law, *When Death Is Sought: Assisted Suicide and Euthanasia in the Medical Context* (New York: New York State Task Force on Life and the Law, 1994), 71.

18. J. Rubenfeld, "The Right to Privacy," *Harvard Law Review* 102 (1989):737–94, 794.

19. *Cruzan,* 497 U.S. at 302–3.

20. See n. 17, New York State Task Force 1994, 75. See also n. 12, Callahan 1993.

21. J. Arras, "News from the Circuit Courts: How Not to Think about Physician-Assisted Suicide," *BioLaw* 2, Special Section (1996): S171–88, S183.

22. *In re* Quinlan, 355 A.2d 647 (N.J. 1976).

23. F. G. Miller, "Legalizing Physician-Assisted Suicide by Judicial Decision: A Critical Appraisal," *BioLaw* 2, Special Section (1996):S136–45, S141.

24. A. M. Capron, "Liberty, Equality, Death!" *Hastings Center Report* 26, no. 3 (1996):23–24.

25. See *Compassion in Dying,* 79 F.3d at 802.

26. *Compassion in Dying,* 79 F.3d at 824.

27. The Ninth Circuit's efforts to conflate the use of opioids to relieve pain with assisted suicide (or active euthanasia) drew heavy fire. See G. J. Annas, "The Promised End: Constitutional Aspects of Physician-Assisted Suicide," *New England Journal of Medicine* 335 (1996):683–87, 685; see also n. 21, Arras 1996, S181; H. Brody, "*Compassion in Dying v. Washington:* Promoting Dangerous Myths in Terminal Care," *BioLaw* 2, Special Section (1996):S154–59, S155–56.

28. *Quill,* 80 F.3d at 729 (quoting the district court, which had found such a distinction significant).

29. See n. 23, Miller 1996, S139.

30. *Quill,* 80 F.3d at 729.

31. *Quill,* 521 U.S. at 800.

32. *Glucksberg*, 521 U.S. at 725.

33. *Quill*, 521 U.S. at 802.

34. Brief for Respondents at 29, *Quill* (No. 95–1858), available in 1996 WL 708912.

35. *Quill*, 521 U.S. at 807.

36. *Glucksberg*, 521 U.S. at 725–26.

37. *Compassion in Dying*, 79 F.3d at 813–14.

38. *Glucksberg*, 521 U.S. at 727.

39. *Glucksberg*, 521 U.S. at 727–28.

40. *Glucksberg*, 521 U.S. at 736 (O'Connor, J., concurring), emphasis added.

41. *Glucksberg*, 521 U.S. at 737, emphasis added.

42. *Glucksberg*, 521 U.S. at 791.

43. Brief for United States as Amicus Curiae Supporting Petitioners at 12, *Glucksberg* (No. 96-110), available in 1996 WL 663186.

44. Transcript of Oral Argument, *Glucksberg* (No. 96-110), available in 1997 WL 13671, at *18, *20–21 (8 January 1997), emphasis added.

45. Transcript of Oral Argument, *Glucksberg* (No. 96-110), available in 1997 WL 13671, at *35–36.

46. See R. H. Fallon, Jr., "The Supreme Court, 1996 Term—Foreword: Implementing the Constitution," *Harvard Law Review* 111 (1997):54–152, 139, n. 616.

47. R. A. Burt, "The Supreme Court Speaks: Not Assisted Suicide but a Constitutional Right to Palliative Care" [sounding board], *New England Journal of Medicine* 337 (1997):1234–36, 1234.

48. Ibid., 47. See also G. J. Annas, "The Bell Tolls for a Right to Suicide," in *Regulating How We Die: The Ethical, Medical, and Legal Issues Surrounding Physician-Assisted Suicide*, ed. L. L. Emanuel (Cambridge, Mass.: Harvard University Press, 1998), 203–33, 230; S. M. Suter, "Ambivalent Unanimity: An Analysis of the Supreme Court's Holding," in Schneider 2000 (see n. 2), 25–35.

49. See H. Brody, "Physician-Assisted Suicide in the Courts: Moral Equivalence, Double Effect, and Clinical Practice," *Minnesota Law Review* 82 (1998):939–63, 960; see also n. 47, Burt 1997.

50. Brief of the American Medical Association, the American Nurses Association, and the American Psychiatric Association et al. as Amicus Curiae in Support of Petitioners at 4, *Glucksberg* (No. 96-110), available in 1996 WL 656263 (citation omitted).

51. To cite one specific example, Dr. Thomas Preston, a well-known proponent of physician-assisted suicide and one of the plaintiffs in the *Glucksberg* case, asserted that "the morphine drip is undeniably euthanasia, hidden by the cosmetics of professional tradition and language." T. A. Preston, "Killing Pain, Ending Life," *New York Times*, 1 November 1994, A27.

52. See n. 49, Brody 1998.

53. Brief of the American Medical Association, the American Nurses Association, and the American Psychiatric Association et al. as Amicus Curiae in Support of Petitioners at 3, *Glucksberg* (No. 96-110), available in 1996 WL 656263.

54. *Glucksberg*, 521 U.S. at 736 (O'Connor, J., concurring).

55. Brief for Respondents at i, *Glucksberg* (No. 95–1858), available in 1996 WL 708925.

56. Transcript of Oral Argument, *Glucksberg* (No. 96-110), available in 1997 WL 13671, at *26–27 (8 January 1997), emphasis added.

57. See Transcript of Oral Argument, *Glucksberg* (No. 96-110), available in 1997 WL 13671, at *27, *29, *33–35, *50–51 (8 January 1997).

58. Transcript of Oral Argument, *Glucksberg* (No. 96-110), available in 1997 WL 13671, at *28, emphasis added.

59. *Glucksberg*, 521 U.S. at 736 (O'Connor, J., concurring).

60. *Glucksberg*, 521 U.S. at 723.

61. *Compassion in Dying*, 79 F.3d at 795–96.

62. See *Singleton v. Wulff*, 428 U.S. 106, 112–13 (1976); *Planned Parenthood v. Ashcroft*, 462 U.S. 476, 478 (1983); *Planned Parenthood v. Danforth*, 428 U.S. 52, 62 (1976); *Doe v. Bolton*, 410 U.S. 179, 188 (1973).

63. See n. 48, Suter 2000, 31.

64. *Glucksberg*, 521 U.S. at 753 (concurring opinion).

65. See n. 46, Fallon 1997, 152; see also "The Supreme Court, 1996 Term—Leading Cases," *Harvard Law Review* 111 (1997):197–439, 248.

66. *Glucksberg*, 521 U.S. at 716.

67. R. A. Burt, "Constitutionalizing Physician-Assisted Suicide: Will Lightning Strike Thrice?" *Duquesne Law Review* 35 (1996):159–81, 179.

68. C. R. Sunstein, "The Right to Die," *Yale Law Journal* 106 (1997):1123–63, 1146 (written before the *Glucksberg* and *Quill* cases).

69. *Glucksberg*, 521 U.S. at 737. Some might argue that, in a system formally prohibiting physician-assisted suicide, those who are wealthy and well connected will still obtain such assistance "underground." But the counterargument is that in a system formally authorizing physician-assisted suicide, the risks of abuse are likely to fall most heavily on members of disadvantaged groups. See generally Y. Kamisar, "Physician-Assisted Suicide: The Problems Presented by the Compelling, Heartwrenching Case," *Journal of Criminal Law and Criminology* 88 (1998): 1121–46, 1127–33.

70. *Glucksberg*, 521 U.S. at 733.

71. Transcript of Oral Argument, *Glucksberg* (No. 96-110), available in 1997 WL 13671, at *49–50 (8 January 1997).

72. See L. Greenhouse, "An Issue for a Reluctant High Court," *New York Times*, 6 October 1996, E3.

73. Ibid.

74. Brief of the American Medical Association, the American Nurses Association, and the American Psychiatric Association et al. as Amicus Curiae in Support of Petitioners at 5, *Glucksberg* (No. 96-110), available in 1996 WL 656263 (citation omitted).

75. L. R. Kass and N. Lund, "Physician-Assisted Suicide, Medical Ethics and the Future of the Medical Profession," *Duquesne Law Review* 35 (1996):395–425, 423.

76. Ibid.

77. F. Miller, H. Brody, and T. E. Quill, "Can Physician-Assisted Suicide Be Regulated Effectively?" *Journal of Law, Medicine, and Ethics* 24 (1996):225–32, 226.

78. See S. A. Law, "Physician-Assisted Death: An Essay on Constitutional Rights and Remedies," *Maryland Law Review* 55 (1996):292–342, 297, n. 13.

79. Transcript of Oral Argument, *Glucksberg* (No. 96-110), available in 1997 WL 13671, at *38–39 (8 January 1997). Justice O'Connor added, "I think there is no doubt that [if those challenging the constitutionality of Washington's anti–assisted suicide law were to prevail] it would result in a flow of cases through the court system for heaven knows how long" at *39. See also n. 48, Suter 2000.

80. See D. J. Garrow, "All Over but the Legislating: There Was a Genuine War over Abortion, These Writers Think, but the Armistice Appears to Be Durable" [book review], *New York Times*, 26 January 1998, 14.

81. See R. Price and T. Mauro, "Advocates Promise to Press the Fight," *USA Today*, 27 June 1997, 4A. See also T. Mauro, "But States Can Enact New Laws," *USA Today*, 27 June 1997, 1A.

82. Transcript of Oral Argument, *Glucksberg* (No. 96-110), available in 1997 WL 13671, at *12 (8 January 1997).

83. See T. Egan, "Assisted Suicide Comes Full Circle, to Oregon," *New York Times*, 26 October 1997, A1; E. J. Emanuel and L. L. Emanuel, "Assisted Suicide? Not in My State," *New York Times*, 24 July 1997, A15.

84. See n. 81, Price and Mauro 1997.

85. See n. 83, Emanuel and Emanuel 1997.

86. T. Egan, "In Oregon, Opening a New Front in the World of Medicine," *New York Times*, 6 November 1997, A26.

87. D. J. Garrow, "The Oregon Trail," *New York Times*, 6 November 1997, A27.

88. W. Gallagher, "Go with the Flow: What We Should Be Doing as We Prepare to Die" [book review], *New York Times*, 30 November 1997, 17.

89. See H. El Nasser and J. Ritter, "Officials: Ore. Suicide Law in Effect," *USA Today*, 6 November 1997, 3A. See also n. 83, Egan 1997.

90. At this point, and in the next five paragraphs, I am relying heavily on two op-ed pieces I wrote at the time Proposal B was defeated. See Y. Kamisar, "Details Doom Assisted-Suicide Measures," *New York Times*, 4 November 1998, A27; and "Devil in the Detail, Not Money, Defeated Assisted Suicide Plan," *Detroit News*, 5 November 1998, 12A.

91. S. Bok, "Physician-Assisted Suicide," in *Euthanasia and Physician-Assisted Suicide*, ed. G. Dworkin et al. (Cambridge: Cambridge University Press, 1998), 83–139, 139.

Chapter 5: The Dutch Experience

1. T. H. C. Bueller, "The Historical and Religious Framework for Euthanasia in the Netherlands," in *Euthanasia: The Good of the Patient, The Good of Society*, ed. R. I. Misbin (Frederick, Md.: University Publishing Group, 1992), 183–88.

2. Ibid.

3. D. Phillips, *De Naakte Nederlander* [The Dutch Exposed] (Amsterdam: Utgeverij, Bert Bakker, 1985).

4. H. Hendin, *Seduced by Death: Doctors, Patients, and Assisted Suicide* (New York: Norton, 1998).

5. See n. 1, Bueller 1992.

6. C. Gomez, *Regulating Death: Euthanasia and the Case of the Netherlands* (New York: Free Press, 1991).

7. Ibid.

8. KNMG, *Medisch Contact* 42 (1986):770–75.

9. P. J. van der Maas, J. J. M. van Delden, and L. Pijnenborg, *Euthanasia and Other Medical Decisions Concerning the End of Life* (New York: Elsevier, 1992).

10. G. van der Wal and P. J. van der Maas, *Euthanasia en Andere Medische Beslissingen Rond het Levenseinde* [Euthanasia and Other Medical Decisions at the End of Life] (The Hague: Staatsuitgeverj, 1996).

11. P. J. van der Maas, G. van der Wal, I. Haverkate, et al., "Euthanasia, Physician-Assisted Suicide, and Other Medical Practices Involving the End of Life in the Netherlands, 1990–1995," *New England Journal of Medicine* 335 (1996):1699–1705; G. van der Wal, P. J. van der Maas, J. M. Bosma, et al., "Evaluation of the Notification Procedure for Physician-Assisted Death in the Netherlands," *New England Journal of Medicine* 335 (1996):1706–11.

12. M. Angell, "Euthanasia in the Netherlands: Good News or Bad?" [editorial], *New England Journal of Medicine* 335 (1996):1675–78.

13. See n. 11, van der Wal et al. 1996, 1705.

14. General Board, Royal Dutch Medical Society, "Vision on Euthanasia," in *Euthanasia in the Netherlands* (Utrecht: Royal Dutch Medical Association, 1994), 12–26.

15. See n. 9, van der Maas et al. 1992.

16. See n. 11, van der Maas et al. 1996, 1703.

17. See n. 6, Gomez 1991.

18. See n. 9, van der Maas et al. 1992, 101–2.

19. See n. 11, van der Wal et al. 1996, 1708.

20. B. D. Onwuteaka-Philipsen, G. van der Wal, P. J. Kortense, and P. J. van der Maas, "Consultants in Cases of Intended Euthanasia or Assisted Suicide in the Netherlands," *Medical Journal of Australia* 170 (1999):360–63.

21. See n. 11, van der Wal et al. 1996, 1708.

22. See n. 11, van der Maas et al. 1996, 1704.

23. See n. 9, van der Maas et al. 1992, 58.

24. See n. 9, van der Maas et al. 1992, 73.

25. See n. 11, van der Maas et al. 1996, 1700.

26. See n. 11, van der Maas et al. 1996, 1704.

27. See n. 11, van der Maas et al. 1996, 1702.

28. See n. 11, van der Maas et al. 1996, 1704.

29. See n. 11, van der Maas et al. 1996, 1704.

30. See n. 11, van der Maas et al. 1996, 1704.

31. H. Hendin, *Seduced by Death: Doctors, Patients, and the Dutch Cure* (New York: Norton, 1996), 79.

32. R. Twycross, "A View from the Hospice," in *Euthanasia Examined: Ethical, Clinical, and Legal Perspectives,* ed. J. Keown (Cambridge: Cambridge University Press, 1995), 141–68, 161.

33. See n. 31, Hendin 1996, 77, 78.

34. H. Hendin, C. Rutenfrans, and Z. Zylicz, "Physician-Assisted Suicide and Euthanasia in the Netherlands: Lessons from the Dutch," *Journal of the American Medical Association* 277 (1997):1720–22.

35. K. L. Dorrepaal, N. K. Aaronson, and F.S.A.M. van Dam, "Pain Experience and Pain Management among Hospitalized Cancer Patients," *Cancer* 63 (1989): 593–98; Z. Zylicz, "The Story behind the Blank Spot: Hospice in Holland," *American Journal of Hospice and Palliative Care* 10 (1993):30–32; Z. Zylicz, "Euthanasia" [letter], *Lancet* 338 (1991):1150; H. Matthews, "Better Palliative Care Could Cut Euthanasia," *British Medical Journal* 317 (1998):617; R. de Wit, F. van Dam, A. Vielvoye-Kerkmeer, C. Mattern, and H. H. Abu-Saad, "The Treatment of Chronic Cancer Pain in a Cancer Hospital in the Netherlands," *Journal of Pain and Symptom Management* 12 (1999):333–50.

36. See n. 9, van der Maas et al. 1992.

37. L. Pijnenborg, P. J. van der Maas, J. J. M. van Delden, and C. W. N. Loonan, "Life-Terminating Acts without the Explicit Consent of the Patients," *Lancet* 341 (1993):1196–1199; L. Pijnenborg, *End-of-Life Decisions in Dutch Medical Practice* (The Hague: CIP-Gegevens Kononklijke Bibliotheek, 1995), 119–35.

38. H. Jochemsen and J. Keown, "Voluntary Euthanasia under Control? Further Empirical Evidence from the Netherlands," *Journal of Medical Ethics* 25 (1999): 16–21, 20.

39. P. J. van der Maas, J. J. M. van Delden, L. Pijnenborg, and C. W. L. Loonan, "Euthanasia and Other Medical Decisions Concerning the End of Life," *Lancet* 338 (1991):669–74.

40. See n. 6, Gomez 1991; n. 11, van der Wal et al. 1996; n. 32, Twycross 1995, 141–68.

41. H. Hendin, "Assisted Suicide, Euthanasia, and Suicide Prevention," *Journal of Suicide and Life-Threatening Behavior* 25 (1995):193–203.

42. H. W. Hilhoorst, *Euthanasie in het Ziekenhuis* [Euthanasia in the Hospital] (Lochem: De Tijdstroom, 1983).

43. See n. 31, Hendin 1996.

44. H. Hendin, "Selling Death and Dignity," *Hastings Center Report* 25, no. 3 (1995):19–23.

45. See n. 34, Hendin et al. 1997.

46. J. Groenwoud, P. J. van der Maas, G. van der Wal, et al., "A Physician-Assisted Death in Psychiatric Practice in the Netherlands," *New England Journal of Medicine* 336 (1997):1795–1807.

47. Figures from the Netherlands Central Bureau of Statistics.

48. M. Simons, "Dutch Doctors to Tighten Rules on Mercy Killings," *New York Times*, 11 September 1995, A3.

49. See n. 20, Onwuteaka-Philipsen et al. 1999.

50. See n. 31, Hendin 1996.

51. See n. 44, Hendin 1995.

52. T. Shelton, *British Medical Journal* 322 (2001): 509.

53. See n. 38, Jochemsen and Keown 1999.

54. J. van Delden, "Slippery Slopes in Flat Countries: A Response," *Journal of Medical Ethics* 25 (1999):22–24.

55. D. Callahan and M. White, "The Legalization of Physician-Assisted Suicide: Creating a Regulatory Potemkin Village," *University of Richmond Law Review* 30 (1996):1–83.

56. See n. 35, Dorrepaal et al. 1989; Zylicz 1991, 1993; Matthews 1998; de Wit et al. 1999.

57. See n. 35, Matthews 1998.

58. E. Borst-Eilers, "Euthanasia in the Netherlands: Brief Historical Review and Present Situation," in Misbin 1992 (see n. 1), 55–68, 68.

59. *The Encyclopedia of Philosophy* (New York: Macmillan, 1972), 2:9.

60. See n. 1, Bueller 1992.

61. J. H. Huizinga, *Dutch Civilization in the Seventeenth Century and Other Essays* (New York: Harper Torchbooks, 1969), 122.

62. B. van Heerikhuizen, "What Is Typically Dutch?" *Netherlands Journal of Sociology* 18 (1982):103–25; A. Hauser, *The Social History of Art* (New York: Knopf, 1952), 1:461.

63. See n. 61, Huizinga 1969.

64. S. Schama, *The Embarrassment of Riches* (New York: Knopf, 1987).

65. See n. 62, van Heerikhuizen 1982.

66. D. Phillips, letter to H. Hendin, 26 April 1995.

67. See n. 6, Gomez 1991, 95; D. Callahan, "When Self-determination Runs Amok," *Hastings Center Report* 22, no. 2 (1992):52–55.

68. See n. 61, Huizinga 1969, 114.

69. See n. 61, Huizinga 1969, 121.

70. Bert Gordijn, "Euthanasia and Palliative Care: The Dutch Experiment," lecture at Congress of the Research Network in Palliative Care, Berlin, Germany, 9 December 2000.

71. Zbigniew Zylicz, personal communication, 18 January 2001.

72. Ibid.

Chapter 6: Palliative Care and Euthanasia in the Netherlands

1. R. J. Janssens, H. A. ten Have, and Z. Zylicz, "Hospice Care in the Netherlands: An Ethical Point of View," *Journal of Medical Ethics* 25 (1999):408–12.

2. Central Bureau of Statistics, *Statistisch Jaarboek, 2000.* CD–ROM.

3. P. J. van der Maas, G. van der Wal, I. Haverkate, et al., "Euthanasia, Physician-Assisted Suicide, and Other Medical Practices Involving the End of Life in the Netherlands, 1990–1995," *New England Journal of Medicine* 335 (1996):1699–1705; H. Hendin, C. Rutenfrans, and Z. Zylicz, "Physician-Assisted Suicide and Euthanasia in the Netherlands: Lessons from the Dutch," *Journal of the American Medical Association* 277 (1997):1720–22; H. Jochemsen and J. Keown, "Voluntary Euthanasia under Control? Further Empirical Evidence from the Netherlands," *Journal of Medical Ethics* 25 (1999):16–21.

4. See n. 2, Central Bureau of Statistics 2000.

5. Z. Zylicz, "The Story behind the Blank Spot: Hospice in Holland," *American Journal of Hospice and Palliative Care* 10 (1993):30–34.

6. Z. Zylicz, "The Netherlands: Status of Cancer Pain and Palliative Care," *Journal of Pain and Symptom Management* 12 (1996):136–38; M. J. Janssens and B. Gordijn, "Palliatieve Geneeskunde in Nederland" [Palliative Medicine in the Netherlands], *Deutsche Medizinische Wochenschrift* 123 (1998):432–35.

7. See n. 2, Central Bureau of Statistics 2000.

8. B. D. Onwuteaka-Philipsen, M. T. Muller, G. van der Wal, et al., "Active Voluntary Euthanasia or Physician-Assisted Suicide?" *Journal of the American Geriatrics Society* 45 (1997):1208–13.

9. F. Martin, D. Poyen, E. Bouderlique, et al., "Depression and Burnout in Hospital Health Care Professionals," *International Journal of Occupational and Environmental Health* 3 (1997):204–9.

10. Y. Rapoport, S. Kreitler, S. Chaitchik, R. Algor, and K. Weissler, "Psychosocial Problems in Head-and-Neck Cancer Patients and Their Change with Time Since Diagnosis," *Annals of Oncology* 4 (1993):69–73.

11. L. Shaiova, "Case Presentation: 'Terminal Sedation' and Existential Distress," *Journal of Pain and Symptom Management* 16 (1998):403–4.

12. J. B. Vander Veer, Jr., "Dutch Euthanasia: Could It Happen Here?" *Western Journal of Medicine* 171 (1999):268–70; H. M. Chochinov, K. G. Wilson, M. Enns, and S. Lander, "Prevalence of Depression in the Terminally Ill: Effects of Diagnostic

Criteria and Symptom Threshold Judgments," *American Journal of Psychiatry* 151 (1994):537–40; H. M. Chochinov, K. G. Wilson, M. Enns, et al., "Desire for Death in the Terminally Ill," *American Journal of Psychiatry* 152 (1995):1185–91.

13. E. H. Verhagen, M. R. Eliel, A. de Graeff, and S. C. Teunissen, "Sedatie in de Laaste Levensfase" [Sedation in the Terminal Phase of Life], *Nederlands Tijdschrift Geneeskunde* 143 (1999):2601–3.

Chapter 7: The Oregon Experiment

1. *The Oregon Death with Dignity Act: A Guidebook for Health Care Providers* (Portland, Ore.: Center for Ethics in Health Care, Oregon Health Sciences University, 1998).

2. Ibid., 59.

3. E. Hoover and G. H. Hill, "Two Die Using Oregon Suicide Law," *Oregonian*, 26 March 1998, A01.

4. D. Gianelli, "Praise, Criticism Follow Oregon's First Reported Assisted Suicides," *American Medical News*, 13 April 1998, 1, 39.

5. See n. 3, Hoover and Hill 1998.

6. See n. 4, Gianelli 1998.

7. E. Hoover, "Two Deaths Add New Angle to Debate," *Oregonian*, 27 March 1998, A01.

8. Ibid.

9. Barbara Coombs Lee, personal communication to Kathleen Foley, April 1998.

10. See n. 3, Hoover and Hill 1998.

11. W. Claiborne, "An Oregon Statute Is Blunting Death's Sting," *Washington Post*, 29 April 1998, A01.

12. See n. 7, Hoover 1998.

13. See n. 3, Hoover and Hill 1998.

14. H. Hendin, K. Foley, and M. White, "Physician-Assisted Suicide: Reflections on Oregon's First Case," *Issues in Law and Medicine* 14 (1998):243–70.

15. Peter Reagan, M.D., personal communication, 23 March 1999.

16. P. Reagan, "Helen," *Lancet* 353 (1999):1265–67.

17. Ibid., 1266.

18. H. M. Chochinov, K. G. Wilson, M. Enns, and S. Lander, "Depression, Hopelessness, and Suicidal Ideation in the Terminally Ill," *Psychosomatics* 39 (1998): 366–70; E. J. Emanuel, D. L. Fairclough, E. R. Daniels, and B. L. Clarridge, "Euthanasia and Physician-Assisted Suicide: Attitudes and Experiences of Oncology Patients, Oncologists, and the Public," *Lancet* 347 (1996):1805–10.

19. See ref. 18, Chochinov et al. 1998; Emanuel et al. 1996.

20. H. Hendin and G. L. Klerman, "Physician-Assisted Suicide: The Dangers of Legalization," *American Journal of Psychiatry* 150 (1993):143–45.

21. G. E. Murphy, "The Physician's Responsibility for Suicide: (1) An Error of Commission and (2) Errors of Omission," *Annals of Internal Medicine* 82 (1975): 301–9.

22. S. D. Passik, W. Dugan, M.V. McDonald, B. Rosenfeld, and S. Edgerton, "Oncologists' Regulation of Depression in Their Patients with Cancer," *Journal of Clinical Oncology* 16 (1998):1594–1600.

23. L. Ganzini, H. D. Nelson, T. A. Schmidt, D. F. Kraemer, M. A. Delorit, and

M. A. Lee, "Physician Experiences with the Oregon Death with Dignity Act," *New England Journal of Medicine* 342 (2000):557–63.

24. Y. Conwell and H. D. Caine, "Rational Suicide and the Right to Die: Reality and Myth." *New England Journal of Medicine* 326 (1992):1100–1103.

25. J. C. Holland, "NCCN Practice Guidelines for the Management of Psychological Distress," *Oncology* 13, no. 5A (1999):113–47.

26. E. Moscowitz, "Difficulties Involved in Identifying the Legal Incapacity to Consent," *American Journal of Forensic Psychiatry* 19 (1998):121–27.

27. L. Ganzini, D. S. Fenn, M. A. Lee, R. T. Heintz, and J. D. Bloom, "Attitudes of Oregon Psychiatrists toward Physician-Assisted Suicide," *American Journal of Psychiatry* 153 (1996):1469–75.

28. L. Ganzini, G. Leong, D. Fenn, et al., "Evaluation of Competence to Consent to Assisted Suicide: Views of Forensic Psychiatrists." *American Journal of Psychiatry* 157 (2000): 595–600.

29. See n. 27, Ganzini et al. 1996, 1474.

30. See n. 23, Ganzini et al. 2000.

31. See n. 23, Ganzini et al. 2000; H. Hendin, "Euthanasia and Physician-Assisted Suicide in the Netherlands" [letter], *New England Journal of Medicine* 336 (1997):1385.

32. J. Lynn, F. Harrell, F. Cohn, D. Wagner, and A. F. Connors, "Prognoses of Seriously Ill Hospitalized Patients on Days before Death: Implications for Patient Care and Public Policy," *New Horizons* 5 (1997):56–61.

33. M. A. Lee, H. D. Nelson, V. P. Tilden, L. Ganzini, T. A. Schmidt, and S. W. Tolle, "Legalizing Assisted Suicide: View of Physicians in Oregon," *New England Journal of Medicine* 334 (1996):310–15.

34. See n. 1, *The Oregon Death with Dignity Act* 1998, 60.

35. D. Callahan and M. White, "The Legalization of Physician-Assisted Suicide: Creating a Regulatory Potemkin Village," *University of Richmond Law Review* 30 (1996):1–83.

36. F. Miller, H. Brody, and T. E. Quill, "Can Physician-Assisted Suicide Be Regulated Effectively?" *Journal of Law, Medicine and Ethics* 24 (1996):225–32.

37. See n. 1, *The Oregon Death with Dignity Act* 1998, 7.

38. E. H. Barnett, "Is Mom Capable of Choosing to Die?" *Oregonian*, 17 October 1999, G1, G2.

39. D. Reinhard, "In the Dark Shadows of Measure 16," *Oregonian*, 31 October 1999, D5.

40. M. D. Reed and J. Y. Greenwald, "Survivor Victim Status, Attachment and Sudden Death Bereavement," *Journal of Suicide and Life-Threatening Behavior* 21 (1991):385–401; N. L. Farberow, D. E. Gallagher-Thompson, N. J. Gilewski, and L. W. Thompson, "Changes in Grief and Mental Health of Bereaved Spouses of Older Suicides," *Journal of Gerontology* 47 (1992):357–66.

41. M. Angell, "Euthanasia in the Netherlands: Good News or Bad?" [editorial], *New England Journal of Medicine* 335 (1996):1675–78.

42. See n. 1, *The Oregon Death with Dignity Act* 1998, 44.

43. Sharon Rice, Manager, Registration Unit, memorandum to staff, Oregon Health Division Center for Health Statistics, 12 December 1997.

44. Sharon Rice, Manager Registration Unit, Center for Health Statistics of the Oregon Health Division, memorandum to funeral home staff, 12 December 1997.

45. See n. 1, *The Oregon Death with Dignity Act* 1998, 59.

46. *Oregon's Death with Dignity Act: The First Year's Experience* (Portland, Ore.: Oregon Department of Human Resources, 1999).

47. A. E. Chin, K. Hedberg, G. K. Higginson, and D. W. Fleming, "Legalized Physician-Assisted Suicide in Oregon: The First Year's Experience," *New England Journal of Medicine* 340 (1999):577–83.

48. K. Foley and H. Hendin, "The Oregon Report: Don't Ask, Don't Tell," *Hastings Center Report* 29, no. 3 (1999):37–42.

49. A. D. Sullivan, K. Hedberg, and D. W. Fleming, "Legalized Physician-Assisted Suicide in Oregon: The Second Year," *New England Journal of Medicine* 342 (2000):598–604.

50. "Legalized Physician-Assisted Suicide in Oregon, 1998–2000," New England Journal of Medicine 344 (2001): 605–607.

51. Ibid, 605.

52. See n. 48, Foley and Hendin 1999.

53. S. Grossman, V. R. Sheidler, and K. Swedeen, "Correlation of Patient and Caregiver Ratings of Cancer Pain," *Journal of Pain* 6 (1993):53–57.

54. S. Ward, N. Goldberg, V. Miller-McCauley, et al., "Patient-Related Barriers to the Management of Cancer Pain," *Journal of Pain* 52 (1993):319–24.

55. E. J. Emanuel, "Report of the ASCO Membership Survey on End of Life Care," *Proceedings of the American Society of Clinical Oncology* 17 (Alexandria, Va.: 1998).

56. S. W. Tolle and K. Haley, "Pain Management in the Dying: Successes and Concerns," *Oregon BME Newsletter*, fall 1998, 1–4.

57. G. Kimsma, "Euthanasia and Euthanizing Drugs in the Netherlands," in *Drug Use in Assisted Suicide and Euthanasia*, ed. M. P. Battin and A. G. Lipman (Binghamton, N.Y.: Haworth Press, 1996), 193–210.

58. J. H. Groenewoud, A. van der Heide, B. D. Onwuteaka-Philipsen, D. L. Willems, P. J. van der Maas, and G. van der Wal, "Clinical Problems with the Performance of Euthanasia and Physician-Assisted Suicide in the Netherlands," *New England Journal of Medicine* 342 (2000):551–56.

59. T. E. Quill, *A Midwife through the Dying Process: Stories of Healing and Hard Choices at the End of Life* (Baltimore: Johns Hopkins University Press, 1996); G. E. Delury, *But What If She Wants to Die?: A Husband's Diary* (Secaucus, N.J.: Birch Lane Press, 1997); A. Wickett, *Double Exit: When Aging Couples Commit Suicide Together* (Eugene, Ore.: Hemlock Society, 1989).

60. E. J. Emanuel, E. R. Daniels, E. L. Fairclough, and B. R. Clarridge, "The Practice of Euthanasia and Physician-Assisted Suicide in the United States: Adherence to Proposed Safeguards and Effects on Physicians," *Journal of the American Medical Association* 220 (1998):507–13.

61. S. B. Nuland, "Physician-Assisted Suicide and Euthanasia in Practice" [editorial], *New England Journal of Medicine* 342 (2000):583–84.

62. See n. 47, Chin et al. 1999, 580.

63. E. J. Emanuel, D. L. Fairclough, J. Slutsman, and L. L. Emanuel, "Understanding Economic and Other Burdens of Terminal Illness: The Experience of Patients and Their Caregivers," *Annals of Internal Medicine* 132 (2000):451–59.

64. D. L. Willems, E. R. Daniels, G. van der Wal, P. J. van der Maas, and E. J. Emanuel, "Attitudes and Practices Concerning the End of Life: A Comparison between Physicians from the United States and the Netherlands," *Archives of Internal Medicine* 160 (Supplement 1) (2000):63–68.

65. K. E. Kovinsky, C. S. Landerfeld, J. Teno, et al., "Is Economic Hardship on the Families of the Seriously Ill Associated with Patient and Surrogate Care Preferences?" *Archives of Internal Medicine* 156 (1996):1737–41.

66. E. H. Barnett, "Dealing with an Assisted Death in the Family: The Adult Children of a Woman Who Used Oregon's Suicide Law Talk about Conflicted Feelings," *Oregonian*, 21 February 1999, G1, G2.

67. Bill Kettler, "Stricken by ALS, Joan Lucas decides to die—then acts," *Medford Mail Tribune*, 25 June 2000, A1 & A8, A1.

68. See n. 67, Kettler 2000, A1.

69. Ibid.

70. Ibid.

71. E. H. Barnett, "Third Known Assisted Suicide Reported," *Oregonian*, 6 May 1998, A1.

Chapter 8: Oregon's Culture of Silence

1. N. G. Hamilton, *Self and Others: Object Relations Theory in Practice* (Northvale, N.J.: Jason Aronson, 1988); *The Self and the Ego in Psychotherapy* (Northvale, N.J.: Jason Aronson, 1996); N. G. Hamilton, P. J. Edwards, J. K. Boehnlein, and C. A. Hamilton, "The Doctor-Patient Relationship and Assisted Suicide: A Contribution from Dynamic Psychiatry," *American Journal of Forensic Psychiatry* 19 (1998):59–75.

2. J. D. Kinzie, J. R. A. Maricle, J. D. Bloom, et al., "Improving Quality Assurance through Psychiatric Mortality and Morbidity Conferences in a University Hospital," *Hospital and Community Psychiatry* 43 (1992):470–74.

3. *Lee v. Oregon*, 869 F. Supp. 1429 (D. Ore. 1995).

4. Brief of Physicians for Compassionate Care as Amicus Curiae in *Lee v. Harcleroad et al.*, U.S. Court of Appeals for the Ninth Circuit, 24 January 1996.

5. L. Ganzini, D. S. Fenn, M. A. Lee, R. T. Heintz, and J. D. Bloom, "Attitudes of Oregon Psychiatrists toward Physician-Assisted Suicide," *American Journal of Psychiatry* 153 (1996):1469–75.

6. New York State Task Force on Life and the Law, *When Death Is Sought: Assisted Suicide and Euthanasia in the Medical Context* (New York: New York State Task Force on Life and the Law, 1994).

7. L. Ganzini, D. S. Fenn, M. A. Lee, R. T. Heintz, and J. D. Bloom, "Dr. Ganzini and Colleagues Reply," *American Journal of Psychiatry* 154 (1997):1327–28; American Medical Association, *Code of Medical Ethics: Current Opinion with Annotations* (Chicago: American Medical Association, 1997).

8. M. Angell, "Caring for the Dying: Congressional Mischief," *New England Journal of Medicine* 341 (1999):1923–25.

9. A. E. Chin, K. Hedberg, G. K. Higginson, and D. W. Fleming, "Legalized Physician-Assisted Suicide in Oregon: The First Year's Experience," *New England Journal of Medicine* 340 (1999):577–83.

10. See also K. Foley and H. Hendin, "The Oregon Report: Don't Ask, Don't Tell," *Hastings Center Report* 29, no. 3 (1999):37–42.

11. H. Hendin, K. Foley, and M. White, "Physician-Assisted Suicide: Reflections on Oregon's First Case," *Issues in Law and Medicine* 14 (1998):243–70; D. M. Gianelli, "Praise, Criticism Follow Oregon's First Reported Assisted Suicides," *American Medical News*, 12 April 1998, 1; N. G. Hamilton and C. A. Hamilton, "Therapeutic

Response to Assisted Suicide Request," *Bulletin of the Menninger Clinic* 63 (1999): 191–201; and see n. 10, Foley and Hendin 1999.

12. E. H. Barnett, "Dealing with an Assisted Death in the Family: The Adult Children of a Woman Who Used Oregon's Suicide Law Talk about Conflicted Feelings," *Oregonian*, 21 February 1999, G1, G2.

13. J. Rojas-Burke, "Oregon's Poor Slip from Safety Net of Health Coverage," *Oregonian*, 29 March 1999, A1, A9.

14. J. Rojas-Burke, "Survey Gives Oregon Health Plan High Marks," *Oregonian*, 3 February 1999, B15.

15. J. Hamby, "The Enemy Within: State Bureaucratic Rules Threaten the Spirit of Oregon Health Plan's Founding Principles," *Oregonian*, 21 January 1998, G1, G2.

16. J. Rojas-Burke, "Insurers Still Unfair with Mentally Ill, Study Says," *Oregonian*, 30 April 1999, D1, D5; "Senate Bill Proposed Increase in Mental Health Benefits," *Oregonian*, 19 June 1999, D1, D9.

17. See n. 10, Foley and Hendin 1999.

18. G. Eighmey, "Oregon's Death with Dignity Act: Health Care Professionals Speak Out on Its Impact," Nineteenth Annual Meeting of Council on Licensure, Enforcement and Regulation, Portland, Oregon, 3 September 1999, audiotape produced by Cambridge Transcriptions, (800) 850–5258, orders@ctran.com.

19. E. Hoover and G. K. Hill, "Two Die Using Suicide Law," *Oregonian*, 26 March 1998, A1, A14.

20. B. Reagan, C. L. Barrett, B. Glidewell, and A. Jackson, "Physician-Assisted Suicide: Counseling Patients/Clients," continuing education class on counseling patients about assisted suicide, Portland Community College, Portland, Oregon, 3 December 1999.

21. C. A. Hamilton, "The Oregon Report: What's Hiding behind the Numbers?" *Brainstorm*, March 2000, 36–38.

22. See n. 18, Eighmey 1999.

23. E. H. Barnett, "Dilemma of Assisted Suicide: When?" *Oregonian*, 17 January 1999, A1, A16, A17.

24. L. Ganzini, H. E. Nelson, T. A. Schmidt, D. F. Kraemer, M. A. Delorit, and M. A. Lee, "Physician's Experience with the Oregon Death with Dignity Act," *New England Journal of Medicine* 342 (2000):557–63.

25. Ibid.

26. E. H. Barnett, "Man with ALS Makes Up His Mind to Die," *Oregonian*, 11 March 1999, D1; J. Filips, "Difficult Suicide Magnifies Debate," *Eugene Register-Guard*, 14 March 1999, 9–10D; R. H. Richardson, "Dr. Hamilton E-mail," e-mail sent to Greg Hamilton and over forty additional medical experts, reporters, ethicists, and legal experts, 22 October 1999.

27. See n. 26, Barnett 1999.

28. S. Jamison, "When Drugs Fail: Assisted Deaths and Not-So-Lethal Drugs," in *Drug Use in Assisted Suicide and Euthanasia*, ed. M. P. Battin and A. G. Lippman (Binghamton, N.Y.: Haworth Press, 1996), 223–43.

29. D. Schuman, official Oregon Department of Justice letter to Senator Bryant, 15 March 1999.

30. "How Assisted Can Suicide Be? Oregon Controversy," *American Medical Association News*, 12 April 1999, 19; "In the Dark Shadows of Measure 16," *Oregonian*, 31 October 1999, D5; N. G. Hamilton, Pain Relief Promotion Act of 1999: Testimony of

Physicians for Compassionate Care before the Judiciary Subcommittee on the Constitution, U.S. House of Representatives, 24 June 1999.

31. See n. 28, Jamison 1996; D. Humphry, "Lethal Drugs for Assisted Suicide: How the Public Sees It," in Battin and Lippman 1996 (see n. 28), 177–82.

32. Royal Dutch Society for the Advancement of Pharmacology, *The Administration of and Preparation for Euthanasia*, translated for and distributed by Physicians for Compassionate Care, Portland, Oregon, September 1997; J. H. Groenewoud, A. van der Heide, B. D. Onwuteaka-Philipsen, D. L. Willems, P. J. van der Maas, and G. van der Wal, "Clinical Problems with the Performance of Euthanasia and Physician-Assisted Suicide in the Netherlands," *New England Journal of Medicine* 342 (2000):551–56; S. B. Nuland, "Physician-Assisted Suicide and Euthanasia in Practice" [editorial], *New England Journal of Medicine* 342 (2000):583–84.

33. B. C. Lee, E. D. Stutsman, and K. T. Hagan, "Physician-Assisted Suicide," in *Oregon Health Law Manual*, Vol. 2 (Salem, Ore.: Oregon State Bar, 1997), 8.1–8.29.

34. See n. 18, Eighmey 1999.

35. See n. 24, Ganzini et al. 2000.

36. See n. 19, Hoover and Hill 1998.

37. E. H. Barnett, "Is Mom Capable of Choosing to Die?" *Oregonian*, 17 October 1999, G1, G2.

38. "Killing Grandma" [editorial], *Brainstorm*, November 1999, 3, 4; D. Phillips, "Doctor-Assisted Suicide Affects Us All—Negatively," *Eugene Register-Guard*, 2 December 1999, 15A; D. Reinhard, "Measure 16: Compassion in Killing," *Oregonian*, 14 March 1999, E5; W. Smith, "Suicide Unlimited in Oregon," *Weekly Standard*, 8 November 1999, 11–14.

39. See n. 38, *Brainstorm* 1999.

40. A. Weiland, "Kaiser Didn't Push Patient's Suicide," *Oregonian*, 18 November 1999, B11.

41. R. H. Richardson and M. Liberson, "When the Diagnosis Is Terminal," Kaiser Permanente Ethics Service Continuing Medical Education Course, Portland, Oregon, 11 June 1999.

42. A. D. Sullivan, K. Hedberg, and D. W. Fleming, "Legalized Physician-Assisted Suicide in Oregon: The Second Year," *New England Journal of Medicine* 342 (2000):598–604; "Legalized Physician-Assisted Suicide in Oregon, 1998–2000," New England Journal of Medicine 344 (2001): 605–7.

43. See n. 41, Richardson and Liberson 1999; see n. 21, Hamilton 2000.

44. See n. 21, Hamilton 2000.

45. See n. 32, Groenewoud et al. 2000.

46. See n. 32, Nuland 2000, 583.

47. See n. 32, Royal Dutch Society 1997; Nuland 2000; Groenewoud 2000.

48. See n. 30, Reinhard 1999.

49. See n. 30, Hamilton 1999.

50. Oregon Revised Statutes 127.800 to 126.897.

Chapter 9: Deadly Days in Darwin

My thanks to Dr. Annette Street for her support and scholarship in review of Nitschke's role and work.

1. D. W. Kissane, A. Street, and P. Nitschke, "Seven Deaths in Darwin: Case Studies under the Rights of the Terminally Ill Act, Northern Territory, Australia," *Lancet* 352 (1998):1097–1102.

2. B. Harrison, *Demography, Northern Territory* (Darwin: Australian Bureau of Statistics, 1994).

3. J. J. Collins and F. T. Brennan, "Euthanasia and the Potential Adverse Effects for Northern Territory Aborigines," *Lancet* 349 (1997):1907–8.

4. Legislative Assembly of the Northern Territory of Australia, *The Right of the Individual or the Common Good? Report of the Inquiry by the Select Committee on Euthanasia* (Darwin: Government Printer, 1995).

5. See n. 4, Legislative Assembly 1995.

6. Rights of the Terminally Ill Act 1995, Northern Territory of Australia.

7. Rights of the Terminally Ill Regulations 1996, Northern Territory of Australia.

8. See n. 1, Kissane et al. 1998.

9. P. Wilkinson, *Euthanasia* (Sydney: Sixty Minutes Television Production, Nine Network, 1995).

10. M. McLaughlin, *The Road to Nowhere* (Sydney: Four Corners' Television Production, Australian Broadcasting Commission, 1966).

11. Ibid.

12. R. B. Dent, Open Letter to Federal Parliamentarians, 21 September 1996. Melbourne: The Age Online. Available at http://www.theage.com.au (also appeared in the newspapers on that day).

13. See n. 1, Kissane et al. 1998, 1099.

14. See n. 1, Kissane et al. 1998, 1101.

15. D. W. Kissane and B. Kelly, "Demoralization, Depression and Desire for Death: Implications of the Dutch Guidelines for Euthanasia of the Mentally Ill," *Australian and New Zealand Journal of Psychiatry* 34 (2000):325–33.

16. J. M. de Figueiredo, "Subjective Incompetence, the Clinical Hallmark of Demoralization," *Comprehensive Psychiatry* 23 (1982): 353–63; J. M. de Figueiredo, "Depression and Demoralization: Phenomenologic Differences and Research Perspectives," *Comprehensive Psychiatry* 34 (1993): 308–11; see n. 15, Kissane and Kelly 2000; D. W. Kissane, D. M. Clarke, and A. Street, "Demoralization Syndrome: A Relevant Psychiatric Diagnosis in Palliative Care," *Journal of Palliative Care*, in press.

17. P. J. van der Maas, J. J. M. van Delden, L. Pijnenborg, and C. W. N. Loonan, "Euthanasia and Other Medical Decisions Concerning the End of Life," *Lancet* 338 (1991):669–74; P. J. van der Maas, G. van der Wal, I. Haverkate, et al., "Euthanasia, Physician-Assisted Suicide, and Other Medical Practices Involving End of Life in the Netherlands, 1990–1995," *New England Journal of Medicine* 335 (1996):1699–1705.

18. A. Street and D. W. Kissane, "Dispensing Death, Desiring Death: An Exploration of Medical Roles and Patient Motivation during the Period of Legalised Euthanasia in Australia," *Omega* 40, no. 1 (1999–2000):229–46.

19. A. E. Curtis and J. I. Furnisher, "Quality of Life of Oncology Hospice Patients: A Comparison of Patient and Primary Caregiver Reports," *Oncology Nursing Forum* 16 (1989):49–53; J. M. Blazeby, M. H. Williams, D. Alderson, and J. R. Farndon, "Observer Variation in Assessment of Quality of Life in Patients with Oesophageal Cancer," *British Journal of Surgery* 82 (1995):1200–1203; K. C. Sneeuw, N. K. Aaronson, M. S. Sprangers, S. B. Detmar, L. D. Wever, and J. H. Schornagel, "Value of

Caregiver Ratings in Evaluation of the Quality of Life of Patients with Cancer," *Journal of Clinical Oncology* 15 (1997):1206–17.

20. Senate Legal and Constitutional Legislation Committee, *Consideration of Legislation Referred to the Committee, Euthanasia Laws Bill 1996, Parliament of the Commonwealth of Australia* (Canberra: Government Printer, 1997).

21. Ibid.

22. Ibid., 47.

23. B. J. Kelly and F. T. Varghese, "Assisted Suicide and Euthanasia: What about the Clinical Issues?" *Australian and New Zealand Journal of Psychiatry* 30 (1996):3–8.

24. F. McInerney and C. Seibold, "Nurses' Definitions of and Attitudes towards Euthanasia," *Journal of Advanced Nursing* 22 (1995):171–82.

25. M. O'Connor, "Palliative Care and the Euthanasia Debate in Australia," *European Journal of Palliative Care* 5 (1998):27–31.

26. H. Kuhse and P. Singer, "Doctors' Practices and Attitudes Regarding Voluntary Euthanasia," *Medical Journal of Australia* 148 (1988):623–27; H. Kuhse and P. Singer, "Euthanasia: A Survey of Nurses' Attitudes and Practices," *Australian Nurses' Journal* 21 (1992):21–22; P. Baume and E. O'Malley, "Euthanasia: Attitudes and Practices of Medical Practitioners," *Medical Journal of Australia* 161 (1994): 137–44; C. Waddell, R. M. Clarnette, M. Smith, L. Oldham, and A. Kellehear, "Treatment Decision-Making at the End of Life: A Survey of Australian Doctors' Attitudes towards Patients' Wishes and Euthanasia," *Medical Journal of Australia* 165 (1996):540–44.

27. S. Aranda and M. O'Connor, "Euthanasia, Nursing and Care of the Dying: Rethinking Kuhse and Singer," *Australian Nursing Journal* 3 (1996):18–21; D. W. Kissane, I. G. Finlay, and R. George, "Euthanasia in Australia," *Progress in Palliative Care* 4 (1996):71–73.

28. C. Seale, "Heroic Death," *Sociology* 29 (1995):597–613.

29. D. Callahan, *The Troubled Dream of Life* (New York: Simon & Schuster, 1993).

30. H. Kuhse, P. Singer, P. Baume, M. Clark, and M. Rickard, "End-of-Life Decisions in Australian Medical Practice," *Medical Journal of Australia* 191 (1997):191–96.

31. Ibid.

32. M. Ashby, "The Fallacies of Death Causation in Palliative Care," *Medical Journal of Australia* 166 (1997):176–77.

33. M. M. Reidenberg, "Barriers to Controlling Pain in Patients with Cancer," *Lancet* 347 (1996):1278.

Chapter 10: Not Dead Yet

1. Combined News Services, "Thirty-One Assisted Suicides/Kevorkian Helps Ohio Woman Die," *Newsday*, 22 June 1996, A8.

2. *Washington v. Glucksberg*, 117 S.Ct. 2258, 138. L.Ed.2d 772 (1997), note 23.

3. D. Coleman, Testimony before the Constitution Subcommittee of the Judiciary Committee of the U.S. House of Representatives, 29 April 1996 and 14 July 1998.

4. M. Johnson, "Right to Life, Fight to Die: The Elizabeth Bouvia Saga," *The Ragged Edge* [serial online], January/February 1997. Available at http://www.ragged-edge-mag.com/archive/bouvia.htm.

5. Plaintiff's Memorandum, *Bouvia v. County of Riverside*, No. 159780 (Cal. Super. Dec. 16, 1983), reported in *Bioethics Report* 458 (1984):14.

6. P. Longmore, "Urging the Handicapped to Die: Bouvia Decision Is Victory for Bigotry Not Self-determination," *Los Angeles Times,* 26 April 1986, 7.

7. *Bouvia v. Superior Court,* 179 Cal. A.3d 1127 at 1143–45, 225 Cal. Rptr. 297 at 305–6 (1986).

8. S. S. Herr, B. A. Bostrom, and R. S. Barton, "No Place to Go: Refusal of Life-Sustaining Treatment by Competent Persons with Physical Disabilities," *Issues in Law and Medicine* 8, no. 1 (1992):3–36.

9. D. Coleman, "Withdrawing Life-Sustaining Treatment from People with Severe Disabilities Who Request It: Equal Protection Considerations," *Issues in Law and Medicine* 8, no. 1 (1992):55–79.

10. *McKay v. Bergstedt,* 801 P.2d 617 (Nev. 1990) at 625.

11. J. Shapiro, *No Pity: People with Disabilities Forging a New Civil Rights Movement* (New York: Random House/Times Books, 1993), 259.

12. J. Shapiro, "Larry McAfee, Invisible Man," *U.S. News & World Report,* 19 February 1990, 60.

13. *Cruzan v. Director, Missouri Department of Health,* 110 S.Ct. 2841 (1990).

14. National Spinal Cord Injury Association, "Spinal Cord Injury Statistics," 1996. Available at http://www.spinalcord.org/resource/Factsheets/factsheet2.html.

15. Brain Injury Association, "The Costs and Causes of Traumatic Brain Injury" (undated). Available at http://www.biausa/costsand.htm.

16. D. S. Wickham, "Paralyzed Woman Is Urged to Live: Quadriplegics Said the Orange Woman's Wish to Die Is a Normal Reaction But That Time Will Change Her Mind," *Orlando Sentinel,* 14 May 1999, A1.

17. D. Sharp and D. Blank, "Woman Allowed to Die; Mom to Be Charged," *USA Today,* 20 May 1999, A1.

18. A. Morrell, "Death Wish Sparks Ethics Debate," *Rochester Democrat and Chronicle,* 5 August 1999, A1.

19. Americans with Disabilities Act, 42 U.S.C. § 12101 *et seq.; Olmstead v. L.C.,* 119 S.Ct. 2176 (1999).

20. K. J. Kaplan, J. O'Dell, O. Uziel, et al., "An Update on the Kevorkian-Reding 93 Physician-Assisted Deaths in Michigan: Is Kevorkian a Savior, Serial-Killer or Suicidal Martyr?" *Omega* 40, no. 1 (1999–2000):209–28; see also K. Cheyfitz, "He Breaks His Own Rules," *Detroit Free Press,* 3 March 1997, A7. "The Suicide Machine: People Assisted in Suicide by Dr. Jack Kevorkian," *Detroit Free Press,* 3–8 March 1997. Available at http://www.freep.com/suicide/assisted/faces.htm.

21. C. J. Gill, "Dating and Relationship Issues," *Sexuality and Disability* 14 (1996):183–90.

22. J. Mathews, *A Mother's Touch: The Tiffany Callo Story* (New York: Henry Holt, 1990).

23. J. Kevorkian, *Prescription Medicide* (New York: Prometheus Books, 1991).

24. J. Kevorkian, "The Last Fearsome Taboo: Medical Aspects of Planned Death," *Medicine and Law* 8 (1998):1–15.

25. J. Kevorkian, Written Statement to Court, 17 August 1990, 11 (emphasis in original).

26. J. Daughterry, "Judith Curren's Last Days Were a Blur of Drugs and Pain," *Detroit News,* 21 August 1996, 5C.

27. B. Harmon, "Paralyzed Man Fulfills Death Wish," *Detroit News,* 27 February 1998, A1.

28. R. Goldberg, "Coroner: Kevorkian Client Mutilated," Associated Press, 9 June 1998.

29. R. Leiby, "Whose Death Is It Anyway?" *Washington Post*, 11 August 1996, F1.1.

30. C. J. Gill, "Health Professionals, Disability, and Assisted Suicide: An Examination of Empirical Evidence," *Psychology, Public Policy, and Law*, forthcoming.

31. U.S. Public Health Service, *The Surgeon General's Call to Action to Prevent Suicide* (Washington, D.C.: U.S. Government Printing Office, 1999).

32. R. H. Gross, A. Cox, R. Tatyrek, et al., "Early Management and Decision Making for the Treatment of Myelomeningocele," *Pediatrics* 72 (1983):450–58.

33. This document was printed as a handout and posted on the Hemlock Society Web site but was later deleted from the site.

34. C. H. Baron, C. Bergstresser, D. Brock, et al., "Statute: A Model Act to Authorize and Regulate Physician-Assisted Suicide," *Harvard Journal on Legislation* 33, no. 1 (1996):1–34.

35. National Death with Dignity Center Web site, http://www.deathwithdignity.org/draft/informed/surveys_opinions/physpers2.html.

36. *Doe and Smith v. Mutual of Omaha Ins. Co.*, 179 F.3d 557 (7th Cir. 1999).

37. Ibid.

38. D. Coleman, "Home Services or Euthanasia: At the Heart of the Debate," *Caring Magazine* 28, no. 7 (1999):16–21.

39. K. A. Gerhart, J. Koziol-McLain, S. R. Lowenstein, and G. G. Whiteneck, "Quality of Life following Spinal Cord Injury: Knowledge and Attitudes of Emergency Care Providers," *Annals of Emergency Medicine* 23 (1994):807–12.

40. Administration on Aging, *The National Elder Abuse Incidence Study: Final Report* (Washington, D.C.: U.S. Department of Health and Human Services, 1998).

41. E. Cox, J. J. Kamakahl, and S. M. Capek, *Come Lovely and Soothing Death: The Right to Die Movement in the United States* (New York: Twayne Publishers, 1999).

42. D. Humphry and M. Clement, *Freedom to Die: People, Politics, and the Right-to-Die Movement* (New York: St. Martin's Griffin, 1998), 313.

43. J. Hardwig, "Is There a Duty to Die?" *Hastings Center Report* 27, no. 2 (1997):34–42.

44. C. Kliewer and S. Drake, "Disability, Eugenics and the Current Ideology of Segregation: A Modern Moral Tale," *Disability and Society* 13, no. 1 (1998):95–111; *Buck v. Bell*, 274 U.S. 200 (1927).

45. F. Kennedy, "The Problem of Social Control of the Congenital Defective: Education, Sterilization, Euthanasia," *American Journal of Psychiatry* 99 (1942):13–16.

46. U.S. Civil Rights Commission, *Medical Discrimination against Children with Disabilities* (Washington, D.C.: U.S. Commission on Civil Rights, 1989), 33.

47. PR Newswire, "Mercy Killing: A Position Statement Regarding David Rodriguez," 3 December 1997.

48. F. J. Girsh, "Clarification of Hemlock Statement on Mercy Killing," *Timelines*, winter 1998, 4.

49. D. Jenish and T. Fennell, "What Would You Do: In Saskatchewan, a Wrenching Verdict of Murder Reignites a Long-Simmering Debate about Mercy Killing," *Maclean's*, 28 November 1994, 16–20.

50. C. H. Farnsworth, "Mercy Killing in Canada Stirs Call for Change in Law," *New York Times*, 22 November 1994, A6.

51. G. Delury, *But What If She Wants to Die?* (Buffalo, N.Y.: Prometheus Books, 1997).

52. See n. 47, PR Newswire 1997.

53. A. Hasbrouck, "Misplaced Mercy: Prosecution and Sentencing of Parents Who Kill Their Disabled Children." Available at http://www.thalidomide.ca/gwolbring/mismercy.htm.

54. H. S. Snyder and T. A. Finnegan, *Easy Access to the FBI's Supplementary Homicide Reports, 1980–1995* [data presentation and analysis package] (Washington, D.C.: Office of Juvenile Justice and Delinquency Prevention, 1997).

55. J. L. Leovy, "Glendale 'Angel' Case Spurs Call to Reform Field," *Los Angeles Times,* 11 May 1998, A1; J. Kelly, "Ex-Nurse Convicted in 6 Ind. Deaths," AP Online, 17 October 1999. Available at http://www.nexis.com.

56. P. Singer, *Rethinking Life and Death: The Collapse of Our Traditional Ethics* (New York: St. Martin's Press, 1995), 180.

57. Ibid., 182.

58. Ibid., 206.

59. W. Raspberry, "Claims against Common Sense," *Washington Post,* 16 November 1998, A25.

60. S. Brown, "Be Careful in Judging Parents of Disabled Boy," *Rocky Mountain News* (Denver), 10 January 2000, 35A.

Chapter 11: Vulnerable People

1. J. D. Lubitz and G. F. Riley, "Trends in Medicare Payments in the Last Year of Life," *New England Journal of Medicine* 328 (1993):1092–96.

2. D. Callahan, "Controlling the Costs of Health Care for the Elderly: Fair Means Foul," *New England Journal of Medicine* 10 (1996):744–46; H. M. Chochinov and K. Janson, "Dying to Pay: The Cost of End-of-Life Care," *Journal of Palliative Care* 14, no. 4 (1998):5–15.

3. N. G. Levinsky, "The Purpose of Advance Medical Planning: Autonomy for Patients or Limitation of Care?" *New England Journal of Medicine* 333 (1996):741–43.

4. J. Hardwig, "Is There a Duty to Die?" *Hastings Center Report* 27, no. 2 (1997): 34–42.

5. E. Emanuel and M. P. Battin, "What Are the Potential Cost Savings from Legalizing Physician-Assisted Suicide?" *New England Journal of Medicine* 339 (1998): 167–72.

6. E. J. Emanuel and L. L. Emanuel, "The Economics of Dying: The Illusion of Cost Savings at the End of Life," *New England Journal of Medicine* 330 (1994):540–44; B. E. Robinson and H. Pham, "Cost-Effectiveness of Hospice Care," *Clinical Geriatric Medicine* 12 (1996):417–28; A. A. Scitovsky, "'The High Cost of Dying' Revisited," *Milbank Quarterly* 72, no. 4 (1994):561–91; E. J. Emanuel, "Cost Savings at the End of Life: What Do the Data Show?" *Journal of the American Medical Association* 275 (1996):1907–14.

7. R. A. Knox, "Poll: Americans Favor Mercy Killing," *Boston Globe,* 3 November 1991, A1; Hemlock Society, *1996 Gallup Poll on Doctor-Assisted Suicide* (Princeton, N.J.: Gallup Organization, 1997); Hemlock Society, *1997 Gallup/CNN/USA Today Poll on Doctor-Assisted Suicide* (Princeton, N.J.: Gallup Organization, 1997).

8. American Medical Association, *AMA End of Life Survey,* December 1996.

9. J. S. Shapiro, "Euthanasia's Home: What the Dutch Experience Can Teach Americans about Assisted Suicide," *U.S. News & World Report,* 13 January 1997, 24–27.

10. See n. 8, American Medical Association 1996.

11. K. Stewart, "Physician Aid in Dying," *Polling Report* 13, no. 15 (1997):1, 6–7.

12. See n. 4, Hardwig 1997.

13. National Hospice Organization, at http://www.nho.org/facts.htm.

14. Ibid.

15. J. Lynn, F. E. Harrell, F. Cohn, et al., for the SUPPORT Investigators, "Defining the 'Terminally Ill': Insights from SUPPORT," *Duquesne Law Review* 25 (1996): 311–36; V. Mor and D. Kidder, "Cost Savings in Hospice: Final Results of the National Hospice Study," *Health Services Research* 20 (1985):407–22.

16. J. Lynn, F. Harrell, F. Cohn, D. Wagner, and A. F. Conners, "Prognoses of Seriously Ill Hospitalized Patients on the Days before Death: Implications for Patient Care and Public Policy," *New Horizons* 5, no. 1 (1997):56–61.

17. J. Lubitz and G. F. Riley, "Trends in Medicare Payments in Last Year of Life," *New England Journal of Medicine* 328 (1993):1092–96.

18. Institute of Medicine, *Approaching Death* (Washington, D.C.: National Academy Press, 1997).

19. See n. 7, Knox 1991.

20. J. L. Bernat, B. Gert, and R. P. Mogielnicki, "Patient Refusal of Hydration and Nutrition: An Alternative to Physician-Assisted Suicide or Voluntary Euthanasia," *Archives of Internal Medicine* 153 (1993):2723–28.

21. J. Lynn and J. Harrold, *Handbook for Mortals* (New York: Oxford University Press, 1999), 113.

22. American Geriatrics Society Ethics Committee, "Physician-Assisted Suicide and Voluntary Active Euthanasia," *Journal of the American Geriatrics Society* 43 (1995):579–80.

23. *Dennis C. Vacco et al. v. Timothy E. Quill, M.D., et al.,* 80 F.3d 716 (2d Cir. 1996), and *State of Washington v. Harold Glucksberg, et al.* (formerly *Compassion in Dying v. Washington*) 79 F.3d 790 (9th Cir. 1996).

24. T. E. Quill, *A Midwife through the Dying Process: Stories of Healing and Hard Choices at the End of Life* (Baltimore: Johns Hopkins University Press, 1996).

25. E. J. Larson, "Seeking Compassion in Dying: The Washington State Law against Assisted Suicide," *Seattle University Law Review* 18 (1995):509–17; New York State Task Force on Life and the Law, *When Death Is Sought: Assisted Suicide and Euthanasia in the Medical Context* (New York: New York State Task Force on Life and the Law, 1994), 102.

26. *Cruzan v. Director, Missouri Dept. of Health,* 497 U.S. 261 (1990).

27. H. M. Chochinov and K. G. Wilson, "The Euthanasia Debate: Attitudes, Practice and Psychiatric Considerations," *Canadian Journal of Psychiatry* 40 (1995): 593–602.

28. J. Lynn, F. Cohn, J. H. Pickering, J. Smith, and A. M. Stoeppelwerth, "American Geriatrics Society on Physician-Assisted Suicide: Brief to the United States Supreme Court," *Journal of the American Geriatrics Society* 45 (1997):489–99.

29. A. Back, "Physician Assisted Death" [editorial], *Journal of the American Medical Association* 276 (1996):1688.

30. D. Meier, C. A. Emmons, S. Wallenstein, et al., "A National Survey of Physician Assisted Death in the United States," *New England Journal of Medicine* 338 (1998):1193–1201.

31. *Quill,* 80 F.3d at 731; *Compassion in Dying v. State of Washington,* 79 F.3d 790, 831 (9th Cir. 1996).

32. W. A. Knaus, D. P. Wagner, E. A. Draper, et al., "The APACHE III Prognostic System: Risk Prediction of Hospital Mortality for Critically Ill Hospitalized Adults," *Chest* 100 (1991):1018–36; W. A. Knaus, F. E. Harrell, J. Lynn, et al., "The SUPPORT Prognostics Model: Objective Estimates of Survival for Seriously Ill Hospitalized Adults," *Annals of Internal Medicine* 122 (1995):191–203.

33. E. Fox, K. Landrum-McNiff, Z. Zhong, et al., "Evaluation of Prognostic Criteria for Determining Hospice Eligibility in Patients with Advanced Lung, Heart, or Liver Disease," *Journal of the American Medical Association* 282 (1999): 1638–45.

34. J. M. Teno, D. Murphy, J. Lynn, et al. for the SUPPORT Investigators, "Prognosis-Based Futility Guidelines: Does Anyone Win?" *Journal of the American Geriatrics Society* 42 (1994):1202–7.

35. Ibid.

36. See n. 16, Lynn et al. 1997.

37. See n. 34, Teno et al. 1994.

38. R. S. Pritchard, E. S. Fisher, J. M. Teno, et al., "Influence of Patient Preferences and Local Health System Characteristics on Place of Death," *Journal of the American Geriatrics Society* 46 (1998):1242–50.

39. J. Lynn, H. R. Arkes, M. Stevens, et al., "Rethinking Fundamental Assumptions: SUPPORT's Implications for Future Reform," *Journal of the American Geriatrics Society* 48 (2000): S214–21.

Chapter 12: Depression and the Will to Live in the Psychological Landscape of Terminally Ill Patients

1. A. Singer, D. K. Martin, and M. Kelner, "Quality End-of-Life Care: Patients' Perspectives," *Journal of the American Medical Association* 281 (1999):163–68.

2. W. Breitbart, B. D. Rosenfeld, and S. D. Passik, "Interest in Physician-Assisted Suicide among Ambulatory HIV-Infected Patients," *American Journal of Psychiatry* 153 (1996):238–42.

3. W. Breitbart, "Suicide in Cancer Patients," *Oncology* 1 (1987):49–53.

4. L. R. Derogatis, G. R. Morrow, J. Fetting, D. Penman, et al., "The Prevalence of Psychiatric Disorders amongst Cancer Patients," *Journal of the American Medical Association* 249 (1983):751–57.

5. See n. 3, Breitbart 1987.

6. M. Lander, H. M. Chochinov, and K. G. Wilson, "Depression and the Dying Older Patient," *Clinics in Geriatric Medicine* 16 (2000):335–56.

7. See n. 4, Derogatis et al. 1983; H. M. Chochinov, K. G. Wilson, M. Enns, and S. Lander, "Prevalence of Depression in the Terminally Ill: Effects of Diagnostic Criteria and Symptom Threshold Judgments," *American Journal of Psychiatry* 151 (1994):537–40.

8. J. Bukberg, D. Penman, and J. C. Holland, "Depression in Hospitalized Cancer Patients," *Psychosomatic Medicine* 46 (1984):199–212.

9. L. Ganzini, M. A. Lee, R. T. Heintz, et al., "The Effect of Depression Treatment on Elderly Patients' Preferences for Life-Sustaining Medical Therapy," *American Journal of Psychiatry* 151 (1994):1631–36.

10. J. H. Brown, P. Henteleff, S. Barakat, et al., "Is It Normal for Terminally Ill Patients to Desire Death?" *American Journal of Psychiatry* 143 (1986):161–65.

11. J. Endicott, "Measurement of Depression in Patients with Cancer," *Cancer* 53 (1998):2243–48.

12. S. Cohen-Cole and A. Stoudemire, "Major Depression and Physical Illness: Special Considerations in Diagnosis and Biologic Treatment," *Psychiatric Clinics of North America* 10 (1987):1–17.

13. See n. 10, Brown et al. 1986.

14. H. M. Chochinov, K. G. Wilson, M. Enns, et al., "'Are You Depressed?' Screening for Depression in the Terminally Ill," *American Journal of Psychiatry* 154 (1997):674–76.

15. M. V. McDonald, S. D. Passik, and N. Coyle, "Addressing the Needs of the Patient Who Requests Physician-Assisted Suicide or Euthanasia," in *Handbook of Psychiatry in Palliative Medicine*, ed. H. M. Chochinov and W. Breitbart (New York: Oxford Press, 2000), 349–56.

16. H. M. Chochinov, D. Tataryn, J. J. Clinch, et al., "Will to Live in the Terminally Ill," *Lancet* 354 (1999):816–19.

17. H. M. Chochinov, K. G. Wilson, M. Enns, et al., "Depression, Hopelessness, and Suicidal Ideation in the Terminally Ill," *Psychosomatics* 39 (1998):366–70.

18. H. M. Chochinov, K. G. Wilson, M. Enns, et al., "Desire for Death in the Terminally Ill," *American Journal of Psychiatry* 152 (1995):1185–91.

19. E. J. Emanuel, D. L. Fairclough, E. R. Daniels, et al., "Euthanasia and Physician-Assisted Suicide: Attitudes and Experiences of Oncology Patients, Oncologists, and the Public," *Lancet* 347 (1996):1805–10.

20. L. Ganzini, H. D. Nelson, T. A. Schmidt, et al., "Physicians' Experiences with the Oregon Death with Dignity Act," *New England Journal of Medicine* 342 (2000):557–63.

21. See n. 1, Singer et al. 1999.

22. D. J. Newport and C. B. Nemeroff, "Assessment and Treatment of Depression in the Cancer Patient" [review], *Journal of Psychosomatic Research* 45 (1998): 215–37.

23. G. Rodin and L. A. Gilles, "Individual Psychotherapy for the Patient with Advanced Disease," in Chochinov and Breitbart 2000 (see n. 15), 189–96.

24. D. Spiegel, J. Bloom, and I. Yalom, "Group Support for Patients with Metastatic Cancer," *Archives of General Psychiatry* 38 (1981):527–33.

25. E. J. Cassell, "The Nature of Suffering and the Goals of Medicine," *New England Journal of Medicine* 306 (1982):639–45, 639.

26. J. L. Spira, "Existential Psychotherapy," in Chochinov and Breitbart 2000 (see n. 15), 197–214; M. Greenstein and W. Breitbart, "Cancer and the Experience of Meaning: A Group Psychotherapy Program for People with Cancer," *American Journal of Psychiatry* 54 (2000): 486–500.

27. M. Viederman, "The Supportive Relationship, the Psychodynamic Life Narrative and the Dying Patient," in Chochinov and Breitbart 2000 (see n. 15), 215–22.

28. V. F. Frankl, *Man's Search for Meaning*, 4th ed. (Boston: Benton Press, 1992).

29. See n. 16, Chochinov et al. 1995; see n. 2, Breitbart et al. 1996.

30. I. D. Yalom, *Love's Executioner and Other Tales of Psychotherapy* (New York: Basic Books, 1989).

31. N. I. Cherny, "The Treatment of Suffering in Patients with Advanced Cancer," in Chochinov and Breitbart 2000 (see n. 15), 375–96.

Chapter 13: A Hospice Perspective

1. L. Colebrook, personal communication, 26 February 1960.

2. D. Clark, "Originating a Movement: Cicely Saunders and the Development of St. Christopher's Hospice, 1957–67," *Mortality* 3, no. 2 (1998):43–63.

3. D. Clark, "'Total Pain: Disciplinary Power and the Body in the Work of Cicely Saunders, 1958–1967," *Social Science and Medicine* 49 (1999):727–36.

4. C. Saunders, "Working at St. Joseph's Hospice, Hackney," in *Annual Report of St. Vincent's Hospital* (Dublin: St. Vincent's Hospital, 1962), 37–39.

5. P. Wall, "25 Volumes of Pain" [editorial], *Pain* 25 (1986):1–4.

6. R. Twycross, "Choice of Strong Analgesic in Terminal Cancer: Diamorphine or Morphine?" *Pain* 3, no. 2 (1977):93–104.

7. C. Saunders, "The Treatment of Intractable Pain in Terminal Cancer," *Proceedings of the Royal Society of Medicine* 56, no. 3 (1963):195–97.

8. C. Saunders and R. Kastenbaum, eds., *Hospice Care on the International Scene* (New York: Springer Verlag, 1997).

9. World Health Organization, *Cancer Pain Relief*, 2nd ed. (Geneva: World Health Organization, 1996).

10. C. Saunders, "In Britain: Fewer Conflicts of Conscience," *Hastings Center Report* 25, no. 3 (1995):44–45.

11. C. Saunders, "Care of the Dying: I. The Problem of Euthanasia," *Nursing Times*, 9 October 1959, 960–61, reprinted in *Nursing Times*, 1 July 1976, 1003–5.

12. See n. 8, Saunders and Kasterbaum 1997.

13. C. Saunders, "The Moment of Truth: Care of the Dying Person," in *Death and Dying: Current Issues in the Treatment of the Dying Person*, ed. L. Pearson (Cleveland: Case Western Reserve University Press, 1969), 49–78.

14. See n. 8, Saunders and Kastenbaum 1997.

15. J. Hinton, "Can Home Care Maintain an Acceptable Quality of Life for Patients with Terminal Cancer and Their Relatives?" *Palliative Medicine* 8 (1994): 183–96.

16. See n. 8, Saunders and Kastenbaum 1997.

17. N. A. Christakis, *Death Foretold: Prophecy and Prognosis in Medical Care* (Chicago: University of Chicago Press, 1999), 199.

18. See n. 8, Saunders and Kastenbaum 1997, 133, 142, 203, respectively.

19. Lord Walton of Detchant, *Medical Ethics: Select Committee Report to the House of Lords* (London: Her Majesty's Stationery Office, May 1944).

20. Z. Zylicz and I. G. Finlay, "Euthanasia and Palliative Care: Reflections from the Netherlands and the U.K.," *Journal of the Royal Society of Medicine* 92 (1999): 370–73.

21. See n. 10, Saunders 1995, 45.

22. See n. 11, Saunders 1959 and 1976.

23. C. Doyle, G. W. Hanks, and N. MacDonald, *Oxford Textbook of Palliative Medicine*, 2nd ed. (Oxford: Oxford University Press, 1998).

24. See n. 3, Clark 1999.

25. D. Barnard, A. Towers, P. Boston, and Y. Lambrinidow, *Crossing Over: Narratives of Palliative Care* (Oxford: Oxford University Press, 2000).

26. Available from St. Christopher's Hospice, 51–59 Lawrie Park Road, Sydenham, London SE26 6DZ, England.

Chapter 14: Compassionate Care, Not Assisted Suicide

1. M. J. Field and C. K. Cassel, eds., *Approaching Death: Improving Care at the End of Life* (Washington, D.C.: Institute of Medicine, 1997).

2. World Health Organization, *Cancer Pain Relief and Palliative Care*, Report of a WHO Expert Committee (Geneva: 1990), 11–12.

3. Ibid.

4. "Protection of the Human Rights and Dignity of the Terminally Ill and the Dying," *Official Gazette of the Council of Europe*, Recommendation 1418, June 1999. Available at http://stars.coe.fr/ta/ta99/erec1418.htm.

5. T. E. Quill, *Death and Dignity: Making Choices and Taking Charge* (New York: Norton, 1993), 203.

6. *Compassion in Dying v. State of Washington*, 79 F.3d 790, at 814 (9th Cir. 1996).

7. *Quill v. Vacco*, 80 F.3d 716, at 729–730 (2nd Cir. 1991).

8. SUPPORT Principal Investigators, "A Controlled Trial to Improve Care for Seriously Ill Hospitalized Patients," *Journal of the American Medical Association* 274 (1995):1591–95.

9. See n. 1, Field and Cassel 1997.

10. D. E. Meier, R. S. Morrison, and C. K. Cassel, "Improving Palliative Care," *Annals of Internal Medicine* 127 (1997):3–25.

11. See n. 1, Field and Cassel 1997.

12. See n. 1, Field and Cassel 1997; n. 10, Meier et al. 1997; n. 2, WHO 1990.

13. N. I. Cherny, N. Coyle, and K. M. Foley, "Suffering in the Advanced Cancer Pain: A Definition and Taxonomy," *Journal of Palliative Care* 10 (1994):57–70.

14. K. M. Foley, "Competent Care for the Dying Instead of Physician-Assisted Suicide," *New England Journal of Medicine* 336 (1997):54–58; K. M. Foley, "Pain, Physician Assisted Suicide and Euthanasia," *Pain Forum* 4 (1995):163–78; K. M. Foley, "The Relationship of Pain and Symptom Management to Patient Requests for Physician-Assisted Suicide," *Journal of Pain and Symptom Management* 6 (1991): 289–97; see also n. 1, Field and Cassel 1997.

15. C. S. Cleeland, R. Godin, A. K. Hatfield, et al., "Pain and Its Treatment in Outpatients with Metastatic Cancer," *New England Journal of Medicine* 330 (1994):592–96; W. Breitbart, B. D. Rosenfeld, S. D. Passik, M. V. McDonald, H. Thaler, and R. K. Portenoy, "The Undertreatment of Pain in Ambulatory AIDS Patients," *Pain* 65 (1996):243–49; R. Bernabei, G. Gambassi, K. Lapane, et al., "Management of Pain in Elderly Patients with Cancer," *Journal of the American Medical Association* 279 (1998):1877–82; J. Wolfe, H. E. Grier, N. Klar, et al., "Symptoms and Suffering at the End of Life in Children with Cancer," *New England Journal of Medicine* 342 (2000):326–33.

16. J. H. Von Roenn, C. S. Cleeland, R. Gonin, A. K. Hatfield, and K. J. Pandya, "Physician Attitudes and Practice in Cancer Pain Management: A Survey from the Eastern Cooperative Oncology Group," *Annals of Internal Medicine* 119 (1993): 121–26.

17. C. Seale and A. Cartwright, *The Year before Death* (Avebury, Great Britain: Aldershot, 1994); N. A. Desbiens, N. Mueller-Rizner, A. F. Connors, Jr., N. S. Wenger, and J. Lynn, "The Symptom Burden of Seriously Ill Hospitalized Patients," *Journal of Pain and Symptom Management* 17 (1999):248–55; R. K. Portenoy, H. T. Thaler, A. B. Komblith, et al., "The Memorial Symptom Assessment Scale," *European Journal of Cancer* 30A (1994):44–46.

18. J. J. Collins, M. E. Byrnes, I. J. Dunkel, et al., "The Measurement of Symptoms in Children with Cancer," *Journal of Pain Symptom Management* 19 (2000):363–77; see also n. 15, Wolfe et al. 2000.

19. K. E. Rosenfeld, N. S. Wenger, R. S. Phillips, et al., "Factors Associated with Change in Resuscitation Preference of Seriously Ill Patients," *Annals of Internal Medicine* 156 (1996):1558–64.

20. D. K. Payne and M. J. Massie, "Depression and Anxiety," *Principles and Practice of Supportive Oncology* 37 (1998):497–511.

21. H. M. Chochinov, K. G. Wilson, M. Enns, and S. Lander, "Prevalence of Depression in the Terminally Ill: Effects of Diagnostic Criteria and Symptom Threshold Judgments," *American Journal of Psychiatry* 151 (1994):537–40.

22. Y. Conwell and H. D. Caine, "Rational Suicide and the Right to Die: Reality and Myth," *New England Journal of Medicine* 326 (1992):1100–1103.

23. H. M. Chochinov, K. G. Wilson, M. Enns, et al., "Desire for Death in the Terminally Ill," *American Journal of Psychiatry* 152 (1995):1185–91.

24. W. Breitbart, "Suicide Risk and Pain in Cancer and AIDS Patients," in *Current and Emerging Issues in Cancer Pain*, ed. C. R. Chapman and K. M. Foley (New York: Raven Press, 1993), 49–65.

25. D. Saltzburg, W. Breitbart, B. Fishman, F. Stiefel, J. Holland, and K. M. Foley, "The Relationship of Pain and Depression to Suicidal Ideation in Cancer Patients," *Proceedings of the American Society of Clinical Oncology* 8 (1989):1215.

26. S. Passik, M. McDonald, B. Rosenfeld, and W. Breitbart, "End of Life Issues in Patients with AIDS: Clinical and Research Considerations," *Journal of Pharmacology in Pain and Symptom Control* 3 (1995):91–111.

27. N. Coyle, J. Adelhardt, K. M. Foley, and R. K. Portenoy, "Character of Terminal Illness in the Advanced Cancer Patient: Pain and Other Symptoms during the Last Four Weeks of Life," *Journal of Pain and Symptom Management* 5 (1990):83–92.

28. L. Ganzini, H. D. Nelson, T. A. Schmidt, D. F. Kraemer, M. A. Delorit, and M. A. Lee, "Physicians' Experience with the Oregon Death with Dignity Act," *New England Journal of Medicine* 342 (2000):557–63.

29. Gallup Institute, *Spiritual Beliefs and the Dying Process: A Report on the National Survey Conducted for the Nathan Cummings Foundation and Fetzer Institute* (Princeton, N.J.: Gallup Institute, 1997).

30. K. E. Steinhauser, E. C. Clipp, M. McNeilly, N. A. Christakis, L. M. McIntyre, and J. A. Tulsky, "In Search of a Good Death: Observation of Patients, Families, and Providers," *Annals of Internal Medicine* 132 (2000):825–32.

31. A. L. Back, J. I. Wallace, H. F. Starks, and R. A. Pearlman, "Physician-Assisted Suicide and Euthanasia in Washington State: Patient Requests and Physician Responses," *Journal of American Medical Association* 275 (1996):919–25.

32. See n. 28, Ganzini et al. 2000.

33. E. J. Emanuel, D. L. Fairclough, J. Slutsman, H. Alpert, D. Baldwin, and L. L. Emanuel, "Assistance from Family Members, Friends, Paid Caregivers and Volunteers in the Care of Terminally Ill Patients," *New England Journal of Medicine* 341 (1999):956–63; E. J. Emanuel, D. L. Fairclough, J. Slutsman, and L. L. Emanuel, "Understanding Economic and Other Burdens of Terminal Illness: The Experience of Patients and Their Caregivers," *Annals of Internal Medicine* 132 (2000):451–59.

34. E. J. Emanuel, "Report of the ASCO Membership Survey on End of Life Care," *Proceedings of the American Society of Clinical Oncology* 17 (Alexandria, Va.: 1998).

35. R. K. Portenoy, N. Coyle, K. M. Kash, et al., "Determinants of the Willingness to Endorse Assisted Suicide: A Survey of Physicians, Nurses, and Social Workers," *Psychosomatics* 38 (1997):277–87.

36. T. P. Hill, "Treating the Dying Patient: The Challenge for Medical Education," *Archives of Internal Medicine* 155 (1995):1265–69; J. A. Billings and S. Block, "Palliative Care in Undergraduate Medical Education: Status Report and Future Direction," *Journal of the American Medical Association* 278 (1997):733–38.

37. See n. 36, Hill 1995.

38. See n. 36, Hill 1995.

39. L. Blank, personal communication, 20 November 1998.

40. A. T. Caron, J. Lynn, and P. Keaney, "End of Life Care in Medical Textbooks," *Annals of Internal Medicine* 130 (1999):82–86.

41. See n. 8, SUPPORT Principal Investigators 1995.

42. See n. 34, Emanuel 1998.

43. J. C. Weeks, E. F. Cook, and S. J. O'Day, "Relationship between Cancer Patients' Prediction of Prognosis and Their Treatment Preferences," *Journal of the American Medical Association* 279 (1998):1709–14.

44. M. Z. Solomon, L. O'Donnell, B. Jennings, et al., "Decisions Near the End of Life: Professional Views on Life-Sustaining Treatments," *American Journal of Public Health* 83 (1993):14–23.

45. A. C. Carver, B. G. Vickrey, J. L. Bernat, et al., "End of Life Care: A Survey of US Neurologists' Attitudes, Behavior and Knowledge," *Neurology* 53 (1999):284–93.

46. J. A. Billings and S. D. Block, "Slow Euthanasia," *Journal of Palliative Care* 12 (1996):21–30; R. K. Portenoy, "Morphine Infusions at the End of Life: The Pitfalls in Reasoning from Anecdote," *Journal of Palliative Care* 12 (1996):44–46; B. Mount, "Morphine Drips, Terminal Sedation, and Slow Euthanasia: Definitions and Facts, Not Anecdotes," *Journal of Palliative Care* (1996):12, 31–37.

47. R. A. Burt, "The Supreme Court Speaks: Not Assisted Suicide but a Constitutional Right to Palliative Care," *New England Journal of Medicine* 337 (1997): 1234–36.

48. F. Brescia, R. Portenoy, M. Ryan, L. Drasnoff, and G. Gray, "Pain Opioid Use and Survival in Hospitalized Patients with Advanced Cancer," *Journal of Clinical Oncology* 10 (1992):149–55.

49. W. D. Wilson, N. G. Smedira, C. Fink, J. A. McDowell, and J. M. Lance, "Ordering and Administration of Sedatives and Analgesics during the Withholding and Withdrawal of Life Support from Critically Ill Patients," *Journal of the American Medical Association* 267 (1992):949–53.

50. S. Chaters, R. Viola, J. Paterson, and V. Jarvis, "Sedation for Intractable Distress in the Dying: A Survey of Experts," *Palliative Medicine* 12 (1998):255–69; N. Sykes, "Opioid Use in the Last Week of Life and Implications for End of Life Decision Making," *Lancet* 356 (2000):398–99.

51. See n. 1, Field and Cassel 1997.

52. R. L. Daut and C. S. Cleeland, "The Prevalence and Severity of Pain in Cancer," *Cancer* 50 (1982):1913–18.

53. See n. 8, SUPPORT Principle Investigators 1995, 1591–95.

54. L. Lagnado, "Hospice's Patients Beat the Odds, So Medicare Decides to Crack Down," *Wall Street Journal*, 5 June 2000, A1.

55. M. A. Lee and S. W. Tolle, "Oregon Assisted Suicide: The Silver Lining," *Annals of Internal Medicine* 124, no. 2 (1996):267–69.

56. S. W. Tolle, V. P. Tilden, S. E. Hickman, and A. G. Rosenfeld, "Family Reports of Pain in Dying Hospitalized Patients: A Structured Telephone Survey," *Western Journal of Medicine* 172 (2000):374–77.

Conclusion

1. R. K. Portenoy, N. Coyle, K. M. Kash, et al., "Determinants of the Willingness to Endorse Assisted Suicide: A Survey of Physicians, Nurses, and Social Workers," *Psychosomatics* 38 (1997).277–87.

2. J. Clements, "Mercy Killing Surge Expected as Dutch Legalize Euthanasia," *Daily Telegraph*, London, 28 November 2000, 18.

3. H. Hendin, *Seduced by Death: Doctors, Patients, and Assisted Suicide* (New York: Norton, 1998).

4. J. Fawcett, W. A. Scheftner, L. Fogg, et al., "Time-Related Predictors of Suicide in Major Affective Disorder," *American Journal of Psychiatry* 147 (1990):1189–94; A. T. Beck, T. R. Streen, R. A. Kovacs, et al., "Hopelessness and Eventual Suicide: A Ten Year Prospective Study of Patients Hospitalized with Suicide Ideation," 142 (1985):559–63.

5. H. Hendin, J. T. Maltsberger, A. Lipschitz, et al., "Recognizing and Responding to a Suicide Crisis," *Journal of Suicide and Life-Threatening Behavior* 31 (2001):115–28.

6. H. Hendin, "Selling Death and Dignity," *Hastings Center Report* 25, no. 3 (1995): 19–23.

7. H. Chochinov, D. Tatryn, K. Wilson, et al., "Prognostic Awareness in the Terminally Ill," *Psychosomatics* 41 (2000):1–5.

8. H. Hendin, "The Psychodynamics of Suicide with Particular Reference to the Young," *American Journal of Psychiatry* 148 (1991):1150–58.

9. L. Thomas, "Dying as Failure," *American Journal of Political Science* 444 (1984):1–4.

10. E. J. Emanuel, "Report of the ASCO Membership Survey on End of Life Care," *Proceedings of the American Society of Clinical Oncology* 17 (Alexandria, Va.: 1998). Also, E. J. Emanuel, personal communication, May 1998.

11. J. Yu, *Breathing Lessons: The Life and Work of Mark O'Brien* (San Francisco: Production of Inscrutable Films with Pacific News Service, 1996).

12. SUPPORT Principal Investigators, "A Controlled Trial to Improve Care for Seriously Ill Hospitalized Patients," *Journal of the American Medical Association* 274 (1995):1591–95.

13. J. Lynn, M. O. O'Connor, J. Duloc, et al., "Medicaring: Development and Test Marketing of a Supportive Care Benefit for Older People," *Journal of the American Geriatrics Society* 47 (1999):1058–64.

14. J. L. Weinstein, "End-of-Life Care Must Improve, Say Victorious Question I Foes," *Portland Herald*, 9 November 2000, 11A.

15. D. S. Broder, *Democracy Derailed: Initiative Campaigns and the Power of Money* (New York: Harcourt, 2000).

16. G. J. Annas, *Some Choice: Law, Medicine and the Market* (New York: Oxford University Press, 1998), 222, 223.

17. *Sampson & Doe v. State of Alaska,* Case No. 3AN-98-11288C1 (3d Sup. Ct., 9 September 1999), 8–9.

18. Associated Press, "Oregon Will Refund $60 after Suicides," 30 March 1999. The Health Care Financing Administration did its own audit, which led to a demand that Oregon refund an additional $1,167.

19. Pain Relief Promotion Act (H.R. 2260, S. 1272).

20. Memorandum from John Ashcroft, Attorney General, to Asa Hutchinson, Administrator, Drug Enforcement Administration, 6 November 2001.

21. *United States v. Oakland Cannabis Buyers' Cooperative,* 523 U.S. 483 (2001).

22. T. Preston, "Whither Peace in Dying?" Paper given at Andrews University conference, The End of Life: Assisted Suicide and the Hospice Movement, 6 April 2000, Berrien Springs, Michigan.

23. *Vacco v. Quill,* 521 U.S. 793 (1997).

24. B. Seaman, "A Call to Action," *Time* 156, no. 12 (2000):1–2.

25. D. Vacco, *Attorney General Dennis Vacco's Commission on Quality Care at the End of Life* (New York: New York State Commission on Quality Care at the End of Life, 1998).

26. M. J. Field and C. K. Cassel, eds., *Approaching Death: Improving Care at the End of Life* (Washington, D.C.: Institute of Medicine, 1997).

27. "Following Through" [editorial], *Bangor Daily News,* 11, 12 November 2000, A12.

Index